Global Health Experiential Education

T0144262

This book presents best practices for ethical and safe international health elective experiences for trainees and the educational competencies and evaluation techniques that make them valuable. It includes commentaries, discussions and descriptions of new global health education guidelines, reviews of the literature, as well as research.

Uniquely, it will include ground-breaking research on perspectives of partners in the Global South whose voices are often unheard, student perspectives and critical discussions of the historical foundations and power dynamics inherent in international medical work.

Global Health Experiential Education is a timely book that will be of interest to academic directors of global health programmes and anyone involved in training and international exchanges across North America.

Akshaya Neil Arya is a family doctor and was founding director of the Global Health Office at Schulich School of Medicine and Dentistry at Western University in Canada. He has also taught global health to masters in public health students at the University of Waterloo and to medical students at McMaster University where he is an assistant clinical professor.

Jessica Evert has been at the forefront of global health education in North America for over a decade. A family physician by training, her undergraduate focus on anthropology and ethnography of health systems and delivery built a deep appreciation for the cultural influences on health and healthcare. She clinically practises inpatient medicine, hospice and palliative care with a focus on underserved, multicultural populations.

This book is dedicated to Dr. Thomas (Tom) Hall, a champion for global health education, who has touched both of us editors, many chapter authors and the field in immeasurable ways. Tom was unconditionally generous with his time, energy, giving to individuals and organizations in peace, global health, environmental protection, democracy, and beyond. He was mentor to many trainees over a career spanning more than half a century, humbly and unconditionally sharing his brilliance from Theory to Practice. Tom will be missed amongst those in our community and we vow to continue his legacy and ensure his passion lives on.

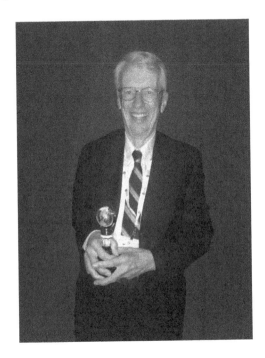

Global Health Experiential Education

From Theory to Practice

Edited by Akshaya Neil Arya and Jessica Evert

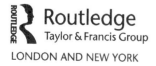

LONDON AND NEW YORK

First published 2018
by Routledge

2 Park Square, Milton Park, Abingdon, Oxfordshire OX14 4RN
52 Vanderbilt Avenue, New York, NY 10017

Routledge is an imprint of the Taylor & Francis Group, an informa business

First issued in paperback 2019

British Library Cataloguing-in-Publication Data
A catalogue record for this book is available from the British Library

Library of Congress Cataloging in Publication Data
Names: Arya, Akshaya Neil, 1962– author. | Evert, Jessica, author.
Title: Global health experiential education : from theory to practice /
edited by Akshaya Neil Arya and Jessica Evert.
Description: Abingdon, Oxon; New York, NY : Routledge, 2018. |
Includes bibliographical references and index.
Identifiers: LCCN 2017011741 | ISBN 9781138236332 (hbk) |
ISBN 9781315107844 (ebk)
Subjects: | MESH: Global Health–education | International Educational
Exchange | Program Development–methods | Health Personnel–education
Classification: LCC RA441 | NLM WA 18 | DDC 362.1–dc23
LC record available at https://lccn.loc.gov/2017011741

ISBN: 978-1-138-23633-2 (hbk)
ISBN: 978-0-367-34153-4 (pbk)

Please visit the eResource at: www.routledge.com/9781138236332

Typeset in Times New Roman
by Out of House Publishing

Contents

Acknowledgements

We would like to thank the following for careful peer review of chapters in the following sections:

Part I: Pedagogies

Leslie Glickman, Brittany Seymour, Phuoc Le, Megan Arthur, William Cherniak, Alison Doucet, Jill Allison, Ian Pereira, Shweta Dhawan, Katy Daniel, Jennifer Kue, Clark Jones, Sahil Angelo, Yassen Tcholakov, Elizabeth Chan, Cody Paris, Kaveh Khoshnood, Rabia Bana.

Part II: Ethics

Kate Standish, Elysée Nouvet, Cody Paris, Mary White, Richard Kiely, Virginia Rowthorn, Manisha Hladio, Sahil Angelo, Leslie Glickman.

Part III: Host perspectives

Jon Dowell, Richard Kiely, Judy Lasker, Kate Standish, Elizabeth Keating, Heather Lukolyo, Michelle Amri.

Part IV: Contemporary conversations

Michelle Amri, Alyssa Smaldino, Heather Lukolyo, Brittany Seymour, Alison Doucet, Elizabeth Chan, Elizabeth Keating, Shailendra Prasad.

Part V: Case studies

Quentin Eichbaum, Chris Mills, Katy Daniels, Brittany Seymour.

Terminology

International Medical Elective (IME)	Medical/Health Professions clinical elective that is abroad.
Short-term Experience(s) in Global Health (STEGH)	Any experience that is diverse/undifferentiated or involves multiple disciplines/levels of trainees.
"Short-term Medical Missions" (STMM)	Experiences that are under the auspices of service and/or volunteering, whether faith-based or secular, can utilise the term. If there is reluctance to use the term "missions" they can be called by a different terms as long as it is defined and explained why the term is preferred in the text.
Global North/South	Terms used vs. developing/developed Western Third underresourced … may not be best term. Sometimes apply low and middle-income countries (LMICs) and high-income countries (HICs).
SMP Social Media Platform	Any experience that is categorised specific to a discipline, such as public health internships or fieldwork, research can be called by discipline-specific term.
Global Health	Discipline field capitalised vs. as a noun improving non-capitalised.
AHA	Anti-homosexuality Act
CBPR	community- based participatory research
GAPS	Global Ambassadors for Patient Safety
HIV	Human Immunodeficiency Virus
HPV	Human Papilloma Virus
LGBT	Lesbian, Gay, Bisexual, and Transgender
MSM	Men who have sex with men
NGO	Non-Governmental Organisation
PBL	problem-based learning
PDT	pre-departure training
PEPFAR	President's Emergency Plan for AIDS Relief

STEGH	short-term experience in global health
STI	Sexually transmitted infections
UNHCR	United Nations High Commissioner for Refugees
WEIGHT	Working Group on Ethics Guidelines for Global Health Training
WHO	World Health Organization
WSW	Women who have sex with women

Contributors

Editors

Akshaya Neil Arya, BASc MD CCFP FCFP D. Litt., has a chemical engineering degree from the University of Toronto, an MD from Queen's University and completed his family medicine residency through McGill University. He was founding director of Global Health Office at Western University managed programming till 2013. He has taught global health in public health and medical schools. As a family physician he has supervised students overseas and in Canada. Neil has written extensively on peace through health and a recently co-edited a volume on health and care of underserved populations in Canada. He has received many awards including a 2009 College of Family Physicians of Canada Geeta Gupta Award for Equity and Diversity. In 2011 he received a D.Litt. (Honorary) from Wilfrid Laurier University and the mid-Career Award in International Health from the American Public Health Association.

Neil served as vice-president of International Physicians for the Prevention of Nuclear War (IPPNW), which won the 1985 Nobel Peace Prize and as president of Physicians for Global Survival (PGS). He is the currently president of the Canadian Physicians for Research and Education in Peace (CPREP) (www.cprep.ca), and of the PEGASUS Global Health Conferences (www.pegasusconference.ca). Neil remains assistant clinical professor in family medicine at McMaster University (part-time) He chaired the Ontario College for Family Physicians Environmental Health Committee from 2013 till 2015 and is an adjunct professor in environment and resource studies at the University of Waterloo. A more detailed CV of the editor is found at www.neilarya.com.

Jessica Evert, MD, has been at the forefront of global health education in North America for over a decade. A family physician by training, her undergraduate focus on anthropology and ethnography of health systems and delivery built a deep appreciation for the cultural influences to health and healthcare. As a medical student, she was vice president of IFMSA–USA, allowing her to lay seeds of collaboration with physician-in-training colleagues from over

120 countries worldwide. Jessica began writing important critiques of global health education and international medical electives as a student. She went on to leadership positions in the Global Health Education Consortium (GHEC) and Consortium of Universities for Global Health (CUGH). As a resident at the University of California, San Francisco (UCSF), Jessica helped develop and participated in one of the first multi-specialty residency tracks in global health, the UCSF Global Health Clinical Scholars Program. Following residency, Jessica joined Child Family Health International (www. cfhi.org), a UN-recognised San Francisco-based non-profit organisation started in 1992 that provides 35+ community-based global health education programmes in ten counties through an asset-based engagement approach with an emphasis on ethics, safety, community empowerment and rigor. CFHI partners with over 200 universities to expand global offerings and oversight of global health experiential education.

Jessica has co-edited and authored multiple books and articles on best practices in global health education at undergraduate through post-graduate levels. She has worked with the American Academy of Family Physicians, World Medical Association, Forum on Education Abroad, NAFSA, Consortium of Universities for Global Health, AAC&U and others to further global health education. Her research has spanned medical anthropological ethnography, health disparities, impacts of service-learning and global health programmes on communities and participants, host perspectives of competencies and the global health employment landscape. Jessica clinically practises inpatient medicine, hospice and palliative care with a focus on underserved, multicultural populations and is the proud mom of two amazing children.

Authors

Ahmed Ali, MD, MRCEM, PGCert, is an emergency medicine registrar in Manchester, United Kingdom and a member of the Junior Doctors Network of the World MEdical Association.

Jill Allison, PhD, is a medical anthropologist and former nurse. She is the global health coordinator in the Faculty of Medicine at Memorial University of Newfoundland.

Michelle Amri, BHSc, MPA, is currently a PhD student in public health at the University of Toronto and has worked previously as a consultant for the World Health Organization in the Philippines and Lao PDR.

Kelly Anderson, MD CCFP(EM) AAHIVS, is a family physician who completed a fellowship in HIV AIDS. She is currently working at St Michael's Hospital and faculty in the Department of Family and Community Medicine at the University of Toronto.

Sahil Angelo is a MD/MPH, candidate at Emory University School of Medicine and former programme manager and research associate at the Center for Strategic and International Studies' Global Health Policy.

Kevin Bergman, MD, is a family and emergency physician who is the co-director of the Global Health Program at the UCSF-affiliated Contra Costa Family Medicine Residency in Martinez, California.

Carolyn Beukeboom, MSc BScN RN(EC), is a nurse practitioner who has worked clinically longer term with Médecins Sans Frontiéres in South Sudan and in a HIV/AIDS clinic in Lesotho; as a health promoter and educator in primary healthcare in Ecuador, in children's homes in India, in evaluation in Liberia; as well as many other short-term missions.

Peter Brown is a professor of anthropology and global health at Emory University, author of *Understanding and Applying Medical Anthropology,* 3rd ed.

Sabrina Butteris, MD, is director of global health education for the Department of Pediatrics at the University of Wisconsin and co-founded the Association of Pediatric Program Directors Global Health Pediatric Education Group.

Elizabeth Chan, BHSc, is a masters of science in public health candidate at Johns Hopkins after finishing her bachelor's thesis research at McMaster University on perceptions of humanitarian healthcare missions.

William Cherniak, MD, MPH, CCFP, is a family and emergency physician, co-founder of Bridge to Health Medical and Dental (www.bridge-tohealth.ca), a Canadian humanitarian organisation working in East Africa. Additionally, he is a lecturer in family medicine at the University of Toronto and a clinical assistant professor at the University of Southern California.

Chih J. Chuang, MD, FAAP, completed a combined residency in internal medicine and pediatrics and is director of global health and education at Wayne State University School of Medicine.

John A. Crump, MB ChB, MD, DTM&H, is professor of global health and co-director, Centre for International Health, University of Otago and adjunct professor of medicine, pathology, and global health at Duke University. He trained as both an internist in infectious diseases and as a pathologist in medical microbiology. Dr Crump co-led efforts to develop the Working Group on Ethics Guidelines for Global Health Training (WEIGHT) guidelines.

Katy Daniels, MBChB, DFSRH, MRCGP, DipMEd, is a general practitioner and a clinical and global health teacher and electives lead at University of Dundee's School of Medicine. Her masters in medical education dissertation evaluates the feasibility and value of south–south medical elective exchanges in Africa.

Katy Davis, MSc, has an interest in gender-based health inequities related to climate change related natural disasters. She currently works at the University of Liverpool.

Matthew DeCamp, MD, PhD, is an assistant professor of general and internal medicine at Johns Hopkins University. Dr DeCamp conducts empirical and conceptual research on ethical issues in the USA and abroad including work to create and evaluate http://ethicsandglobalhealth.org, an online training program for ethics and short-term global health experiences.

Ginny DeFrank is programme manager at the Keck School of Medicine of the University of Southern California where she assists with the development and administration of undergraduate, masters and professional programmes.

Jan De Maeseneer, MD, PhD, is head of department of family medicine and primary healthcare, vice-dean for strategic planning and director of the department's WHO Collaborating Center on Primary Health Care at Ghent University. From 2007 until 2015, he was the secretary-general of the Network: Towards Unity of Health (www.thenetworktufh.org).

Roopa Dhatt, MD, MPA, is an internist and director and co-founder of Women in Global Health. She previously served as the president of the International Federation of Medical Students' Associations (IFMSA).

Shweta Dhawan, HBSc, MPH, is now studying medicine at Dalhousie University. She has diverse global health-related experience in non-profit, research and government settings in Canada, India, the Philippines and Cambodia including with the World Health Organization and is co-director of the Canadian Society for International Health's MentorNet programme.

Ashti Doobay-Persaud, MD, is an assistant professor of medicine in the Division of Hospital Medicine and the associate director of global health graduate education at Northwestern University's Feinberg School of Medicine. She has served as a clinician-educator in several countries and focuses on medical education.

Alison Doucet, BSc, MD, CCFP, FCFP, is a family physician and assistant professor of family medicine at McGill University where she has served as director of the Global Health Division. Currently, she is the principal investigator of the TEACH project, a 5-year train-the-trainer programme for Indigenous community health workers in Ecuador.

Jon Dowell, BMSc, MBChB, MRCGP, MD, FHEA, is a general practitioner and head of undergraduate medicine at the University of Dundee,

Scotland. Having worked and studied in a number of countries he sought to revise medical electives and develop a more responsible approach that includes meaningful reciprocity within typical north–south attachments.

Quentin Eichbaum, MD, PhD, MPH, was born and raised in Namibia and South Africa where he studied law and worked on human rights during apartheid. An MD MPH PhD/postdoctoral graduate of Harvard Medical School and MIT in Boston, he is currently associate professor of pathology, microbiology and immunology as well as of medical education at Vanderbilt University. He works in global health education in several African countries.

Mei Elansary, MD, MPhil, is a pediatric global health fellow and pediatric resident of the Boston Combined Residency Program. Dr Elansary has worked in Egypt, Indonesia and Tanzania.

Matthew Fentress, MD, was a co-founder of the global health track at Contra Costa Family Medicine Residency (CCFMR). He has worked with Medecins Sans Frontieres in Myanmar and South Sudan, and later worked with Last Mile Health in Liberia during the 2014–15 Ebola epidemic and spent clinical time in India.

Leslie Glickman, PT, PhD, is adjunct faculty, Department of Physical Therapy and Rehabilitation Science at the University of Maryland and an independent educational consultant. She has a Fullbright grant to provide educational and programmatic consultation as well as faculty and staff development for the Kachere Rehabilitation Centre and conducted funded research in Malawi.

Thomas Hall, MD, DrPH, is lecturer in UCSF's Department of Epidemiology and Biostatistics, with previous faculty positions at schools of public health including Puerto Rico, Johns Hopkins, UNC/Chapel Hill, and the University of Washington. He was the Global Health Education Consortium executive director (2002–11) and has consulted with WHO, the World Bank and many countries on health workforce planning.

Mary Halpine, MD, is a resident in the Division of Physical Medicine and Rehabilitation. She was active in the Canadian Federation of Medical Students in developing global health competencies and predeparture training.

Dan Hayhoe, OD FAAO, is an optometrist, teaching as adjunct clinical faculty at the University of Waterloo and coordinating primary care clinical rotations for optometry interns in Malawi. Dan also helped establish the School of Optometry at the University of Benin in Nigeria in 1976.

Adam Hoverman, DO DTMH, is a family physician and preventive medicine resident and MPH candidate in health management and policy at

Portland State University and has taught as the director of global health and research at Pacific Northwest University.

James Hudspeth, MD, is a internal medicine hospitalist at Boston University, where he is director of global health programmes. He also works on nursing and medical education with EqualHealth in Haiti, and with the Consortium of Universities in global health on improving graduate medical bilateral exchanges.

Caity Jackson, MSc, is a global health consultant, co-founder and director of Communications for Women in Global Health and founder of the MentorNet mentorship programme, the annual Global Health Student and Young Professional Summit and This Week in Global Health.

Gabrielle A. Jacquet, MD, MPH, is the director of global health for the Boston Medical Center Emergency Medicine Residency Program and the assistant director of global health at Boston University School of Medicine. She is the founding course director of *The Practitioner's Guide to Global Health*, and serves as the medical director for Child Family Health International.

Neil Jayasekera, MD, is a family and emergency physician and the founder of the current global health programme at the Contra Costa Family Medicine Residency Program in Martinez, California. He is an associate clinical professor in family and community medicine at UCSF and has worked in India, Sri Lanka, South Sudan, Haiti, Kenya and Malawi.

Elizabeth M. Keating, MD, is a senior resident in pediatrics and global child health at Baylor College of Medicine, with international experience in Tanzania, Nepal, India, Cambodia and Lesotho. She is beginning a combined paediatric emergency medicine and global health fellowship at the University of Utah.

Kaveh Khoshnood, PhD, is an infectious disease epidemiologist and an Associate professor and director of undergraduate studies at the Yale School of Public Health where he teaches courses in public health ethics, global health and violent conflict and health and is involved in providing pre-departure ethics training for research.

Richard Kiely, MA, PhD, is a senior fellow in the Office of Engagement Initiatives at Cornell University. Richard continues to be an active scholar in the area of service-learning and community engagement in higher education.

Emily Kocsis, BSc MSc, has a master's in global health, is a research officer with the Canadian Coalition for Global Health Research (CCGHR) and co-directs the Canadian Society for International Health's programme, MentorNet.

Lisa Kuhn, MSc, is the executive director of the Foundation for Sustainable Development and has provided training, assessment, and capacity-building services to more than 35 organisations in 22 countries in Africa, Asia, Europe and Latin America.

Judith N. Lasker, PhD, is NEH distinguished professor in sociology at Lehigh University and author of *Hoping to Help; The Promises and Pitfalls of Global Health Volunteering* (Cornell University Press, 2016).

Désirée Lichtenstein, MD, is co-founder and the gender specialist of women in global health and currently interning at Karolinska Hospital in Sweden.

Amy Lockwood, MS, MBA, is chief of staff at UCSF's Global Health Sciences and has a background spanning business, non-profit and academic sectors.

Samuel Luboga, MB ChB, M,Med (Surgery), PhD, is a professor, a church minister and (now retired) deputy dean education for the Makerere University College of Health Sciences in Kampala, Uganda, where he hosted medical trainees and facilitated numerous north–south collaborations.

Heather Lukolyo, MD, MHS, is completing her residency in a combined pediatrics and child global health programme at Baylor College of Medicine; she also holds a graduate degree in international public health and has lived and worked extensively in Uganda where she co-founded and runs a non-profit organisation for disadvantaged girls.

Keith Martin, MD, PC, is the founding executive director of the Consortium of Universities for Global Health (CUGH) after serving as a Canadian member of parliament for over 17 years. Dr Martin has been on numerous diplomatic missions to areas in crisis and served as a physician on the Mozambique border during that country's civil war.

Janice McMillan, MEd, PhD, has a Master's in Education from the University of the Western Cape and PhD in Sociology from the University of Cape Town where she is director of the global citizenship programme.

Ryan Meili is a family physician in Saskatoon, an assistant professor in the College of Medicine at the University of Saskatchewan where he serves as the head of the Division of Social Accountability. He was director of Making the Links from 2005 to 2016. He is the author of *A Healthy Society* and founder of Upstream.

Neil Merrylees, MBChB, FRCGP, FHEA, MMed, is a GP and clinical teacher in the Department of General Practic, University of Dundee, Scotland. In total he has spent the better part of 10 years working overseas, mainly in developing countries.

Simone Mohrs, MSc, is a public relations consultant with a focus on healthcare and programme coordinator of the Global Health Mentorships Program.

Jeanne Moseley, MPH, is a lecturer in the Division of Nutritional Sciences (DNS) and the associate director for the Global Health Program at Cornell.

Catherine Myser, PhD, is professor and director of global health and ethics at Rosalind Franklin University. She has conducted education, research and clinical ethics consulting in medical schools and hospitals in Africa, Asia, Australia, the Caribbean, Europe, Latin America, the Middle East and North America and edited the book *Bioethics Around the Globe* (Oxford University Press, 2011).

Elahe Nezami, PhD, is associate professor of clinical preventive medicine at the Keck School of Medicine of the University of Southern California where she also serves as associate dean for undergraduate, masters, and professional programmes and has directed programmes of global health at bachelor's and master's level.

Kristin Neudorf, MSc, is a public health researcher who works with research institutions and non-profit organisations around the world.

Elysée Nouvet is a medical anthropologist and an assistant professor (global health) in the Faculty of Health Sciences at Western University with research in Latin America, Canada and West Africa centered on social dimensions of distress and disease and perceptions, ethics and politics of trans-national care and research.

Shawna O'Hearn, MA, MSc (OT), is an occupational therapist and director for the Global Health Office at Dalhousie University, which includes social accountability in local and international collaborations.

Jody Olsen, PhD, MSW, is co-director of the Baltimore Center for Global Education Initiatives and visiting professor at Baltimore School of Social Work at the University of Maryland. Before joining the faculty, she was deputy director and acting director of the US Peace Corps.

Cody Morris Paris, PhD, is the deputy director of Middlesex University Dubai and an associate professor in the law and business schools. Cody serves on the board of Amizade (www.amizade.org), a global-service learning and community development NGO with UN consultative status.

Michael Peluso, MD, MPhil, MHS, is a resident in medicine and the Division of Global Health Equity, Brigham and Women's Hospital. He works with local partners on postgraduate medical education programme development in Botswana.

Ian Pereira, BASc, MD, is a radiation oncology resident and past director of education for the World Medical Association Junior Doctors Network.

Tracy L. Rabin, MD, SM, is an assistant professor of internal medicine and assistant director of the Office of Global Health at the Yale School of Medicine, as well as associate residency programme director for global and community health and co-director of the Makerere University–Yale University (MUYU) collaboration.

Mena Ramos, MD, graduated from the Latin American School of Medicine and is currently working as a family and emergency physician in Martinez, California.

Kris Ronsin, BSc, is a master of public health candidate at the University of Haifa in Israel, co-founder and director of Women in Global Health.

Virginia Rowthorn, JD, LLM, is co-director of the UM Baltimore Center for Global Education Initiatives and managing director of the law and health-care programme at Maryland Carey Law.

Brittany Seymour, DDS, MPH, is assistant professor of oral health policy and epidemiology, Harvard School of Dental Medicine and a Harvard Medical School academy fellow in medical education.

Alyssa Smaldino is the executive director of GlobeMed.

Becky L. Spritz, PhD, is professor of psychology and the director of the honors programme at Roger Williams University.

Kate Standish, MD, is a family medicine resident at Boston Medical Center who prior to beginning her medical studies at Yale University worked in community-based health research in Nicaragua, Mexico and New York City.

Jennifer Staple-Clark is founder and chief executive officer of Unite For Sight, a non-profit global health organisation.

Rebecca Stoltzfus, PhD, is a professor in the Division of Nutritional Sciences (DNS), and director for the Global Health Program and vice provost for undergraduate education at Cornell University.

Roger Strasser, AM, professor of rural health, dean and CEO, Northern Ontario School of Medicine, Lakehead and Laurentian Universities, Canada.

Jeremy Sugarman, MD, MPH, MA, is Professor of Bioethics and Medicine at the Berman Institute of Bioethics and Department of Medicine at Johns Hopkins University; he co-led development of the working group on Ethics Guidelines for Global Health Training (WEIGHT) guidelines.

Yassen Tcholakov, MD, MIH, is a public health resident at the McGill University and officer of the Junior Doctors' Network of the World Medical Association.

Kelly Thompson, MBBS, MLitt, MPhil, is a postgraduate trainee in Australia, global health consultant and a programming specialist/gender advisor with Women in Global Health.

Tricia Todd, MPH, is assistant director of the Health Careers Center at the University of Minnesota and instructor for the School of Public Health.

Cynthia Toms-Smedley, PhD, is associate professor of global studies and director of the Global Health Minor at Westmont College, and has lived/worked in China and Uganda.

María del Carmen Valdivieso is the director of a non-profit-Nexos Comunitarios, has a law degree and 14 years of development work experience in the Sacred Valley of the Incas (Peru).

Anvar Velji, MD, FRCP (C), FACP, FIDSA, is a professor of medicine and medical education, associate dean of global health, California University of Science and Medicine, Colton, CA.

Xaviour Walker, MD, MPH, DTM&H, is a geriatric fellow at the University of California, Irvine and public health and preventive medicine physician. He is a past chair and co-founder of the Junior Doctors Network, World Medical Association.

Mary White, PhD, is professor and director of medical humanities at the Boonshoft School of Medicine, Wright State University, where she teaches medical and public health ethics, global health and electives in medical humanities.

1   Introduction

Jessica Evert and Akshaya Neil Arya

Increasing visibility of global realities and disparities coupled with pop culture drive demand for global health education, research and service experiences. Meanwhile, grossly inadequate educational paradigms, perhaps challenged by cultural, geopolitical and social heterogeneity of communities where global health delivery takes place, create unique tensions at institutions and challenges within professional circles to developing a community of practice focused on global health education. Educators are often concerned about overconfident programme graduates without any demonstrated aptitudes. The aim of this book is to assist those creating and improving global health education programmes. Instigating programmes representing the full scope of global health competencies (skills/knowledge/attitudes), involves breaking down longstanding silos on campus and between disciplines. We explore the theoretical underpinnings, as well as the practical implementation, of global health education with in-depth exploration of experiential learning.

A spectrum of global health experiential education

A variety of terms is used to refer to global health experiential educational offerings. These include service-learning, short-term experiences in global health (STEGH), international medical electives (IME), fieldwork and internships. Although service-learning has established a strong foothold in undergraduate (bachelor's) education and is increasingly gaining traction at graduate and professional education levels, there is a lack of appreciation of how it differs from stand-alone volunteering or service. The umbrella term STEGH can take a variety of forms. For example, during the summer after first year medical school, STEGH includes preclinical activities termed electives, internships, fieldwork, research, service and volunteering. STEGH has utility as a "catch-all" shared taxonomy to discuss standards and ethics and is less attached to an academic pedagogy than service learning.

Pitfalls of global health "missions"

Global health fieldwork experiences should differ whether under the auspices of education or service. Ethical blunders are frequent when students and faculty act in service before they have sufficient education and understanding of complex global health contexts. Historically, the basic form of interaction in the field of international health, that of missions and brigades, premised on emotionally based neocolonial motivations glorified in the media and popular culture, involves those from higher resource settings uprooting themselves to "help" and "serve" those they perceive to be less fortunate in other parts of the world. Research, community service or medical electives are to this day often based on this legacy.

While disparities in health and economic resources are stark between and within regions, shortsighted, misguided efforts to act immediately in a completely foreign setting risk giving global health "volunteers" and service providers a false sense of accomplishment. While we wish to nurture the idealism that students embody, and as global health educators are uniquely positioned to do so, we must balance this with developing foundational elements and a realistic recognition of the complexities of global health challenges. The formalisation of global health as an academic pursuit can be seen as a countercurrent to poorly designed and ethically tenuous ventures.

Concerns are multiple. A set up to see large numbers of patients in short periods of time in itself risks individual patients getting incomplete attention or treatment. This danger is magnified many fold when healthcare workers from outside the community or country lack language expertise, and do not appreciate cultural influences to care or nuances. Moreover, many missions/brigades operate in parallel, or tangential to existing health systems which they ignore or integrate very superficially. Some allow students to provide healthcare services usually reserved for licensed healthcare workers including history/physicals, invasive physical exams, dispensing medications and providing patient instructions. Such efforts done in the name of "global health" are a sham, disregarding basic tenets of health equity and evidenced-based medicine. As educators, we can establish institutional processes and regulations to prevent students from engaging in experiential settings that do not adhere to best practices and thus prevent our students from getting mis-educated.

From theory to practice

This book considers many aspects of global health education relevant to the classroom, although we dive deep into the paradigms, ethical challenges and conversations relevant to experiential learning in global health. A common challenge is that even when rigor is applied to university-sanctioned programming, many more student-driven and civil society initiatives (either secular or faith-based) may operate with campus support (perhaps the use of meeting rooms or advertising outlets), but without careful oversight and attention to patient and participant safety. So classroom learning in global health majors, minors and certificates can be well thought-out and appropriately supported with faculty and administrator time. However, fieldwork or experiential component is a "free for all" in which students are given credit for service experiences that defy best practices and do not do justice to the learning objectives achieved in the classroom. The number of students in programmes may be too large to allow adequate faculty and staff time to oversee the quality, safety and rigor of fieldwork. Our intention is to provide faculty, staff and programme administrators with an overview of relevant pedagogies, ethical considerations and a diversity of perspectives. In addition, we embrace the critiques with which we must engage in constructive dialogue, due to the complex nature of resource differentials, partnership dynamics, power imbalances, institutional agendas and colonial legacies.

Principles: humility, reflection, transdisciplinarity

As communities around the globe are diverse in their cultural, geopolitical and social realities, there are a few personal qualities and ethical principles that, if imbued, can serve learners regardless of context, remedying individual and institutional missteps. A first principle is humility. "(C)ountercultural though it is, humility need not suggest weakness or lack of confidence. On the contrary, humility requires toughness and emotional resilience" (Coulehan 2010). Humility in global health education and practice faces an uphill battle against predominant cultures such as helping/aid, and healthcare that traditionally has not emphasised humility. Working within complex community and nation-state realities that contextualise challenges to human wellness and thriving requires humility that is often antithetical to academic accolades. We often ask learners to embrace humility (broadly and culturally), when our own institutions and initiatives are full of hubris, at times unable to acknowledge the degree of capability and impacts. Humility beyond a concept or principle should be a tangible tool for global health education and practice.

Trudging ahead with passion and purpose, we run the risk of leaving little time or space for reflection. Without reflection, harms may go unrecognised and our teaching can lack authenticity. To optimise our role as global health actors, educators and mentors, we must engage in critical reflection, to attempt to scratch the surface of complex relationships we have with people, as well as with intoxicating sentiments such as success, power and control.

Definitions of global health vary; however, all of them reflect a concept that spans multiple disciplines and communities of practice. While the term "health" conjures up white coats and stethoscopes, global health demands that we examine realities upstream of hospitals and clinics, and more complex than biology or pathophysiology. As global health defies a single discipline or community of practice, it requires us as educators to go beyond our discipline-specific comfort zones and integrate other fields of study into our knowledge base and teaching. While mastering all disciplines that are required to achieve global health (think for example – engineering, law, medicine, anthropology, public health, biomedical research, economics, political science, law, ecology) is impossible, we can impart to trainees a sense of appreciation and respect for other professions and build a foundation of teamwork and partnership skills. Global health transcends our collective professional acumens. While higher education excels at exploring theories, data and critical thinking, many of the successes or failures in global health depend on grassroots, community-based realities, that can defy our academic frameworks (and all their culturally informed "logic").

Creating a community of practice

Beyond professional and academic frameworks, global health spans multiple communities of practice – including international development, trade, medicine, environmental stewardship, community-based engagement, politics, global finance and Indigenous rights. This expansiveness creates a challenge for developing shared gathering spaces and optimal inter-sector collaborations. At its worse this can lead to policies and practices in one arena that are damaging to goals and ideals in another. It can also feed the phenomenon of "recreating the wheel" and ignoring established guidelines and best practices.

A community of practice allows us to have shared understanding of the field and educational discipline which reflects it. This includes shared concepts of what to teach, best ways to teach and tools to shape learner development in a meaningful and appropriate way. This book furthers the creation of a community of practice that begins to recognise the complex Venn diagram of fields and sectors contributing to global health practice, and thus education about that practice. As a community of practice that is essential to preparing the current and future generations to continue to make inroads into human wellness and thriving, we encourage ongoing reflection, information sharing and pedagogical creativity. With this book we aim to build a foundation that does justice to the potential benefits if we are to succeed as educators in creating the leaders that usher in a better tomorrow.

What this book contributes

The global health field is fraught with ethical hazards. This book is intended to creating shared understanding and ethical codes of global health education as we develop a community of practice. It highlights the interdependence of pedagogy, ethics and diverse voices. It is no coincidence that ethics has a dedicated part and is mentioned in nearly every chapter. Even for the most expert practitioner, ethical missteps are a constant concern. However, when inexperienced trainees are thrown into the mix, often hailing from a different culture than where they are working or learning, the result is an ethical minefield, affecting the health, lives and conditions of individuals and communities.

Ethics is patient safety. Ethics is life or death. Ethics is the difference between learners gaining an appreciation of true realities and false constructs heralded by outsiders.

A companion Practical Guide volume is meant for trainees and those choosing such experiences. While many of the values underlying the two volumes are the same, the knowledge and skills for those on field experience will necessarily be different. This volume may be considered higher level, or reflective as well as for those directly engaged in design and education of programmes.

Our backgrounds: the path to this book

Guiding our desire to create a community of educators with shared understanding, syntax and collaboration are personal motivations. Our backgrounds span academia and community-based global health experiential learning. We have each taught in formal classroom settings and facilitated community-based immersion, and each experienced "the great deflation" during our exposure to global health.

Jessica Evert was a first year medical student in Kenya when she was handed a 5 inch long needle and asked to do a spinal tap on a 7-year-old child. In the moment between that offer and her acceptance the assumptions that flashed through her brain represent all that is wrong with global health education and practice. She was "there to help," saying yes to do things you have never done and had no proper training to do "is what you do when you want to be a doctor." The poor, black, Kenyan child "had no other options." After an unsuccessful procedure delaying diagnosis, subjecting the child to unimaginable pain, while an expertly capable local physician sat beside her, Jessica began to re-evaluate her assumptions.

As she gained more experience she developed an appreciation that even the most seemingly benign intervention such as aspirin could cause unintended harms. The fact that thousands of students (often with the encouragement of licensed physicians and sanctioned institutions), masqueraded as with requisite expertise, were picking themselves up from high-income countries (HICs) and landing in low and middle-income countries (LMICs) and diving into taking histories, doing physicals and prescribing/dispensing medication became an outrage and Jessica decided to speak out. As she toured the country, students and faculty alike would approach her, confessing the harms they had committed when they "drank the koolaid" of global health. This misrepresentation of global health was distressing on multiple levels, antithetical to global health principles including health equity, professionalism, human rights and social justice needed to be unveiled. She also saw a need to balance the prestige differential between international and local global health and joined the ranks of family medicine, a discipline aligned with "Health for All." Jessica found practitioners and researchers who were glorified for serving abroad, while their careers seemed to turn their back on local global health, including underserved communities and injustices in our own backyard. This book can thus be seen through the lens of authenticity, Jessica's quest for representation of impacts of global health practice, research and education, as well as to achieve health equity and justice.

Neil Arya abandoned a fledgling career in chemical engineering to study medicine out of a perhaps misguided, effort to "help." As an elective student in Tanzania, he was struck with the limited impact of medicine, witnessing disparities in health and healthcare access related to accidents of birth. Presenting to sponsoring church and service groups on his return, although he had gone merely to learn, he found himself placed among the pantheon of colonial heroes such as Florence Nightingale, David Livingstone and Albert Schweitzer. The next year, he returned to the land of his birth on elective at Mother Teresa's Missionaries of Charity in Delhi. Upon arrival he was told his role was to tend to children, changing diapers, cleaning, entertaining. He realised that he actually had developed no specific peda- gogical goals. There was a tacit assumption that he would somehow learn something of value and the onus was on him to seek out opportunities and develop goals. Feeling guilt at voyeuristic experiences in Africa and India, doing a delivery at a high-risk tertiary care institution and taking pictures at a leprosy centre, and a culture which considered such experiences as not just desirable but compulsory, left him so discomforted he foreswore over- seas work for more than a decade, choosing instead to be active locally, as clinician, teacher, writer and advocate.

He relented when asked to assist a friend supervising an interprofes- sional group of students going to Guatemala, noting what good connec- tions with a local community, an ethical approach and adequate training might do, but also the importance of principles of respect, relationships and communication. Teaching medical and public health students locally and globally, he noticed not just parallels between local work he was doing with refugees and others on the margins of Canadian society, but also the value of experiential learning for students to link day to day experience to macro-level determinants. Through their reflection papers and debriefing, he began to appreciate the life changing nature of such experiences for the positive and negative.

Recruited to an administrative role as director of an academic global health office, he approached the opportunity eagerly. Here students helped guide him developing objectives and curricular guidelines. Sometimes the disconnect between the principles he wished to respect and academic pres- sures, desires to publicise work, discordance in the measures of success and the principles of engagement led to stress. The challenges and opportunities developing programming for structured learning, building relationships in North America and abroad, made him understand that respectful communi- cation needed to be intrinsic in all interactions, lest colonial assumptions and behaviurs be allowed to dominate.

Organisation

This volume is meant to fill gaps, largely unaddressed in the literature and current teaching. Medical practitioners often learn with the axiom – "see one, do one, teach one." This would be problematic if we were dealing with inanimate objects but is of particular concern when our concerns are vulnerable human beings, whether trainees or hosts. We begin with a large part on pedagogy, examining curricula, objectives and competencies, interprofessionalism, the links between local and global, preparation and best practices. What disturbed us personally, as we sought to "do no harm," were ethical issues of participation, equity, beneficence and justice. We address issues of power and culture and highlight recent standards. The next part includes perspectives of the host, those administrators, trainees and people "served" from the Global South, whether recipients of clinical electives, short-term medical missions, research or international volunteer programmes, often neglected from global health discourse. This includes a literature survey and what we feel is landmark original research. Our final partss deal with critical contemporary conversations, of interest recently to many in the global health community, including issues of women and the lesbian, gay, bisexual and transgender community in global health and challenges in the digital age, concluding with case study examples of best or novel practices from major institutions and of less known players.

As you reflect on your own learning or require a guide in your teaching, whatever your background, we trust that you will find common ground with many of our contributors as we seek to further our global health community of practice.

Reference

Coulehan J. 2010. "On humility." *Annals of Internal Medicine* 153(3):200–201.

Part I
Pedagogies

2 Global health pedagogy

The art and science of teaching global health

Ashti Doobay-Persaud, Chih J. Chuang and Jessica Evert

Website: www.routledge.com/9781138236332

This online chapter is dedicated to global health educational pedagogy, the art and science, or the theory and practice, of teaching global health. There is now widespread acceptance and recognition that this field requires specialised knowledge and skill beyond that can be acquired by experience. Leaders and learners of global health programmes agree that a codified body of knowledge to produce the next generation of experts in the field is needed. The intent of this chapter is to provide you with a broad array of educational tactics and approaches as well pedagogical perspectives that are available to global health educators. Our aim is to highlight the rich landscape of tools, frameworks and theories that educators use to teach their diverse groups of global health students. The subsequent chapters will explore many of these topics in greater depth. We conclude with a list of suggested pedagogical resources for areas not covered in this book.

3 Objectives and competencies of international electives for medical trainees

Michael J. Peluso and William Cherniak

Introduction

International medical electives (IMEs) are finite clinical experiences characterised by immersion in a culture and medical system outside of the context of the health system at a trainee's home institution. Each year, significant proportions of medical school graduates participate in experiences related to global health, many of which are IMEs (Dowell *et al.* 2009). IMEs are also undertaken by physician assistants, allied health professionals and other clinical disciplines. It is important to recognise that IMEs are appropriate for clinical-level trainees. When experiences that mirror IMEs are undertaken by students who are not yet accepted to professional schools, or are preclinical, they are fraught with ethical and safety issues. Thus, what follows should be applied to appropriate clinical level, professional school trainees.

One of the first sets of guidelines for IMEs was by the American Academy of Pediatrics (Torjesen *et al.* 1999). More recently, IME programmes have made efforts to delineate goals and objectives for participants as health professional education has shifted to focus on competencies (Frenk *et al.* 2010). Global health, like other fields, has begun to explore links between competencies and objectives in order to meet standards of accrediting organisations and to clarify the expected outcomes of training activities. Here, we utilise definitions of goals, objectives and competencies, as laid forth by the Accreditation Council for Graduate Medical Education (Mullan and Lypson 2011).

The standard lens for approaching the objectives and competencies of IMEs has been from high-income countries, whose students are often participating in IMEs with institutional partners in low and middle-income country (LMIC) settings. As global health has matured as a field, sustainable partnerships and diverse input into desirable learning outcomes, with IME objectives and competencies framed from the perspectives of all partners, have been emphasised (Bozinoff *et al.* 2014).

In this chapter, we review the current landscape of objectives and competencies in IMEs, including examples from specific organisations, as well as best practices from the literature.

Key concepts

Timed objectives and competencies

Just as learning during a medical school rotation extends beyond the time spent in the clinical setting, it is helpful to frame IMEs as encompassing experiences before, during and after the clinical experience. While the clinical experience at the away site is the centerpiece of the IME, it is important for institutional partners to consider the educational value of the time preceding and following the time a student spends away.

A recent study exploring competencies for IMEs found that the majority of attention was paid to the intra-elective objectives, that is, the objectives framing the time that students spend away from their home institution (Cherniak *et al.* 2013). This study identified 15 intra-elective objectives derived from 11 articles describing IMEs. The most common intra-elective objectives included "enhancing clinical skills," "understanding different healthcare systems," "understanding cultural differences in treating patients," "increasing cultural awareness" and "learning to manage diseases rarely seen at home."

While programmes seem to place significant emphasis on the intra-elective period, the learner development preceding and following the time spent away are relatively poorly described. In the same study, pre-elective objectives were found to focus primarily on logistical factors related to travel to the site of the IME. While these are important considerations, the lack of focus on pre-departure training may represent a missed opportunity for harnessing the educational value of this time period. In addition to promoting cultural awareness and building a foundation of background knowledge to prepare students for an IME, more research is necessary to determine how the pre-IME period might be formulated to focus on trainees' preparation for their IME while also priming them to maximise their educational experience (Anderson *et al.* 2012).

The description of desired learner development during the post-elective/ post-return period is similarly limited. One common objective during this period focuses on reflection, which is an accepted method by which trainees can organise the content of their IME (Brugner and Duke 2012, Howe *et al.* 2009, Naidu and Kumagi 2016, Sandars 2009). Further research is needed to determine how reflection can best be optimised following IMEs, in addition to determining whether there are other objectives that can be achieved during this time period.

Levels of proficiency

Recent work led by the Consortium of Universities for Global Health (CUGH) has proposed a framework for increasing levels of global health and differing nature of proficiency (Jogerst *et al.* 2015). This work recognises that a career in global health can take many different forms, ranging from a few weeks a year working outside of the context of one's primary practice to spending the majority of one's time practising in a global health setting. As career paths in global health have broadened, and as postgraduate fellowship programmes in global health have begun to multiply, leaders in academic global health have recognised that a "one size fits all" model for planning IMEs no longer suffices. In the same way that a medical student pursuing a residency in surgery is expected to participate in an advanced clinical rotation with graduated responsibility (i.e., a so-called "sub-internship" in US medical schools) while still a student to develop more advanced skills, different levels of training are needed in order to allow students and residents seeking specialisation in global health to enhance their preparation for such a career.

The CUGH competencies propose the following objective levels: global citizen, exploratory, basic operational (including practitioner-oriented and programme-oriented) and advanced. Each level is aimed to meet the needs of different participants in IMEs – for example, a participant learning at the exploratory level might aim to achieve objectives meant to provide a broad orientation to global health, while a different participant who is specifically interested in developing skills necessary to implement oncology programmes in resource-restricted settings may be learning at the programme-oriented operational level during an IME.

Context-free versus context-linked

Echoing other chapters in this textbook, whether competencies should be linked to specific contexts remains an important point of debate in global health education. *Chapter 4* expands on this discussion. Briefly, context-free competencies may describe an activity where one's performance in a particular situation is generalisable to other situations, such as evaluating a blood smear for malaria parasites. While a student could attain such a competency in a setting where malaria is common, this skill is theoretically translatable to reading blood smears in a place where it is not, or where other parasites such as babesia might be common.

On the other hand, global health in general and IMEs in particular are defined by the varying contexts in which they occur. As a result, some have argued that competencies and context in global health are inextricably linked (Eichbaum 2015), and that assumptions that local educational standards should be contorted to fit frameworks developed elsewhere are misdirected (Gruppen *et al.* 2012). An example of a context-linked competency could include providing culturally appropriate HIV screening for married women in Botswana; some of the questions asked and the approach to the patient are likely to be different in this setting than they would be for a similar screening initiative in Thailand. In part, this is due to cultural and linguistic differences between the contexts.

Context-linked competencies are likely to be more labour-intensive in that they must be developed for each site in which an IME is occurring with specific attention paid to the context of the site; in contrast, context-free competencies are convenient, but may be too generic to be useful or achievable across a broad swatch of different cultural and health systems contexts. The context-linked competencies also challenge home institution based faculty who may have understanding of global health principles and practices broadly, but not intimate knowledge of unique practices in the locations where learners go for IMEs.

The current landscape of objectives and competencies

Considerations from the academic literature

A number of studies have explored the current approaches to global health objectives and competencies in the medical education literature. Taken together, these studies demonstrate a growing trend towards programmes displaying the objectives and competencies of IMEs in publications, but also reveal variability between institutions developing competencies for their specific IMEs. Competencies articulated or reviewed in four studies are listed in Table 3.1. While not all of the competencies described here are specific to IMEs, they provide a useful illustration of the diversity of content and level of detail regarding objectives and competencies in global health education.

Recommendations from professional organisations

Over the last decade, a number of groups have attempted to delineate objectives and competencies for global health education (Table 3.2).

In 2010, the Global Health Education Consortium (GHEC) and the Association of Faculties of Medicine of Canada's Global Health Resource Group undertook an effort to delineate global health competencies for undergraduate medical education (Arthur *et al.* 2011). The result was a list of essential core competencies for global health, which GHEC argued were relevant to all medical graduates worldwide. These competencies included six domains, and included specific direction with regard to how a student could demonstrate such competencies.

Also in 2010, the United Kingdom's Global Health Learning Outcomes Working Group laid out objectives for British medical students engaged in global health experiences (Johnson *et al.* 2012). These objectives were based on a report from the General Medical Council, and focused specifically on compulsory teaching in global health (not optional training for students with a career interest or pre-elective training). These learning outcomes included six themes, each with several sub-components; the details of teaching and assessment were specifically delegated to each individual institution.

Subsequently, in 2011 a group of academic family physicians from Ontario, Canada developed a set of curricular guidelines in global health for family medicine residency programmes (Redwood-Campbell *et al.* 2011).

Table 3.1 Domains/themes for objectives and competencies adapted from various publications

Author	Method	Goals/Objectives/Competencies
Houpt et al. 2007	Survey of professional and academic groups	• Global burden of disease • Traveller's medicine • Immigrant health
Battat et al. 2010	Literature review	• Skills to interface better with different populations, cultures, and healthcare systems • An understanding of immigrant health • Primary care within diverse cultural settings • Understand healthcare disparities between countries • An understanding of the burden of global disease • An understanding of travel medicine • Develop a sense of social responsibility • Appreciate contrasts in healthcare delivery systems and expectations • Humanism • Scientific and societal consequences of global change • Evolving global governance issues • Cost of global environmental change • Taking adequate patient histories and physical examinations in resource-poor settings • Cost-consciousness; using physical diagnosis without high technological support
Peluso et al. 2012	Nominal group technique among a group of experts in global health education	• Cross-cultural competence • Communication and linguistic skills • Understanding the geographical burden of disease • Problem solving with limited resources • Identifying social and environmental determinants of health • Recognising health inequities and their effect on individual health • Teamwork and collaborative problem solving • Professionalism and ethical behaviour • Awareness of requirements for global health workers • Conducting a limited, population or community-based study • Applying knowledge of preventive care

| Cherniak et al. 2013 | Literature review | • Understanding the impact of migration and marginalisation on health
• Understanding key global health "players"
• Knowledge of local history, culture, social structure, politics
• Understanding local healthcare service structure
• Knowledge of local medical terminology
• Increasing cultural awareness
• Building knowledge of tropical medicine
• Learning about resource availability
• Understanding culture shock
• Learning a new language
• Enhancing clinical skills
• Understanding different healthcare systems
• Understanding cultural differences in treating patients
• Learning to manage diseases rarely seen at home
• Learning about common health concerns in the developing world
• Maintaining and reviewing data entry logs
• Understanding differences in medical education
• Functioning in low resource settings
• Gaining surgical experience
• Understanding clinical ethics
• Attending lectures
• Engaging in research projects
• Learning research methodology
• Reflecting on experiences |

Table 3.2 Domains/theme areas for objectives and competencies from professional societies and organisations focused on global health education

Group	Theme areas
Global Health Education Consortium	• Global burden of disease • Health implications of travel, migration and displacement • Social and economic determinants of health • Population, resources and environment • Globalisation of health and healthcare • Healthcare in low resource settings • Human rights in global health
Global Health Learning Outcomes Working Group	• Global burden of disease • Socioeconomic and environmental determinants of health • Health systems • Global health governance • Human rights and ethics • Cultural diversity and health
Consortium of Universities for Global Health	• Global burden of disease • Globalisation of health and healthcare • Social and environmental determinants of health • Capacity strengthening • Collaboration, partnering and communication • Ethics • Professional practice • Health equity and social justice • Programme management • Sociocultural and political awareness • Strategic analysis

These guidelines were structured to match the Canadian Medical Education Directives for Specialists (CanMEDS), with an ultimate goal of producing a "global health expert." This framework was underpinned by values and principles such as reciprocity, respect and humility (among others).

Since that time, the CUGH has also developed global health competencies, which it has divided into different levels (as discussed above; Jogerst *et al.* 2015, Wilson *et al.* 2014); specifically, it has articulated eight domains for the global citizen level and three additional domains for the programme-oriented basic operational level. Each domain has a subset of competencies, and each competency is categorised with a knowledge, skill, or attitude classification. CUGH's classification seeks to develop a broad, unifying set of competencies, but at the same time recognises that it is unlikely that any one programme would be able to achieve all of the competencies. CUGH's competencies are, at the current time, the most exhaustive and comprehensive list available and represent a major step towards standardisation of global health curricular goals.

Diverse perspectives: the voice of low and middle-income countries

In general, voices from high-income countries (HICs) have outnumbered perspectives from LMICs in the published literature on objectives and competencies for IMEs. However, authors representing LMICs have explored academic partnerships broadly, and in doing so have noted concerns with inequitable agendas, transitory relationships and lack of adequate supervision and objectives for trainees (Kolars *et al.* 2012, Kumwenda *et al.* 2015). These authors have proposed objectives by which collaborations can be evaluated, but the focus is on an institutional level rather than a trainee level.

In particular, Kumwenda *et al.* conducted semi-structured interviews with leaders at seven host sites in sub-Saharan Africa (Kumwenda *et al.* 2015). They noted great variability in the motivations that hosts described for providing elective experiences, and reviewed key themes including how IMEs are organised, the pros and cons of hosting IMEs, issues with supervision and perspectives on how systems for electives could be improved. In particular, they focus on the importance of enlisting institutions from LMICs as partners in the design and implementation of IMEs, at the same time noting that these institutions may rely on support and investment from sending institutions to ensure that trainees can achieve whatever objectives are put in place.

Other authors representing LMICs have suggested that an approach that lacks rigid structure or preplanned tasks might be the most optimal, because the focus on optimising the experience for the student may actually detract from mutual benefit (Ouma and Dimaras 2013). It is unclear whether such a philosophy could apply to medical trainees participating in IMEs, who will likely be involved in the provision of patient care and whose training in other non-IME contexts would be subject to the standards put in place by accrediting organisations.

Controversy and challenges

Some authors argue that the development of competencies in global health is particularly problematic, citing, for example, challenges already noted – lack of adequate input from LMIC host partners and lack of appropriate attention to the details of the local context (Eichbaum 2015). Eichbaum also notes some unique challenges to competencies in global health. These include the disjunction between "individualist" and "collectivist" approaches to clinical medicine and healthcare delivery and challenges with regard to adequate methods of assessing the achievement of objectives and competencies due to limited capacity for evaluation in many of IME settings. These concepts are explored further in *Chapter 4*.

An additional perspective is that when asking partners in the Global South to describe their impression of "global health" competencies, they may be likely to reply, "it's just called health where I live." While an important perspective to consider, we believe that global health is in fact informed by a uniform set of novel principles, and is not simply medicine in a different setting. A global health perspective to IMEs can be thought of as a unique way of engaging in medical work abroad, that shifts focus from the pure clinical management of disease to more broadly defined global health principles. Ethical considerations must also be central for IMEs to do more good than harm. These considerations are discussed in depth in *Chapters 12–18*.

Recommendations and conclusions

Based on this review, we put forth the following considerations for the development and revision of global health programmes:

1. Frame the IME not just as the time spent away, but rather as consisting of at least three distinct periods – the pre-departure period, the away period and the return period.
2. Consider specific objectives and competencies for each of the three periods of time, not just the away period.
3. Consider specific objectives and competencies that can be achieved at the "home" site or sending institution and at the "away" site or receiving institution.
4. Goals for the IME should likely include some combination of context-free and context-linked objectives and competencies, and these should be specifically noted as such. Context-linked objectives and competencies, in particular, should be constructed with significant input from the receiving site.
5. Objectives and competencies should be constructed in the context of professional society recommendations reviewed in this chapter, but a single IME need not achieve all of these recommendations, nor should it strive to achieve recommendations that are not achievable, or would put considerable strain on the receiving institution in the local context.
6. Specific thought and planning must be given ahead of time to how each objective or competency can be demonstrated or assessed. Objectives or competencies that cannot be assessed should be reconsidered, or framed in a way that can be evaluated.
7. There is more value in focusing on what is unique to an IME (i.e., "Learn about the cultural context of traditional healers as they relate to the Ugandan healthcare system"), than articulating objectives or competencies that can be assumed based on what is known about these experiences in general (i.e., "improve clinical skills"). The development of such objectives and competencies might be iterative, depend upon input from both the local site and students who have previously completed the IME, and may likely be context specific.

In this chapter, we have reviewed principles related to objectives and competencies for IMEs. It is ultimately the efforts of individual programmes that will shift the focus of IMEs from general experiences to specific actionable items. This shift will also reflect increasingly authentic and achievable (and more modest) learning objectives for IMEs. In this way we also decrease the risk of inappropriately exaggerating the abilities of HIC trainees who have participated in an IME. For global health to grow as a field, it will be crucial for IMEs to be held to similar standards as traditional medical school rotations and for objectives and competencies to capture what is unique to global health education. This will require significant thought and creativity on the part of educational leaders, but will yield tangible results for generations of students to come.

References

Anderson KC, Slatnik MA, Pereira I, Cheung E, Xu K, Brewer TF. 2012. "Are we there yet? Preparing Canadian medical students for global health electives." *Academic Medicine* 87(2):206–209.

Arthur MA, Battat R, Brewer TF. 2011. "Teaching the basics: core competencies in global health." *Infectious Disease Clinics of North America* 25(2):347–358.

Battat R, Seidman G, Chadi N, *et al.* 2010. "Global health competencies and approaches in medical education: a literature review." *BMC Medical Education* 10:94.

Bozinoff N, Dorman KP, Kerr D, *et al.* 2014. "Toward reciprocity: host supervisor perspectives on international medical electives." *Medical Education* 48(4):397–404.

Brunger F, Duke PS. 2012. "The evolution of integration: innovations in clinical skills and ethics in first year medicine." *Medical Teacher* 34(6):e452–458.

Cherniak WA, Drain PK, Brewer TF. 2013. "Educational objectives for international medical electives: a literature review." *Academic Medicine*. 88(11):1778–1781.

Dowell J, Merrylees N. 2009. "Electives: isn't it time for a change?" *Medical Education* 43(2):121–126.

Eichbaum Q. 2015. "The problem with competencies in global health education." *Academic Medicine* 90(4):414–417.

Frenk J, Chen L, Bhutta ZA, *et al.* 2010. "Health professionals for a new century: transforming education to strengthen health systems in an interdependent world." *Lancet* 376(9756):1923–1958.

Gruppen LD, Mangrulkar RS, Kolars JC. 2012. "The promise of competency-based education in the health professions for improving global health." *Human Resources for Health* 10:43.

Houpt ER, Pearson RD, Hall TL. 2007. "Three domains of competency in global health education: recommendations for all medical students." *Academic Medicine* 82(3):222–225.

Howe A, Barrett A, Leinster S. 2009. "How medical students demonstrate their professionalism when reflecting on experience." *Medical Education* 43(10):942–951.

Jogerst K, Callender B, Adams V, *et al.* 2015. "Identifying interprofessional global health competencies for 21st-century health professionals." *Annals of Global Health* 81(2):239–247.

Johnson O, Bailey SL, Willott C, *et al.* 2012. "Global health learning outcomes for medical students in the UK." *Lancet* 379(9831):2033–2035.

Kolars JC, Cahill K, Donkor P, *et al.* 2012. "Perspective: partnering for medical education in Sub-Saharan Africa: seeking the evidence for effective collaborations." *Academic Medicine* 87(2):216–220.

Kumwenda B, Dowell J, Daniels K, Merrylees N. 2015. "Medical electives in sub-Saharan Africa: a host perspective." *Medical Education* 49(6):623–633.

Mullan PB, Lypson ML. 2011. "Communicating your program's goals and objectives." *Journal of Graduate Medical Education* 3(4):574–576.

Naidu T, Kumagai AK. 2016. "Troubling muddy waters: problematizing reflective practice in global medical education." *Academic Medicine* 91(3):317–321.

Ouma BD, Dimaras H. 2013. "Views from the Global South: exploring how student volunteers from the Global North can achieve sustainable impact in global health." *Globalization and Health* 9(1):32.

Peluso MJ, Encandela J, Hafler JP, Margolis CZ. 2012. "Guiding principles for the development of global health education curricula in undergraduate medical education." *Medical Teacher* 34(8):653–658.

Redwood-Campbell L, Pakes B, Rouleau K, *et al.* 2011. "Developing a curriculum framework for global health in family medicine: emerging principles, competencies, and educational approaches." *BMC Medical Education* 11:46.

Sandars J. 2009. "The use of reflection in medical education: AMEE Guide No. 44." *Medical Teacher* 31(8):685–695.

Torjesen K, Mandalakas A, Kahn R, Duncan B. 1999. "International child health electives for pediatric residents." *Archives of Pediatrics & Adolescent Medicine.* 153(12):1297–1302.

Wilson L, Callender B, Hall TL, *et al.* 2014. "Identifying global health competencies to prepare 21st century global health professionals: report from the global health competency subcommittee of the Consortium of Universities for Global Health." *The Journal of Law, Medicine & Ethics* 42 (Suppl 2):26–31.

4 Challenging paradigms of global health education

Examining critiques of competency-based education

Quentin Eichbaum, Virginia Rowthorn,
Jill Allison and Catherine Myser

Introduction

The marked proliferation of global health (GH) programmes in high-income countries (HICs) over the past couple of decades has resulted in a haphazard and uncoordinated development of associated educational curricula. During the same period but starting earlier, a vigorous debate was occurring in medical schools across North America about competency-based education in the curriculum. Preoccupied with developing other components of their own curricula, GH programmes were late entering this debate, partly because they are new programmes, and partly because competency issues are more complex across the variable range of GH topics and contexts (Eichbaum 2015).

While numerous GH programmes – both within academic institutions and in public and GH organisations – have since developed models incorporating lists of specific domains and competencies, several complex issues relating to GH competencies remain unresolved. In this chapter, we present four such unresolved perspectives challenging competency-based education in GH.

Contexts: grounding principle

A current paradigm in GH education in HICs features students and trainees taking part in experiential learning in low resource settings of low and middle-income countries (LMICs). It is in these settings that many of the advocated competencies apply and ought to be assessed. However, the approach that HIC GH programmes have taken in developing these competencies is problematic, in that they have often taken insufficient account of local host LMIC contexts, and have failed to elicit and include LMIC health worker and community member perspectives.

Contexts vary widely in GH settings, where different disease profiles, geographies, climates, cultures and/or sociopolitical environs may substantially affect healthcare and delivery. However, competency-based health education has not fully appreciated the significance of these widely varying contexts. Competencies can be either context linked or context free. Competencies that are context free can be learned any place or time independent of a specific context, and can be applied generically across different contexts. An individual who has acquired such a competency can be predicted to be competent across such different contexts with regard to that particular competency. Context-linked competencies, on the other hand, are inextricably linked to specific contexts and are not transferable across contexts.

Some GH programmes have adopted "ready-made" lists of competencies developed by external organisations, while other GH programmes develop their own specific lists of competencies. It has seemed convenient for programmes to provide students and trainees with generic lists of competencies that can be applied in any of the varied LMIC sites in which they may seek to learn and work. Developing competencies for a range of differing, yet also specific, contexts takes additional effort and time. Experienced field workers in GH understand, however, that being competent in one context does not necessarily transfer or predict competence in another context. The failure to take sufficient account of contexts has been a major shortcoming of GH education, and has compromised effective assessment of such competencies.

The perspective of assessment

An important distinction in GH education is the difference between the "individualist" cultures of HICs and "collectivist" cultures of LMICs (Hofstede 1980). Understanding the parameters of this distinction is particularly important, given the educational paradigm in which students and trainees from HICs do elective work of varying periods in LMICs.

Individualist cultures focus on attributes of the individual and are generally competitive. They view learning as something that the individual can "acquire" and "possess" independently of contexts. Collectivist cultures tend to be group-oriented and view learning as "situated" within specific contexts and arising dynamically through group participation. Sfard (1998) drew the distinction between "acquired" and "participatory" learning with regard to approaches to learning in the individualist cultures of HICs and collectivist cultures of LMICs (Sfard 1998).

Competencies too may be viewed as "acquired" or "participatory" (Eichbaum 2016). Acquired competencies include those learnable as knowledge or skills. An individual can "acquire" and possess such competencies and they are, so to speak, "housed within" the individual. Such competencies are therefore not linked to specific contexts but can be applied across different contexts. Examples of acquired competencies are the ability to use a stethoscope or possessing the knowledge to interpret viral loads and CD4 cell counts in HIV infections. Participatory competencies, on the other hand, are those that arise dynamically in social settings and are inextricably linked to contexts. Examples include the American College of Graduate Medical Education (ACGME) core competency domains of communication and collaboration.

Acquired or participatory competencies need to be assessed differently. We can assess individually acquired competencies through direct observation and by standard psychometric methods. Participatory competencies are "situated" and learned through social participation, and cannot be effectively assessed through direct observation or psychometric methods. We have not as yet determined the most effective modality for assessing participatory competencies.

One suggested modality for assessing participatory competencies is self-directed assessment seeking (Eva and Regehr 2008, Eichbaum 2014, Eichbaum 2016). This method involves the student/trainee proactively seeking feedback (and being encouraged by faculty and mentors to do so) from a range of pertinent sources – then translating this feedback into improving performance. Sources from whom such feedback might be obtained include peers, teachers, team members and others connected with the student's or trainee's learning. Involvement of others in this assessment has been shown to be more reliable than that of single assessor preceptors. This approach to assessment, which may also include allied health professionals and community workers who have worked with the student/trainee, is also consonant in its inclusiveness with the collectivist cultures of LMICs. Furthermore, its inclusion of ancillary health workers is consonant with the notion of transprofessionalism as presented in the landmark 2010 *Lancet* report, Health Professionals for a New Century (Frenk *et al.* 2010).

Other previously described challenges in assessing competencies of HIC trainees working in LMICs include the following (Eichbaum 2015): (1) faculty shortages and workload demands in overcrowded LMIC hospitals and rural clinics that curtail time available for effective assessment of visiting HIC trainees; (2) absence of a valid "frame of reference" against which LMIC faculty can assess visiting HIC trainees who have trained in high tech tertiary care settings that differ substantially from LMIC low resource settings; (3) inadequacy of the "checkbox" assessment format that has resulted in "trivialised and mechanistic types of assessment" (Schuwirth and van der Vleuten 2012), also spurring overconfidence in HIC trainees; (4) limitations of medical microsystems in resource-constrained settings, themselves perhaps not yet sufficiently "competent" to develop and assess competency in visiting HIC trainees (Asch *et al.* 2009, Eichbaum 2015). Effective assessment of competencies in GH education thus remains an unresolved issue requiring significant additional discussion and research.

The perspective of ethics

There is a lexicon in the field of GH that routinely advances – and distinguishes, if only by implication – "competencies" to which HIC students and practitioners ought to aspire and achieve, and "capacities" to which LMIC students and practitioners should aspire and be helped to build. This lexicon is evident, for example, in discussions relating to GH education, research and grants. It is important to begin to problematise these contrasting concepts and aspirations; as well as their "geographical" location, i.e., mostly originating from the Global North, conceding inadequate consultation with the Global South; and associated, perhaps unconscious, epistemological assumptions of HIC normativity and even superiority. All the above might reveal a "hidden curriculum" of colonialism or neocolonialism that would benefit from examination and possible redress.

To begin exploring possible underlying assumptions, it is worth considering the following. "Competency" generally carries the sense of being well qualified, of being able to do something successfully or efficiently. "Capacity," by contrast, refers to the ability to receive, hold, or absorb something, for example, learning or retaining knowledge. "Capacity" thus appears more passive and preliminary, and "competency" seems more active and robust. If this is true, after "capacity" is "built" by HIC teachers and/or "received" by LMIC learners, can and do aspirations to LMIC "competency" follow? Furthermore, why is there not more acknowledgement highlighting the many contexts and topics for which LMIC teachers are the ones who possess local and regional knowledge and skills, on which basis HIC learners are the ones who need help "building capacity," assisted by LMIC teachers? We need to be more explicit about these concepts and their relationships, especially in the GH context, where discussions of "competency attainment" usually attach to HIC learners, and discussions of "capacity building" usually attach to LMIC learners taught by HIC teachers.

In other words, who can or should "build capacity," and who can or should "achieve competency?" Who should be doing the teaching ("capacity building") and who should be doing the learning (whether "receiving capacity" or "acquiring competency")? For example, LMIC hosts have a better understanding of local and regional contexts and are therefore better placed to develop the requisite associated competencies, and are in these contexts therefore also best equipped to "build capacity" in HIC learners.

Authors from the Global South object that the "existing... GH [literature] – its evolving definitions, scope, and, very importantly the values and *competencies* required for ethical practice – reveals a troubling imbalance: there is little contribution from southern authors based in the South" (Sanchez and Lopez 2013). At the same time, authors from the Global North issue caveats that "it is these [experts/power brokers] prominent researchers from the most prestigious HICs and a very select group of elite researchers from LMICs that have the [epistemological] power [to] set agendas, frame issues, identify problems, and propose solutions" within GH (Crane 2010). Without more egalitarian Global South input to challenge and "decenter" HIC and Global North concepts – such as the above concepts and perspectives on "competency" and "capacity," – remarkably intransigent and structurally enduring colonial relations are maintained, and HIC and Global North learners and teachers remain in a position of positional superiority with respect to their LMIC and the Global South counterparts.

The perspective of interprofessionalism

Over the past 15 years, interest in GH among undergraduate and graduate students in all professions has reached unprecedented levels (Merson and Page 2009). At the first meeting of the Consortium of Universities for Global Health (CUGH) in 2008, many academics in the field argued that rapid expansion of GH programmes at the university level led to haphazard growth of the field, a lack of agreed-upon definitions, and failure to standardise curricula and competencies (CUGH 2008). To remedy these concerns and promote standardisation, much work has been done in recent years in a number of individual professions, such as nursing and medicine, to develop GH competencies (Wilson *et al.* 2012, Battat *et al.* 2010). However, as awareness of GH has expanded, so too has the realisation that addressing the complex factors that contribute to the health of individuals and communities requires participation by a broad range of professionals from health and non-health disciplines. Although individual professions are making strides in developing and measuring discipline-specific competencies, less has been done in the area of interdisciplinary or interprofessional GH education.

Working from the understanding that GH is an interprofessional collaborative field, GH programmes are faced with the imperative of teaching students *how* to be collaborative. Within the universe of what is considered interprofessional GH education are two separate areas of learning – shared substantive content (often called cognitive or "hard skills") and non-cognitive individual and interpersonal skills, such as perseverance, openness and ability to work as part of a team (often called social/relational or "soft" skills) (Bloom 1956). A major first step towards addressing the need for a standardised interprofessional GH curriculum in the area of substantive content was taken by the Association of Schools and Programs of Public Health (ASPPH) in 2011 when it published a GH competency model for schools of public health and other GH educational programmes (Association of School of Public Health 2011). The model defines essential competencies for students specialising in GH such as capacity strengthening collaborating and partnering, and ethical reasoning and professional practice. The ASPPH model was explicitly designed to be used in both graduate schools of public health and beyond, e.g., "schools of international relations/affairs, business schools, law schools and, of course, other health professions' schools, such as those in medicine and nursing, as well as programs in the biological and social sciences." In a related vein, in 2013, CUGH commenced a project headed up by Dr Lynda Wilson to define the interdisciplinary core content expected of all GH programmes (Jogerst *et al.* 2015). This multi-year effort resulted in a comprehensive list of cross-cutting competencies created with input from a range of professional school faculty.

Another global competency initiative that focused solely on non-cognitive, interpersonal and team competencies from an interprofessional perspective uses the well-known Interprofessional Education Collaborative

(IPEC) *Competencies for Interprofessional Collaborative Practice* model as the framework for a team skills competency domain for GH students (Rowthorn and Olsen 2015). The IPEC competencies, which are focused on healthcare providers and clinical care, were adapted for use in GH settings which typically include non-health professionals and often place students and practitioners in team settings where the interpersonal aspects of teamwork may be harder to achieve because of unfamiliar work and cultural settings. As noted by one GH scholar, "[i]n a global and complex environment, the ability to cooperate between professions and work across cultures is vitally important. Sharing knowledge is a crucial component of this process, yet in many cases the greatest challenge to the success of interprofessional education is the collaborative component." (Rowthorn and Olsen 2015).

A significant problem with GH competencies from the interprofessional perspective is that GH interventions often involve skills that are difficult to assess, especially for non-health students, such as law, ethics, social work and social science students, whose participation in GH often relates to policy or regulatory or ethnographic work.

The perspective of critical social science

Culture is not a static concept: it cannot be enumerated or packaged as a skill to be learned, or assessed. Culture moves and shifts, absorbs and changes, as new ideas, political realities and economic elements shape its edges. GH programmes incorporate cultural competency training, often in pre-departure orientations, as a means of preparing learners to be appropriately responsive to different cultural contexts. The challenge lies in the complexity of culture and the implications of competency, as outlined above.

Cultural competency has become a "fashionable term" but lacks the precision enabling it to be put into practice (Ogbu 1981, Kleinman and Benson 2006). While accounting for culture in healthcare is crucial, there has been little research to guide pedagogy more robustly for skill building around cultural competency (Ogbu 1981, Kleinman and Benson 2006). Achieving cultural competency in GH is not only context dependent but experience dependent. Accordingly, one aim in GH education is to enrich knowledge through experience in order to increase understanding of the relationship between culture, health and wellbeing in all contexts. A superficial approach to cultural competency risks empowering learners and practitioners to make assumptions while reducing their capacity to see the depth of cultural influence. Health inequalities may be attributed to cultural differences rather than political, economic and structural inequalities and relations of power (Kirmayer 2012, Pon 2009, Sakamoto 2007).

Lila Abu Lughod reminds us that culture, as a concept, is akin to "race" in its potential to convey politicised meanings (Abu Lughod 1999). Suggestions that culture resides in others can serve to consolidate notions of superiority endorsed by privilege in the Global North. More important is the cultivation of "structural competency," through which practitioners recognise that downstream healthcare challenges are often the result of upstream social determinants (Metzl and Hansen 2014). How to teach learners to distinguish between culture and structural inequalities is linked again to creating conditions that foster experiential learning and the process of attaining cultural competence in context.

The skill that must be acquired is not how to respond to one cultural behaviour or another, but how to assess the way cultural differences shape an experience, for both provider and patient. A critical dialogue around what actually defines cultural competency will help position it within both GH education and health sciences education more broadly. It will also ensure that competency is a tool for advocacy towards health equity locally and globally.

Conclusion

We present four different perspectives on competency-based education in GH. The issues each perspective raises are complex, and it is not apparent how to align or reconcile them – or whether indeed that is necessary? The grounding principle is that of context. Assessment, ethics, interprofessionalism and critical perspectives in social sciences all have contextual constraints in GH.

Each of the perspectives we present also, however, provides a unique angle on the competency debate. The assessment perspective makes the distinction between the individualist and collectivist approaches to learning and suggests that competencies be classified as either (individually) "acquired" or "participatory" (and situated in social dynamics); the ethical perspective draws attention to the linguistic distinction between "capacities" and "competencies" that complicates the education debate between the "Global North and South;" the interprofessionalism perspective insists that GH is increasingly an interdisciplinary or interprofessional collaboration that often involves teams, and that competencies be devised and assessed to reflect such shared knowledge; the critical social science perspective reminds us of the challenges of defining, teaching and assessing "cultural competency;" emphasising more importantly the crucial skill of "structural competency," i.e., perceiving and addressing root political, economic and structural determinants and inequalities.

In developing competencies for students and trainees in GH, training programmes in HICs have not only taken insufficient account of contexts, but have also frequently failed to understand the different perspectives on competency-based training. It is our hope that this chapter will stimulate further debate and research on these perspectives on competency-based training in GH.

References

Abu Lughod, L. 1999. "Comment in response to writing for culture: why a successful concept should not be discarded." *Current Anthropology* 40(S1):S1–S27. doi: 10.1086/200058.

Asch, D.A., S. Nicholson, S. Srinivas, J. Herrin, and A.J. Epstein. 2009. "Evaluating obstetrical residency programs using patient outcomes." *JAMA* 302(12):1277–1283. doi: 10.1001/jama.2009.1356.

Association of School of Public Health. 2011. "Global Health Competency Model – Final Version 1.1." Association of Schools & Programs of Public Health. Accessed 06/10/16. www.publichealth.pitt.edu/Portals/0/Main/ASPH GH Competencies.pdf.

Battat, R., G. Seidman, N. Chadi, M.Y. Chanda, J. Nehme, J. Hulme, A.N. Li, N. Faridi, and T.F. Brewer. 2010. "Global health competencies and approaches in medical education: a literature review." *BMC Medical Education* 10. doi: Artn 9410.1186/1472-6920-10-94.

Bloom, B. 1956. "Taxonomy of educational objectives, Handbook I: Cognitive domain." *Journal of Interprofessional Care* 19(S1):49–59.

Crane, J.T. 2010. "Unequal 'partners'. AIDS, academia, and the rise of global health." *Behemoth A Journal on Civilisation* 3(3):78–97.

Eichbaum, Q. 2016. "Acquired and participatory competencies in global health education: definition and assessment." Academic Medicine in press.

Eichbaum, Q. 2015. "The problem with competencies in global health education." *Academic Medicine* 90(4):414–417. doi: 10.1097/ACM.0000000000000665.

Eichbaum, Q.G. 2014. "Thinking about thinking and emotion: the metacognitive approach to the medical humanities that integrates the humanities with the basic and clinical sciences." *The Permanente Journal* 18(4):64–75. doi: 10.7812/TPP/14-027.

Eva, K.W., and G. Regehr. 2008. ""I'll never play professional football" and other fallacies of self-assessment." *Journal of Continuing Education in the Health Professions* 28(1):14–19. doi: 10.1002/chp.150.

Frenk, J., L. Chen, Z.A. Bhutta, J. Cohen, N. Crisp, T. Evans, H. Fineberg, P. Garcia, Y. Ke, P. Kelley, B. Kistnasamy, A. Meleis, D. Naylor, A. Pablos-Mendez, S. Reddy, S. Scrimshaw, J. Sepulveda, D. Serwadda, and H. Zurayk. 2010. "Health professionals for a new century: transforming education to strengthen health systems in an interdependent world." *Lancet* 376(9756):1923–1958. doi: 10.1016/S0140-6736(10)61854-5.

Hofstede, G.H. 1980. *Culture's consequences: international differences in work-related values.* Cross-cultural research and methodology series. Newbury Park; London: Sage.

Jogerst, K., B. Callender, V. Adams, J. Evert, E. Fields, T. Hall, J. Olsen, V. Rowthorn, S. Rudy, J.B. Shen, L. Simon, H. Torres, A. Velji, and L.L. Wilson. 2015. "Identifying interprofessional global health competencies for 21st-century health professionals." *Annals of Global Health* 81(2):239–247. doi: 10.1016/j.aogh.2015.03.006.

Kirmayer, L.J. 2012. "Rethinking cultural competence." *Transcultural Psychiatry* 49(2):149–164. doi: 10.1177/1363461512444673.

Kleinman, A., and P. Benson. 2006. "Anthropology in the clinic: the problem of cultural competency and how to fix it." *Plos Medicine* 3(10):1673–1676. doi: ARTN e29410.1371/journal.pmed.0030294.

Merson, M.H., and K.C. Page. 2009. The Dramatic Expansion of University Engagement in Global Health: Implications for U.S. Policy. Washington, D.C.: CSIS/ Center for Strategic & International Studies.

Metzl, J.M, and H. Hansen. 2014. "Structural competency: theorizing a new medical engagement with stigma and inequality." *Social Science & Medicine* 103:126–133.

Ogbu, J.U. 1981. "Origins of human competence – a cultural-ecological perspective." *Child Development* 52(2):413–429. doi: 10.1111/j.1467–8624.1981.tb03064.x.

Pon, G. 2009. "Cultural competency as new racism: an ontology of forgetting." *Journal of Progressive Human Services* 20(1):59–71. doi: 10.1080/ 10428230902871173.

Rowthorn, V., and J. Olsen. 2015. "All together now: developing a team skills competency domain for global health education." *Journal of Law, Medicine & Ethics* 42(4):550–563. doi: 10.1111/jlme.12175.

Sakamoto, I. 2007. "An anti-oppressive approach to cultural competence." *Canadian Social Work Review* 24(1):105–118.

Sanchez, A., and V.A. Lopez. 2013. "Perspectives on global health from the South." In: *An introduction to global health ethics*, edited by A.D. Pinto and R.E.G. Upshur, 129–135. New York: Routledge.

Schuwirth, L.W.T., and C.P.M. van der Vleuten. 2012. "Assessing competence: extending the approaches to reliability" In: *The question of competence: reconsidering medical education in the twenty-first century*, 113–130. IRL Press.

Sfard, A. 1998. "On two metaphors for learning and the dangers of choosing just one." *Educational Researcher* 27(2):4–13.

Wilson, L., D.C. Harper, I. Tami-Maury, R. Zarate, S. Salas, J. Farley, N. Warren, I. Mendes, and C. Ventura. 2012. "Global health competencies for nurses in the Americas." *Journal of Professional Nursing* 28(4):213–22. doi: 10.1016/ j.profnurs.2011.11.021.

5 Engendering interprofessionalism in global health education

Virginia Rowthorn, Peter Brown, Leslie Glickman, Amy Lockwood, Jody Olsen and Brittany Seymour

Background: developing interprofessional global health competencies

Over the past decade, interest in global health among undergraduate and graduate students has reached unprecedented levels (Merson and Page 2009). As awareness of global health has expanded, so too has the realisation that addressing the complex factors that contribute to the health of individuals and communities requires the participation of a broad range of professionals from health and non-health disciplines.

The importance of interprofessional collaboration has been emphasised by the World Health Organization (WHO) which, in 2006, encouraged stakeholders in global health endeavours to "…work together through inclusive alliances and networks – local, national, and global – across health problems, professions, disciplines, ministries, sectors, and countries" (World Health Organization (WHO) 2006). Strong professional skills are not useful if they cannot be deployed as part of a bigger whole; sometimes the necessary knowledge or resources rest with another – perhaps an individual, agency, or even a community – that could be mobilised in an effective way (Collaborative Justice 2015).

While many professionals working in the global health arena appreciate the value of an interprofessional approach, colleges and universities have been slow to adopt effective interprofessional education (IPE) methods, especially outside of the health sciences. The challenge is how to create interprofessional global health education programmes in training systems predicated on single disciplines. Even among universities that offer campus-wide global health programmes, administrators of these programmes report substantive and logistical barriers because professional education is largely provided through schools that focus on ensuring that students acquire the skill base required by a specific profession and its licensing requirements (Knapp *et al.* 1993). Much work has been done in recent years in a number of individual professions, such as nursing (Wilson *et al.* 2012) and medicine (Battat *et al.* 2010) to develop global health competencies and the academic rigor and standards that competency frameworks encourage. However, less has been done in the area of interdisciplinary or interprofessional global health competencies.

A major step towards addressing the need for a standardised interprofessional global health curriculum was taken by the Association of Schools and Programs of Public Health (ASPPH) in 2011 when it published a global health competency model. The ASPPH model was explicitly designed to be used in graduate schools of public health and beyond, including "schools of international relations/affairs, business schools, law schools and, of course, other health professions' schools, such as those in medicine and nursing, as well as programmes in the biological and social sciences" (Association of Schools and Programs for Public Health (ASPPH) 2011).

In a related vein, in 2013, the Consortium of Universities for Global Health (CUGH) commenced a project to define the interdisciplinary core content expected of all global health programmes at both the undergraduate and graduate level. This multi-year effort resulted in a comprehensive list of cross-cutting competencies created with input from a range of professional school faculty (Jogerst *et al.* 2015). The competency domains in this framework include the global burden of disease and the globalisation of health and healthcare.

The value of teamwork in global health

In addition to shared knowledge and skills, to bolster the field of global health, students need to be taught the value of teamwork, as well as the development and management of relationships that are key to making any well-designed endeavour possible. This is particularly important in the field of global health where teamwork takes many forms, including teams comprising students, community members, healthcare practitioners, government officials, civil society, researchers, faculty members and any combination thereof.

To work towards interprofessional collaboration in the field of healthcare, the field of IPE was developed as a way to teach students the knowledge, skills and attitudes necessary for effective and ethical teamwork. The field of IPE was greatly advanced by the publication in 2011 of "Core Competencies for Interprofessional Collaborative Practice," a massive effort by the Interprofessional Education Collaborative (IPEC), a group composed of six prominent health professional organisations. The IPEC competency model was designed to promote "interprofessional collaborative practice as key to the safe, high quality, accessible, patient-centered care desired by all" (Interprofessional Education Collaborative (IPEC) 2011). However, the field of IPE and the IPEC competency model are directed almost exclusively to the education of health professional students and are most frequently framed as a way to improve clinical care. This makes the IPEC competencies slightly less useful for global health which, in addition to clinical care, often involves public health, technology, regulatory and policy work. Furthermore, the field of global health encompasses clinical, service, advocacy and research initiatives with host country partners, which limits the utility of the US domestic version of IPE envisioned by IPEC.

To address this shortfall, in 2014, Rowthorn *et al.* used the IPEC model to create a team skills competency domain for global health (Rowthorn and Olsen 2014).

Business and organisational skills: critical for all global health practitioners

One critical area of learning that has still not been widely adopted in global health education is training in business principles, specifically management and leadership skills. Well-functioning health systems require strong leadership and management in order to put policies and structures in place that allow them to deliver quality care and to respond to changing circumstances. Many of the aspects of delivering care are not clinical, but instead are related to information, communication, supply chains, logistics, human resources, finances and regulations. It is often the way in which these issues are addressed that determines the success of a global health intervention.

According to Bill Foege, the former CDC director and a senior advisor to the Bill and Melinda Gates Foundation, lack of management skills appears to be the single most important barrier to improving health throughout the world (Foege *et al.* 2005). As evidenced by efforts to contain Ebola in West Africa (World Health Organization (WHO) 2015), scale-up of antiretroviral therapy in sub-Saharan Africa (Curran *et al.* 2005) or eradicate polio in India (United Nations Children's Fund 2003), the final barriers to equitably delivering healthcare are often not scientific, but managerial, including: collecting and analysing data, modelling demand for and securing supplies of essential medicines, and developing communication and social marketing efforts. Crafting public health messages and disseminating information and results to the lay public is important to change behaviours. The shortage of staff with appropriate skills, weak systems for planning and monitoring performance, and a workplace without proper support for ongoing training or performance incentives all contribute to the management challenge faced by those responsible for delivering health services and public health in low-income countries (Egger *et al.* 2005, Oliveira-Cruz *et al.* 2003).

Barriers to implementing interprofessional global health programmes at the university level

When universities and programmes try to incorporate IPE into their curriculum, it is difficult to do so for multiple reasons, including university-level logistical barriers, disincentives for faculty participation and professional silos. It is also difficult to measure the value of an interprofessional approach because there is no consensus about evaluation frameworks, analytical methods or impact metrics. Educational methods that are unmeasurable often find little administration-level support (Rowthorn and Olsen 2014). Furthermore, most IPE evaluation tools are strictly designed to evaluate clinical education and outcomes, not public health, community health or advocacy outcomes as are often pursued by interprofessional teams in global health.

However, there are notable exemplars of IPE evaluation tools that merit mention. They include the Canadian Interprofessional Health Collaborative (CIHC) competency framework; the Collaborative Practice Assessment Tool (CPAT); the Interprofessional Collaborative Organizational Map and Preparedness Assessment (IP-COMPASS); the Interprofessional Collaborator Assessment Rubric (ICAR); the Performance Assessment Communication and Teamwork Tools Set (PACT); and the Assessment of Interprofessional Team Collaboration Scale (AITCS) (Canadian Interprofessional Health Collaborative (CIHC) 2009, National Center for Interprofessional Practice and Education (NCIPE) 2016). Faculty implementing interprofessional global health programmes should make an effort to evaluate their programmes at least for student interprofessional learning and, as resources allow, work towards evaluating behaviour and project results (if the training programme incorporates patient/community outcome goals). The global health community as a whole – including funders – should support development and implementation of a broad range of evaluation tools for interprofessional global health.

Interprofessionalism in education: an experiential learning model

Lessons learned from the global health grant programme at the University of Maryland Baltimore (UMB) offer one perspective on overcoming barriers to IPE to prepare students to approach the practice of global health collaboratively. CGEI is premised on an experiential learning approach to train global health students early in their professional career how to work with other professions in pursuit of shared global health goals (Rowthorn 2013).

Between 2010 and 2013, the UMB Center for Global Education Initiatives (CGEI) organised multiple 6-week long interprofessional experiential learning programmes in Malawi involving faculty and students from all six UMB professional schools – dentistry, law, medicine, nursing, pharmacy and social work. In 2013, CGEI redesigned the programme to push responsibility for the creation of interprofessional programmes out of the centre and into the hands of faculty. Under this programme, individual faculty members apply for small grants and then students from all campus schools apply to participate in any of the advertised faculty projects. Faculty who apply for these grants typically have ongoing international research projects into which they incorporate students with logistical support from CGEI. To be eligible for funding, the proposed project must be interprofessional and include at least two participating students representing at least two, and often more, different schools on campus. The student role in the project must relate to the overall goal of the project AND in some way to the student's future profession to ensure that the project is truly interdisciplinary and not simply a vehicle to hire student research assistants or one in which students work in silos in the same setting. As such, some topics are more appropriate for interprofessional teams and those include public health, health policy and behavioural intervention projects (Rowthorn and Olsen 2015). An example of such a project was the "Communication of end-of-life issues: an interprofessional approach" project in 2015 during which Dr Mei Ching Lee of the University of Maryland School of Nursing included students from nursing, dentistry, social work and medicine in a project in Hong Kong during which time the team interviewed Chinese healthcare professionals as part of a bigger project regarding effective communication methods to engage Chinese Americans in the discussion of end-of-life issues.

Benefits from the revised project model include more student and faculty participation, more research projects in countries on all continents, more faculty/student mentoring based on their familiarity with the research topic and country, and more post-project presentation opportunities for both faculty and students together (Olsen and Chatterjee, 2017).

Interprofessionalism in education: preparation for interprofessional immersion experiences

To prepare students to engage in interprofessional experiential learning, a framework of structured and unstructured activities should be used to prepare students, engage them while onsite, and follow up on their return from travel. Research has demonstrated that adequate student preparation is key to a project's success and to cohesion of a team and that team-building activities must continue into and even after the immersion experience (Eckhert 2006).

Pre-immersion activities consist of coursework preparation, team building experiences (informal and formal), informational discussions, orientation meetings, review of cultural expectations, safety/security requirements, details for the specific project and Institutional Review Board proposal processes with preliminary data collection if indicated. The pre-immersion time frame is also when students should be taught critical themes of cultural humility, cross-cultural communication, power and privilege and bioethical concepts. Although these themes are important for all global health participants – not just those in interprofessional teams – the interprofessional perspective adds a great deal of value to these discussions. Immersion activities consist of on-the-ground planning meetings, continuous opportunities to reflect on the interprofessional nature of the team and the project, implementation of client-focused research projects, cultural experiences in the local communities, and presentation of project results/recommendations to local leaders, partners and other interested parties. Post-immersion activities consist of detailed work on the dissemination projects, reflection journaling, university-related reports, initiation of scholarly papers, completion of school/programme requirements and future planning (Rowthorn and Olsen 2015, Glickman 2016).

Interprofessionalism and culture

Moving beyond the model of a mixed profession university team, consideration must be given to the concept of interprofessionality across cultures. Because global health projects are generally located in low or middle-income countries with different cultures, the field of medical anthropology has proved to be a very important addition to a wide range of health and development programmes (Nichter 2008). Anthropologists are particularly interested in understanding diverse cultures and counteracting the endemic ethnocentrism and intercultural miscommunications that often plague international programmes. In this regard, it is possible to say that *every global health project is a cross-cultural interaction.* It is unfortunately the case that students often go into field situations with very little knowledge of local history, culture and politics; moreover, they can show little curiosity about local people, their culture and knowledge – preferring only to interact with one another. Basic knowledge and appreciation are relatively simple to learn and, in fact, such knowledge is crucial both for the design of projects, as well as the creation of true partnerships with local people.

This means that it is important for practitioners to be cognisant of culture on both sides of the equation – being aware of the presuppositions of the culture of global health itself as well as the culture of the local people. Students must engage in self-reflection about the role of their own culture as they process their global health training experience and their interactions with local partners. Local counterparts must also learn to understand the culture of research and global health programming (as conceptualised in high-income countries).

Recently, Closser and Finley have summarised five lessons for working in interprofessional global health contexts with members of a team whether the team members are from the same university or international collaborators. These skills include: (a) communicating clearly without jargon; (b) being transparent about methodologies; (c) being factually correct; (d) being aware of anthropological biases; and (e) making concrete recommendations for action. With regard to interprofessional training, such suggestions are valuable for all participants (Closser and Finley 2016).

Interprofessionalism in practice: oral health example

The mouth is a mirror of the body, reflecting signs and symptoms of systemic disease, such as HIV/AIDS, malnutrition, and non-communicable diseases (FDI World Dental Federation 2015, Seymour *et al.* 2014). Many systemic conditions worsen oral diseases, and vice versa. For example, diabetes and periodontal disease are closely associated; having one makes controlling the other more difficult. Oral diseases and systemic conditions also share common risk factors, including sugar, tobacco and alcohol. This relationship between oral health and overall health is becoming increasingly complex due to the shared health impacts of emerging trends such as our ageing global population; urbanisation; demographic, epidemiological, and nutrition transitions; and other social determinants such as the environment. It simply is not possible to control the burden of oral diseases and their impact on systemic health without an interprofessional approach to prevention and health promotion, including integration into primary care services (Donoff *et al.* 2014).

The Rwanda Human Resource for Health (HRH) programme is an example of an interprofessional global health partnership. The WHO's recommended minimum provider to population density is 2.3 providers to 1000 population. In 2011, Rwanda had a density of merely 0.84 physicians, nurses and midwives, and only 92 public oral healthcare providers for its population of approximately 11 million (Binagwaho *et al.* 2013). Thus, the HRH programme was designed to train and retain high-quality healthcare professionals in order to improve the health of Rwandans. Oral diseases were the leading cause of morbidity in district hospitals, but dentistry was initially not a planned part of HRH. Thus, oral health professionals advocated for a "diagonal approach" to curriculum design for the HRH programme. This design combined vertical disease-specific training (such as treating dental caries) with horizontal methods for broader health system strengthening and common risk factor approaches (such as dietary sugar reduction) to break down educational silos, maximise limited resources, and integrate interprofessional educational opportunities (Seymour *et al.* 2013). The proposal was well received and currently, dental, medical and nursing students are being trained together at the new University of Rwanda College of Medicine and Health Sciences. Medical and dental students are now successfully trained together for the first 2 years of their programmes, prior to breaking out into more specialised training programmes for the latter years. The new dental school is in its fourth year of operation, of a 5-year degree programme, and is currently training approximately 65 future dentists for the country. The first class of 15 dentists, with 2 years of education with their medical school colleagues, is scheduled to graduate in 2018. This landmark year will mark the first time practising dentists in Rwanda will have been fully trained in Rwanda.

Conclusion

In this chapter, we present different perspectives on how to understand, value and encourage interprofessionalism in global health programmes. Although one would be hard pressed to find a global health faculty member or practitioner who did not agree that working collaboratively is essential to success in global health endeavours – doing so is not easy. Professional, structural and funding barriers stand in the way, but inroads are being made across the range of professions that play a role in global health. Each of the perspectives we present are designed to provide background and concrete models to assist faculty members and practitioners with moving forward in this area. Engendering interprofessional collaboration in global health is possible but more importantly, it is essential to realising the lofty goals of the field.

References

Association of Schools and Programs of Public Health (ASPPH). 2011. "Global Health Competency Model –Final Version 1.1." University of Pittsburgh Graduate School of Public Health. Accessed June 1, 2016. www.publichealth.pitt.edu/Portals/0/Main/ASPH%20GH%20Competencies.pdf.

Battat, R., G. Seidman, N. Chadi, M. Chanda, J. Nehme, J. Hulme, A. Li, *et al.* 2010. "Approaches in Medical Education: A Literature Review." *BMC Medical Education* 10(94):1–7. doi: 10.1186/1472-6920-10-94.

Binagwaho, A, P. Kyamanywa, P.E. Farmer, T. Nuthulaganti, B. Umubyeyi, J.P. Nyemazi, A. Asiimwe, *et al.* 2013. "The human resources for health program in Rwanda—new partnership." *New England Journal of Medicine* 369:2054–2059. doi: 10.1056/NEJMsr1302176.

Canadian Interprofessional Health Collaborative (CIHC). 2009. "Program Evaluation for Interprofessional Initiatives: Evaluation Instruments/Methods of the 20 IECPCP Projects: A report from the Evaluation Subcommittee." Accessed December 1, 2016. www.cihc.ca/files/CIHC_EvalMethods_Final.pdf.

Closser, S., and Finley E. 2016. "A new reflexivity: why anthropology matters in contemporary health research and practice, and how to make it matter more." American Anthropologist Accessed June 1, 2016. doi:10.1111/aman.12532.

Collaborative Justice. 2015. "How to Collaborate: A Working Definition of the Term 'Collaboration.'" Accessed June 6, 2016. www.collaborativejustice.org/how.htm, quoted in C. Larsen and F. LaFasto. *TeamWork: What Must Go Right/ What Can Go Wrong.* Newbury Park, CA: Sage Publications, 1989.

Curran J, H. Debas, M. Arya, *et al.*, editors. 2005. *Scaling Up Treatment for the Global AIDS Pandemic: Challenges and Opportunities.* Institute of Medicine (US) Committee on Examining the Probable Consequences of Alternative Patterns of Widespread Antiretroviral Drug Use in Resource-Constrained Settings. Washington, DC: National Academies Press.

Donoff, B., J.E. McDonough, and C.A. Riedy. 2014. "Integrating oral and general health care." *New England Journal of Medicine* 371(24):2247–2249. Accessed June 7, 2016. doi: 10.1056/NEJMp1410824.

Eckhert, N.L. 2006. "Getting the most out of medical students' global health experiences." *Family Medicine* S38–S39.

Egger, D., P. Travis, D. Dovlo, and L. Hawken. 2005. "Making Health Systems Work: Working Paper No.1, Strengthening Management Low-Income Countries," *Department of Health System Policies and Operations, World Health Organization.* Accessed June 6, 2016 www.who.int/management/general/overall/Strengthening%20Management%20in%20Low-Income%20Countries.pdf.

FDI World Dental Federation. 2015. *The Challenge of Oral Disease – A call for global action: The Oral Health Atlas.* Geneva: FDI World Dental Federation. www.fdiworldental.org/media/77552/complete_oh_atlas.pdf.

Foege, W.H., N. Daulaire, R. Black, and C. Pearson. 2005. *Global Health Leadership and Management*. San Francisco, CA: Jossey-Bass.

Glickman, L. B., Rambob, I., and Lee, Mei Ching. 2016. "Global learning experiences, interprofessional education, and knowledge translation: Examples from the field." *Annals of Global Health* 82(6):1048–1055. Accessed June 2, 2017. doi: 10.1016/j.aogh.2016.11.005.

Interprofessional Education Collaborative (IPEC). 2011. *Core Competencies for Interprofessional Collaborative Practice*. Washington, DC: Interprofessional Education Collaborative. www.aacn.nche.edu/education-resources/ipecreport.pdf.

Jogerst, K., Wilson, L., B. Callender, V. Adams, J. Evert, E. Fields, T. Hall, V. Rowthorn, *et al.* 2015. "Identifying interprofessional global health competencies for 21st-century health professionals." *Annals of Global Health* 81(2):239–247. Accessed June 7, 2016. doi: 10.1016/j.aogh.2015.03.006.

Knapp, M.S., K. Barnard, R.N. Brandon, N.J. Gehrke, A.J. Smith, and E.C. Teather. 1993. "University-based preparation for collaborative interprofessional practice." *Journal of Education Policy* 8(5):137–151. Accessed June 7, 2016. doi: 10.1080/0268093930080510.

Merson, M.H., and K.C. Page. 2009. *The Dramatic Expansion of University Engagement in Global Health: Implications for U.S. Policy*. Washington, DC: Center for Strategic and International Studies. www.ghdonline.org/uploads/Univ_Engagement_in_GH.pdf.

National Center for Interprofessional Practice and Education (NCIPE). 2016. Assessment and Evaluation Database. Accessed December 1, 2016. https://nexusipe.org/advancing/assessment-evaluation.

Nichter, M. 2008. *Global Health: Why Cultural Perceptions, Social Representations, and Biopolitics Matter*. Tucson: University of Arizona Press.

Oliveira-Cruz, V., K. Hanson, and A. Mills. 2003. "Approaches to overcoming constraints to effective health service delivery: A review of the evidence." *Journal of International Development* 15(1):41–65. Accessed June 7, 2016. doi:10.1002/jid.965.

Olsen, J., and A. Chatterjee. "Integrating social work students into short-term global health interprofessional education projects University of Maryland." *Practicing as a Social Work Educator in International Collaboration*. Alexandria, VA: CSWE Press, forthcoming.

Rowthorn, V. 2013. "A place for all at the global health table: a case study about creating an interprofessional global health project." *The Journal of Law, Medicine & Ethics* 41(4). Accessed June 9, 2016. doi: 10.1111/jlme.12100.

Rowthorn, V., and J. Olsen. 2014. "All together now: developing a team skills competency domain for global health education." *The Journal of Law, Medicine & Ethics* 42(4):550–563. Accessed June 7, 2016. doi: 10.1111/jlme.12175.

Rowthorn, V., and J. Olsen. 2015. "Putting the pieces together: creating and implementing an interprofessional global health grant program." *Health Care: The Journal of Delivery Science and Innovation* 3(4):258–263. Accessed June 7, 2016. doi: 10.1016/j.hjdsi.2015.09.008.

Seymour, B., L. Simon, and B. Nelson. 2014. *Essential Global Health Medicine*. United States: Wiley-Blackwell.

Seymour, B., I. Muhumuza, C. Mumena, M. Isyagi, J. Barrow, and V. Meeks. 2013. "Including oral health training in a health system strengthening program in Rwanda." *Global Health Action* doi: 10.3402/gha.v6i0.20109.

United Nations Children's Fund. 2003. *A Critical Lead to Polio Eradication in India.* Accessed July 22, 2016. www.unicef.org/rosa/critical.pdf.

Wilson, L., D.C. Harper, I. Tami-Maury, R. Zarate, S. Salas, J. Farley, N. Warren, *et al.* 2012. "Global health competencies for nurses in the Americas." *Journal of Professional Nursing* 28(4):213–222. Accessed June 7, 2016. doi: 10.1016/j.profnurs.2011.11.021.

World Health Organization (WHO). 2006. *World Health Report 2006: Working Together for Health.* Geneva: World Health Organization. Accessed June 3, 2016. www.who.int/whr/2006/ whr06_en.pdf?ua=1.

World Health Organization (WHO). 2015. *Ebola response: What needs to happen in 2015.* Geneva: World Health Organization. Accessed July 22, 2016. www.who.int/csr/disease/ebola/one-year-report/response-in-2015/en/.

6 Best practices in global health graduate and postgraduate medical education

James Hudspeth, Neil Jayasekera, Kevin Bergman and Matthew Fentress

Introduction

This chapter will address best practices for global health in graduate medical education (GME) training, dividing the topic between residency programmes and post-residency fellowships within the United States. We use the term GME interchangeably with postgraduate medical education, the preferred term in many other countries. For a comprehensive review on this topic, we refer readers to the 2011 Global Health Training in Graduate Medical Education: A Guidebook (2nd edition), available online as a book or PDF.

A surge of global health interest parallels the increase of global health programmes in undergraduate and graduate medical education (Morrison *et al.* 2016). Although comprehensive data on GME trainees are limited, surveys conducted in surgery (Powell *et al.* 2007), family medicine (Bazemore *et al.* 2007), and primary care (Bauer *et al.* 2009) show that while 50–80 percent of residents have interest in rotations in low resource settings at the start of residency, only 10–20 percent will actually complete one. These results likely reflect the paucity of global health opportunities (Kerry *et al.* 2013), the time constraints inherent to residency training, and the lack of funding for resident/fellow international work and travel expenses.

Given the strong interest in global health training, what is the rationale for global health programming within a GME context? Although definitive studies are lacking we do know from survey data that medical students or residents who choose to undergo global health training are more likely to do primary care, general medicine or public health as a career choice (Umoren *et al.* 2015, Ramsey *et al.* 2004). Potential benefits of global health education include: understanding healthcare disparities and the impact of the social determinants of health; quality improvement training; a better knowledge of health systems, stemming from comparisons between high and low resource locations; a deeper appreciation of the struggles faced by patients and healthcare practitioners in low resource settings; and the ability to practice medicine with limited resources, with more attention to the costs of care.

Global health in residency training

We divide residency global health programmes into three broad categories: residencies, pathways and informal programmes. Global health residencies are programmes entered via the national match process as well as programmes that add additional funded time to residency. Residents choose pathways (interchangeably called tracks) after matching into residency, and pathways do not extend residency. Informal programmes lack an overarching curriculum or selection process.

Global health residencies

A residency programme focused on global health is a resource-intensive process. Examples such as the Brigham and Women's Global Health Equity Residency, the Massachusetts General Hospital Global Primary Care Residency (now recast into a fellowship), or the Duke Global Health Residency involve adding a year to training, either scattered throughout the residency or as a single year after completion of the usual schedule. Most include master's degrees, and split the additional year between intensive didactics in global health paired with large amounts of time in affiliated low resource settings.

Such programmes require a significant investment from faculty as well as salary support for an additional year of residency, as Medicare does not fund international work. These programmes require a grant or charitable donation to cover a year of resident salary, faculty and administrative support and travel expenses to international sites. The graduates of such programmes leave with the highest level of global health training available within GME, comparable to a global health fellowship. The long-term impact of these opportunities remains unclear; ongoing studies on graduates will be completed in the coming years.

Global health pathways

A global health pathway or track in a residency programme will provide education in global health topics and typically the opportunity for an elective rotation in a low resource setting. The level of didactics, skill training, support, and away elective time varies widely between programmes.

The process of starting a pathway depends heavily on the number of residents involved as well as the amount of support available for the pathway. Pathways can be multidisciplinary, with shared didactics or a single residency pathway. The amount of interest from residents, support from the programme, and dedication of the programme organisers constitute the key three factors to consider when pondering the level of pathway to build. Cross-residency programmes allow faculty from multiple departments to combine resources and provide cross-specialty exposure to trainees.

Scheduling and logistical challenges posed by the involvement of multiple residency programmes can be managed by a university sponsored global health centre or institute.

Informal global health programmes

Given the lack of interested faculty and financial support most residencies support an informal global health programme. These programmes will allow trainees to do self-funded elective work abroad but will not have the resources to provide global health didactics or education. To ensure that the elective sites are safe and provide educational value we recommend developing a list of vetted programmes, especially those from third parties who have longitudinal relationships with a low resource setting site. These programmes typically are more expensive than an *ad hoc* experience, but are usually safer, more educational, and on firmer ethical footing. Providing a standardised approach to pre-departure preparation and post-return debriefing is an important part of any such programme and is further discussed in *Chapter 9*.

Curriculum

Curricular structure and content for global health in residencies vary, and there are no widely accepted norms, although a number of publications provide frameworks, as further discussed in Chapter 3 by Peluso. ACGME core competencies have been created by Anspacher and colleagues and can be used for residency supported global health programmes in internal medicine, paediatrics and obstetrics/gynaecology. The key structural elements of global health curricula in residency training includes didactics, scholarly work and local or international field experience. Specific content will vary by specialty, but usually includes global burden of disease, social determinants of health, environmental health, ethics and human rights. There are multiple sources of online global health lecture material that can be used to supplement the didactic portion of the curriculum, with notable examples including Consortium of Universities for Global Health (CUGH) and Unite for Sight.

ACGME and RRC requirements for international rotations

All global health programmes in a residency setting are subject to the guidelines of the Accreditation Council of Graduate Medical Education (ACGME) and the Residency Review Committee (RRC) for that specialty. The requirements vary considerably between specialties. Internal medicine requires approval from the residency programme, the institution's GME office, and compliance with ACGME requirements including an appropriate site advisor, appropriate learning objectives, and a letter of agreement between the sites. General surgery is more restrictive and requires written approval from the RRC for surgery and the American Board of Surgery for an international elective. General surgery also mandates compliance with RRC and ACGME requirements, access to educational resources at the international site and appropriate licensure for practice within the host country. For residencies starting global health programmes of any nature, we recommend reviewing the ACGME and RRC requirements for your specialty to determine what constraints are placed on rotations abroad. In situations in which constraints are overly burdensome, domestic global health rotations can provide compelling alternatives.

Global health fellowships

A global health fellowship acts as a logical extension of the global health pathway in residency. As described, a global health pathway provides basic global health knowledge, often with some scholarly work and several global health clinical electives. A global health fellowship curriculum can provide a diploma/certificate training in tropical medicine, faculty development, capacity building, public health and systems development and advanced scholarly work. Global health fellows usually spend approximately 6 months at an international site and 6 months at the home institution per year. Most global health fellowships are 1 to 2 years in length, with 2-year fellowships usually offering a masters in public health (Nelson *et al.* 2012a). No fellowships are presently ACGME certified, and so applications are performed outside of the match. The first global health fellowship was established in 1994. A 2012 survey found 83 global health fellowships in all major fields of medicine including emergency medicine (34), family medicine (14), internal medicine (11), pediatrics (ten), interdisciplinary (eight), surgery (three) and women's health (three) (Nelson *et al.* 2012a). Global health fellowships are usually small, often taking only one to three fellows per year – although larger interdisciplinary fellowships have developed in the past few years, namely the UCSF Heal Initiative and the Peace Corp/Global Health Service Partnership.

Considerations for starting a global health fellowship

As discussed above, a strong global health programme can be a recruiting tool for institutions to attract applicants who are interested in the care of underserved populations (Drain *et al.* 2007). Fellowships have the benefit of being better supported than residencies; typically fellows will work as attendings during their domestic period, and the revenue they generate pays for both their salary and some of the administrative aspects of the programme. As a global health fellow usually works 6 months abroad they have sufficient time to work on projects of mutual benefit. Barriers to creating a global health fellowship can include liability issues, difficulties with faculty support, lack of curriculum, absence of scholarship opportunities, or missing connections with an appropriate Global South partner (Nelson *et al.* 2012b). In particular, providing adequate mentorship both domestically and at the international site can be challenging, given the typically small amounts of support for supervising faculty.

Post-fellowship

Global health work is guided by the principles of social justice, overcoming healthcare disparities, and providing low resource medical care in any setting. Upon graduation, the global health fellow may find career opportunities domestically or abroad. Local global health work (i.e., "glocal") may include work in a refugee clinic, a federally qualified health centre (FQHC) that serves a large immigrant population or an academic centre that supports research or education in global health; see Chapter 24 for further discussion. A 2016 study showed that the primary motivation for a programme director to support a global health programme was not to "prepare physicians to serve in developing countries," but to, "prepare physicians to practice underserved medicine in the United States" (Hernandez *et al.* 2016). Graduates of a global health fellowship may choose to do local global health work because of high debt burden, lack of high paying international global health experiences, or favourable loan repayment for physicians who work in an FQHC. International global health work may include capacity building, research and systems or public health development. Service and programme delivery for governmental groups can include work with the CDC Epidemic Intelligence Service, United Nations, World Bank, or USAID. Humanitarian work with a non-governmental organisation (NGO) can include work with World Vision and Catholic Relief Services (faith based) or one of the thousands of NGOs worldwide that include Doctors without Borders, Partners in Health, the International Red Cross, Oxfam, CARE and Save the Children.

Competencies/milestones and global health fellowships

Broad competencies to guide and evaluate global health fellowships are difficult to derive, given differences between sites and specialties. One model was recently published for family medicine global health fellowships (El Rayess *et al.* 2017). The guidelines have been adapted, with permission, to assess the efficacy of any global health fellowship programme and/or fellow.

The six key competencies are:

1. Patient Care: the ability to care for patients in diverse circumstances throughout the world.

    The type of patient care delivered by the fellow is specific to their residency training and the needs of the communities they serve. A global health fellow will need appropriate supervision by experienced faculty at home and abroad.

2. Medical Knowledge: specific to global health.
   a. Demonstrates care of immigrants and refugees.
   b. Prepares for international travel including stress management, recognition and response to culture shock and pre and post work debriefing.
   c. Demonstrates knowledge of tropical medicine including malaria, tuberculosis, HIV, other communicable diseases and the global and local burdens of disease.
   d. Employs World Health Organization (WHO) protocols for clinical care in low resource settings.
   e. Understands country-specific resource availability.
   f. Develops an ethical approach to healthcare in low resource settings including consideration of impact of power, privilege and structural violence.
   g. Demonstrates an understanding and integrates measures to address public health and the social determinants of health in a global health context. (i.e., complete a masters in public health).
   h. Demonstrates an understanding of:
      1. the organisation and financing of healthcare systems.
      2. the role of NGOs like the WHO, International Monetary Fund and other similar organisations.
      3. the different healthcare models including horizontal and vertical approaches and private versus government run delivery systems.
      4. non-western medical training programmes.
3. Professionalism: the ability to immerse oneself in a different culture and operate with humility and respect to promote learning and collaboration.
   a. Demonstrates capacity for compassion (desire and commitment to address human suffering).
   b. Employ self-care, work–life balance in low resource settings.
   c. Demonstrates commitment to service, equity and principles of social justice.
   d. Demonstrates commitment to self-directed learning and engaging in a plan to overcome personal limitations.
4. Communication and Leadership: the ability to develop communication and leadership skills to facilitate collaboration with interdisciplinary teams.
   a. Develop advanced language adaptation skills (ability to work in a setting where you are not a native speaker).
   b. Demonstrate transcultural competency (ability to move beyond understanding the differences between two cultures to focusing on similarities).
5. Teaching: the ability to use teaching methods to educate healthcare providers and to teach others to teach.
   a. Develop and employ teaching skills for all medical professionals in a global health setting. Utilise multiple teaching techniques (small group, 1:1, lectures, precepting).

    b.   Demonstrate an approach to curriculum design, educational modules development and curriculum evaluation.

    c.   Develop an approach to faculty development (training the trainers).

    d.   Demonstrate advanced mentoring skills/modelling skills.

    e.   Tailor educational strategies to local educational system, includes performing an educational needs assessment with cultural sensitivity.

6.   Scholarship: demonstrate (1) a critical, intellectually rigorous approach in clinical and teaching activities, (2) proficiency in the application of basic principles of research.

    a.   Develop functional skills in research methods (needs assessment, design, implementation, evaluation).

    b.   Recognise the need for a tailored approach to community-based research in international settings.

    c.   Cite examples of ethical considerations needed while engaging in international research.

    c.   Demonstrate exposure to basic funding strategies for global health including grant-writing skills.

Ethics in global health GME

Part II of this book discusses the ethical considerations of global health work in greater detail. The WEIGHT guidelines provide a helpful summary of key considerations for global health training experiences (Crump *et al.* 2010). From the programmatic perspective of GME and global health, we focus primarily on the question of equity in educational opportunities. The costs of hosting US-based trainees vary, but typically include substantial time on the part of host faculty and administrators. As such, it is important to ask what benefits they reap from hosting trainees, and to ask what subsequent opportunities the trainee's institution can provide to the hosting institution. Although limited data exist, there are clear benefits of robust bilateral exchange programmes for trainees and faculty of both institutions (Pitt *et al.* 2016, Umoren *et al.* 2014). In order to have an equitable partnership both parties will need excellent communication, longitudinal involvement and an awareness of the power imbalance that typically exists between institutions in the Global North and Global South.

Conclusion

The role of global health in GME has steadily increased over the preceding years, and given the increasing support for global health combined with the large, unmet demand for global health experiences, we suspect global health programmes in GME will continue to expand in the short term. While the complexities of arranging ethical, equitable and educational experiences for residents and fellows are not trivial, the benefits reaped by trainees, faculty and host sites can be substantial. Key challenges for the field include developing expected competencies for graduates of global health training programmes; dissemination of model curricula to lower the difficulty for new programmes; and promoting equity in training programmes, such that partners in the Global South reap equal benefits from these arrangements.

We encourage programmes interested in global health GME training to join the larger discussion through CUGH and their specialty organisations. The authors welcome questions, and can be reached via their institutional emails.

References

Bauer T, Sanders J. 2009. "Needs assessment of Wisconsin primary care residents and faculty regarding interest in global health training." *BMC Medical Education* 9:36.

Bazemore AW, Henein M, Goldenhar L, Szaflarski M, Lindsell C, Diller P. 2007. "The effect of offering international health training opportunities on family medicine residency recruiting." *Family Medicine* 39:255–260.

Crump JA, Sugarman J, and Working Group on Ethics Guidelines for Global Health Training (WEIGHT). 2010. "Ethics and best practice guidelines for training experiences in global health." *The American Journal of Tropical Medicine and Hygiene* 83(6):1178–1182.

Drain PK, Primack A, Hunt DD, Fawzi WW,Holmes KK, Gardner P. 2007. "Global health in medical education: a call for more training and opportunities." *Academic Medicine* 82(3):226–230.

El Rayess F, Filip A, Doubeni A, Wilson C, Haq C, Debay M, Anandrajah G, Heffron W, Jayasekera N, Larson P, Dahlman B, Valdman O, Hunt V. 2017. "Family medicine global health competencies: a modified Delphi study. *Family Medicine* In Press.

Hernandez R,Sevilla Martir J,Van Durme D,Faller M,Yong-Yow S, Davies M, Achkar M. 2016 "Global health in family medicine residency programs: a nationwide survey of US residency directors: a CERA study." *Family Medicine* 48(7):532–537.

Kerry VB, Walensky RP, Tsai AC, Bergmark RW, Rouse C, Bangsberg DR. 2013. "US medical specialty global health training and the global burden of disease." *Journal of Global Health* 3(2).

Morrison, SJ. 2016. www.csis.org/analysis/global-health-programs-and-partnerships. Last accessed 12 December 2016.

Nelson BD, Izadnegahdar R, Hall L, Lee PT. 2012a. "Global health fellowships: a national, cross-disciplinary survey of US training opportunities." *Journal of Graduate Medical Education* 4(2):184–189.

Nelson B, Kasper J, Hibberd P, Thea D, Herlihy J. 2012b. "Developing a career in global health: considerations for physicians-in-training and academic mentors." *Journal of Graduate Medical Education* 301–306.

Pitt MB, Gladding SP, Majinge CR, Butteris SM. 2016. "Making global health rotations a two-way street: a model for hosting international residents." *Global Pediatric Health* 3:1–7.

Powell A, Mueller C, Kingham P, Berman R, Pachter HL, Hopkins MA. 2007. "International experience, electives, and volunteerism in surgical training: a survey of resident interest." *Journal of the American College of Surgeons* 205:162–168.

Ramsey AH, Haq C, Gjerde CL, Rothenberg D. 2004 "Career influence of an international health experience during medical school." *Family Medicine* 36(6):412–416.

Umoren RA, Gardner A, Stone GS, Helphinstine J, Machogu EP, Huskins JC, Johnson CS, Ayuo PO, Mining S, Litzelman DK. 2015. "Career choices and global health engagement: 24-year follow-up of U.S. participants in the Indiana University–Moi University elective." *Healthcare (Amsterdam)* 3(4):185–189.

Umoren RA, Einterz RM, Litzelman DK, Pettigrew RK, Ayaya SO, Liechty EA. 2014. "Fostering reciprocity in global health partnerships through a structured, hands-on experience for visiting postgraduate medical trainees." *Journal of Graduate Medical Education* 6(2):320–325.

7 A profile of global health curricula at Canadian medical schools

Akshaya Neil Arya, William Cherniak, Kristin Neudorf, Mary Halpine and Ian Pereira

Global health education is of increasing interest to medical trainees, faculty and administrators throughout North America. However, varied appreciation and understanding of global health and its competencies have led to disparate programmes, curricula, implementation and evaluation. This chapter presents a study that examines the spectrum of global health education delivery at medical schools across Canada with a specific focus on undergraduate medical education (UME). To ensure clarity, UME is medical students, as opposed to graduate medical education, which refers to residency.

Summary of this study

Collecting information from all 14 English-speaking Canadian medical schools through an online survey administered to both faculty and students, and follow up interviews with faculty in early 2013, we found that all schools offered some component of global health education in the preclinical curriculum, with less offered during the clinical curriculum. Programmes varied considerably with regard to time allotted to global health. Only half of the schools confirmed formal assessment of students through exams or assignments. At the time of the survey, efforts towards developing a comprehensive global health certificate or concentration were underway.

For global health truly to find its rightful place in medical curricula, there must be institutional support from universities, development and acceptance of standardised competencies by accreditation bodies, and evaluation of global health knowledge by the schools and the licensing authorities.

Introduction

In 2006, Izadnegahdar and colleagues conducted a survey of Canadian medical schools to map the global health education landscape (Izadnegahdar *et al.* 2008). They found a considerable range in the quantity and quality of global health curricula offered across the country. At some medical schools global health education was offered through well-developed, multi-year electives that included didactic and experiential learning. At other schools such learning opportunities were extremely limited, with neither required nor elective courses available. Moreover, 44 percent of the schools surveyed allowed international health electives (IHEs) with no clear faculty oversight or input. There was no consensus on what global health content should be covered, when it should be introduced in the curriculum, which aspects of global health were elective or required components, or how much training in global health was needed.

The following years saw a shift from piecemeal efforts in global health education to coordinated approaches. A global health resource group struck by the representative body for medical schools across Canada established the case for global health education (Kittler *et al.* 2006). The benefits to society were numerous, demand was growing from medical educators and students, and accreditation and licensing bodies were already calling for integration. Medical educators and students worked with Canadian and American organisations to agree on the general components of global health education (Evert *et al.* 2008, Brewer 2007, Jogerst *et al.* 2015), gain acceptance by all medical schools (Busing *et al.* 2010, Watterson *et al.* 2015, Moineau *et al.* 2015), ensure accountability through accreditation standards (Liaison Committee on Medical Education (LCME) 2015), provide evaluation by licensing bodies (Dauphinee and Mandin 2015) and develop standards for national competencies (Brewer and Hall 2010, Gao *et al.* 2015). One of the first examples was pre-departure training (PDT) for IHEs (Anderson *et al.* 2012). After students and educators developed national PDT guidelines (Anderson *et al.* 2008), deans of medicine agreed to provide opportunities for global health electives, training, preparation and support (Busing *et al.* 2010). This guided new accreditation criteria that mandated PDT, improved elective supervision and post-return debriefing (Liaison Committee on Medical Education (LCME) 2015). Work has also been done to develop the content and structure of of these experiences to ensure they maximise benefit and minimise harm (Cherniak *et al.* 2013, Loh *et al.* 2015, Gao *et al.* 2015). This mirrored the growth of global health offices across Canada, which would play an increasing role in national, coordinated and cooperative approaches to global health education including IHEs and PDT.

Drain and colleagues found that while residents in the USA were increasingly interested in international experiences, guidance and support from most residency programmes and accreditation organisations remained inadequate (Drain *et al.* 2009). While structured opportunities for experiential and didactic components are fewer in postgraduate medical education than in UME, with less flexible schedules, some resident educators, global health associations, and national specialty associations have pushed to develop educational objectives and competencies (Redwood-Campbell *et al.* 2011, Cherniak *et al.* 2013, Chase and Evert 2011, Jogerst *et al.* 2015).

Global health experts generally accept that coordinated and cooperative approaches are needed in global health education. Despite advances in the past decade, it was unclear how much Canadian medical schools agreed on global health education standards. We thus decided to map the level of concordance of global health integration into UME.

Study methods

Instrument

Thirty-five survey questions were designed to assess global health education in UME. These were based on two previous Canadian surveys (Izadnegahdar *et al.* 2008, Anderson *et al.* 2012). LimeSurvey was used to develop and publish the survey, collect responses and export data for analysis (Schmitz 2013). Consent was obtained electronically at the start of the survey.

Faculty interviews were designed to clarify survey responses and resolve any discrepancies between faculty and student responses through a standard set of questions. Interviews were done through an hour-long semi-structured process by phone and transcribed. Verbal consent was obtained at the start of the interviews.

Consistent with a comprehensive view of global health, we defined global health education to include local health initiatives aimed at vulnerable and marginalised populations (Koplan *et al.* 2009).

Both the survey and interviews were approved for use by the Research Ethics Board at Western University.

Study participants

One faculty member and one student representative who were self and peer-identified as leaders in global health education were selected from each medical school in Canada. Selected faculty were the lead of a global health office or programme, IHEs or pre-departure training. Selected students were their schools' representatives to the Canadian Federation of Medical Students (CFMS) as either a global health liaison or local officer for global health education. Surveys were distributed to selected faculty and students between September to December 2012. The same faculty member was later invited to participate in the interview between February and March 2013.

Analysis

The survey results and quantifiable interview results were analysed by the authors through descriptive statistics using Microsoft Excel. Interviews were also thematically analysed by techniques based on other studies (Xu *et al.* 2011).

Results

Faculty from all 14 English-speaking medical schools and ten students responded. No faculty or students responded to the English survey from the three francophone schools. Our analysis was restricted to English-speaking schools.

Global health as part of core curriculum

All schools (14/14) indicated that global health was part of the core curriculum and integrated at various places throughout the medical school experience. Twenty-one per cent (3/14) had global health education in the clerkship curriculum and 86 percent (12/14) had it in the preclinical curriculum. Eighty-six percent (12/14) of schools also had elective or extracurricular opportunities.

The time devoted to global health ranged from a 2-hour introductory lecture in the first year to 20 hours of lectures and small group discussions throughout UME. Thirty-six per cent (5/14) of schools were restructuring their UME and faculty reported using this as an opportunity to examine how and where global health could be taught. Twenty-one per cent of schools (3/14) indicated that they already had a global health track or certificate, and an additional seven (50 percent) indicated an interest in, or plans, to develop one.

Curricular topics (see Table 7.1)

All schools (14/14) included the global burden of disease, social and economic determinants of health, and healthcare in low resource settings in their curriculum. Eighty-six per cent (12/14) included the health implication of travel, migration and displacement. Only 14 percent of schools (2/14) included disaster relief, humanitarian aid, or HIV/AIDS.

Table 7.1 Topics covered in global health curriculum in the English-speaking Canadian medical schools in the 2012–13 academic year (*N*=14)

Topics	Percentage
Global burden of disease	100
Social and economic determinants of health	100
Healthcare in low resource settings	100
Health implications of travel, migration and displacement	93
Globalisation of health and healthcare	57
Human rights in global health	57
Aboriginal peoples' health	36
Refugee health	29
Law and ethics	29
Cultural competency	21
Disaster relief and/or humanitarian aid	14
HIV/AIDS	14

Other topics mentioned in survey and interview results included international surgery, working in low resource settings, working with marginalised populations, water and sanitation, tuberculosis, pandemics and outbreaks, non-communicable diseases, injuries and prevention, environmental determinants of health, health advocacy, children and armed conflict, health equity, child and maternal health, international adoption, emerging infectious diseases and northern and rural health.

Assessment and evaluation

Half of the medical schools (7/14) reported that global health was included in examinations at some point during medical school. Most reported the inclusion of a few questions related to global health as part of the evaluation of another course. In many schools, content experts in global health were not involved with the design and evaluation of these questions. Fewer than half of schools had dedicated global health evaluations. Forty-three per cent (6/14) had a specific written assignment or presentation and 14 percent (2/14) used a quiz or survey.

Half of schools (7/14) had no specific recognition for the global health involvement by students, although 29 percent (4/14) had plans to move towards recognition. Twenty-one percent (3/14) recognised global health course work, either through credits or on the dean's letter.

Discussion

Global health implementation

In 2010, medical schools agreed to provide opportunities for global health and licensing bodies set objectives. Medical schools across Canada have moved towards providing global health in their curriculum (Kittler *et al.* 2006, Anderson *et al.* 2012). We found that all schools had some global health in their UME and over 80 percent (12/14) offered additional education through elective experiences. This had increased since 2006 when Izadnegahdar and colleagues found that only 60 percent (10/17) of schools included global health lectures or modules in their curriculum and only 40 percent (7/17) offered elective courses (Izadnegahdar *et al.* 2008). Global health education is now taught to medical students across Canada and additional experiences are available to help meet the growing demand from students and faculty. From high above, it appears as if we are almost there.

However, a recent update from medical schools provided limited descriptions of and varied progress on global health commitments over the last 5 years (Battat *et al.* 2010, Busing *et al.* 2010, Moineau *et al.* 2015). More than a third (5/14) were redeveloping their curricula, and as part of this process were reviewing how and where global health should be taught. Much is still in flux.

Common educational approaches have been didactic teaching or experiential learning (Battat *et al.* 2010). Unfortunately, inconsistencies in approaches remain. We found substantial variation in the delivery of global health education, timing, number of hours and teaching methods varied between and within medical schools. This pointed to a lack of consensus on how best to teach global health. Additionally, there is no consistency in the number of hours devoted to global health or its guiding principles. No schools offered more than 20 hours of formal curricula. Houpt and colleagues recommended that medical schools provide a 30-hour curriculum on topics such as global burden of disease, traveller's medicine, immigrant health and cultural awareness (Houpt *et al.* 2007), whereas the resource group of the faculties of medicine recommended guiding principles rather than a specific time criteria (Brewer 2007). From the ground, it appears that schools are still far apart and may have a ways to go before reaching consistent, evidence-based, and high resolution educational approaches.

Curricular time allocation does not have to be a zero sum game; indeed global health teaching can be done simultaneously and facilitate other, often hard to teach, aspects of the curricula such as ethical issues, social determinants of health and language competencies. In an increasingly globalised world, global health as an entity is becoming more widely accepted and students are encountering new circumstances or patients important to their training. Formalised oversight and training best to equip students for these experiences needs to be integrated into mainstream medical training.

Elective opportunities are an important complement to mandatory training, allowing students to steer their career to follow their goals. The apparent increase in global health elective courses does not necessarily translate into improvement in the quality of elective education. Some reported that opportunities were arranged and supported mainly by students without clear faculty support or supervision (Izadnegahdar *et al.* 2008, Anderson *et al.* 2012). Furthermore, many schools reported that capacity was limited and admission to elective courses was highly competitive. As such, the quality and quantity of elective opportunities should be further assessed to ensure that supply is meeting demand and the desired outcomes are achieved.

Domains and competencies

To address society's emerging health-related needs, the medical education community has worked over the past several years to describe the global health domains and competencies of increasing importance to the development of all physicians. A joint US/Canadian committee built on work of the Global Health Resource Group of the Association of Faculties of Medicine (AFMC) to develop consensus on essential core competencies for formal integration into medical curricula (Kittler *et al.* 2006, Brewer 2007, Brewer and Hall 2010). Arthur and colleagues described the development of these competencies (Arthur *et al.* 2011). However, for many years the development of global health curricula has existed separately from other medical curricula. The Association of Schools of Public Health developed similar aspects for public health (Ablah *et al.* 2014, Shortell and Curran 2006) and Jogerst and colleagues, guided by these efforts, developed inter-professional competencies for the Consortium of Universities for Global Health (CUGH) (Jogerst *et al.* 2015). Jogerst and colleagues developed 13 competencies across eight domains at a global citizen level and 39 competencies across 11 domains at a basic operational programme-oriented level. In addition, frameworks have been developed for global health training and competencies in particular medical specialties such as family medicine (Redwood-Campbell *et al.* 2011) and paediatrics (Torjesen *et al.* 1999, Howard *et al.* 2011), and other fields such as nursing (Wilson *et al.* 2012) and dentistry (Benzian *et al.* 2015). Brewer and colleagues have also suggested a universal global health curriculum that includes high, middle, and low-income countries (Brewer *et al.* 2015).

In Canada, the national CanMEDS framework and MCC objectives drive traditional curricula. CanMEDS outlines the roles of a physician and the competencies needed. The MCC administers two Canadian licensing exams. More recently, topics such as the recognition of inequality (Frank 2005, Frank *et al.* 2015), enhancement of social justice (Brewer 2007, World Federation on Medical Education (WFME) 2003, World Federation on Medical Education (WFME) 2015), cultural diversity (Medical Council of Canada (MCC) 2005), and impact of environmental issues on health (Kittler *et al.* 2006, Medical Council of Canada (MCC) 2005, Frank *et al.* 2015) have been added. These new topics have considerable overlap with the domains and competencies of global health.

Although a medical education topic of particular importance in Canada, approaches and philosophy vary among schools regarding whether Indigenous peoples' health is included under the mandate of global health. Many schools have a distinct department or office that addresses this area of medical training due to unique needs and sensitivities. Therefore, the five schools identified in our survey that include this topic in their global health curricula may be an under-representation of its overall inclusion in medical education programmes across Canada. Indeed, accreditation standards (Liaison Committee on Medical Education (LCME) 2015) and initiatives by the faculties of medicine, the accreditation council (Medical Council of Canada (MCC) 2005, Dauphinee and Mandin 2015), and the regulatory college (Royal College of Physicians and Surgeons of Canada (RCPSC) 2013) suggest that this is an important curricular topic in Canada. As part of their work on social accountability, in 2004 the faculties of medicine identified aboriginal health as important for medical schools to meet societal needs (Maclellan 2005). The faculties of medicine worked with the Indigenous Physicians Association of Canada to collect evidence and develop competencies (Lavallee *et al.* 2009). The regulatory college developed resources for educators including a values and principles statement based on the CanMEDS framework (Royal College of Physicians and Surgeons of Canada (RCPSC) 2013). In addition, a First Nations Toolkit for working with Indigenous communities has been developed to address more effectively this important component of global health within Canada (Medical Council of Canada (MCC) 2005). This approach towards identifying, developing and implementing competencies may serve as a model for a broader global health education framework within medical schools.

In our study, we found wide variation in the global health topics taught at medical schools. This echoes the results of Battat and colleagues in their global literature search of competencies (Battat *et al.* 2010). This suggested a lack of national coordination. Recently, the CFMS Global Health Program and AFMC Global Health Working Group merged CanMEDS and global health competencies to develop a national consensus on global health core competencies (Gao *et al.* 2015). The competency domains from Battat (Battat *et al.* 2010), Arthur (Arthur *et al.* 2011), Jogerst (Jogerst *et al.* 2015) and the CFMS/AFMC (Gao *et al.* 2015) are summarised in Table 7.2. We are optimistic that this national, coordinated approach will help schools cooperate and converge on a way forward that integrates traditional and global health curricula best to match society's needs.

Assessment and evaluation

As the medical education community reaches consensus on global health content and delivery in UME, how quality will be measured and improved remains a question. Our study revealed little agreement on assessment and evaluation. Most schools assessed elements of their global health curriculum as part of other curricula rather than giving specific recognition for global health education. This may be related to the limited inclusion of global health topics in accreditation criteria and licensing objectives. Furthermore, the introduction of global health topics in licensing exams is relatively new. Global health is not included in licensing exam objectives as a discipline and some suggested and taught domains and competencies are still not included (Dauphinee and Mandin 2015). Although the recent development of national competencies in global health education may set a standard in global health education (Gao at al. 2015), without alignment of what is taught and what is tested, it will continue to be difficult to improve the global health curriculum. A way forward is for the medical education community including schools and licensing bodies to work together to recognise global health, set objectives and measure them.

Limitations and management

Although we distributed surveys to all 17 Canadian medical schools, we had no suitable French translation and only obtained responses from the 14 English-speaking schools. As we mainly relied on CFMS global health liaisons to establish contact and francophone schools did not have global health liaisons, we might have been better contacting Quebec's medical school representative association (FMEQ).

Follow up was therefore directed to English-speaking medical school faculty. Although we believe that many of our findings may be applicable to other countries, e.g., the USA and UK, we cannot even generalise to French-speaking Canadian schools. On the other hand, clarification by follow up telephone interviews with faculty, unlike previous work to verify discrepancies between faculty and students, also allowed a better understanding of interpretation of questions, nuances and granular detail to be obtained which is partly reflected in the following chapter.

The lower student response rate (10/14) may have resulted from the busy student schedule and the lack of a process to identify alternative contacts. This may also have been a result of survey fatigue, compared to Izadnegahdar (Izadnegahdar *et al.* 2008) and Anderson (Anderson *et al.* 2012). Our survey was much more comprehensive, covering both formal and informal global health education, where and when training occurred, international partnerships and local global health for example. Future studies may benefit from methods that assess and encourage progress while providing alternative contacts if needed.

Due to the diverse nature of global health curricula and oversight at schools across Canada, it is often difficult to understand fully what is taught from a school's website, and equally difficult to survey such issues thoroughly and comprehensively. Knowledge is often not housed in a single person, be it faculty or student. The faculty member chosen was the most senior physician or administrator responsible for global health or their designate, often the global health office director. The student chosen was the global health liaison or their designate. These individuals, respectively, may be at arm's length from the general medical curriculum or uninvolved with the content and delivery of global health education. Furthermore, domestic global health experiences for students often fall outside the mandate of global health offices and are separately administered. However, once national global health education standards are adopted, aligned with other curricula, assessed and evaluated, this knowledge should be better understood.

Conclusion

Global health education is clearly a growing priority for students, medical educators, medical accreditation bodies, licensing councils and society. Some progress has been made over the past 10 years, but we are not there yet. Global health education is in flux. Delivery, content, assessment and evaluation among Canadian medical schools still varies considerably. Recognising that there are many factors contributing towards an optimal global health education, a coordinated, consistent and comprehensive approach is needed best to meet the growing demand. This includes increased commitments to global health education by medical schools, continued support by accreditation standards and licensing requirements, and effective advocacy.

All medical schools must commit to global health education for it to work. This should include accepting national guidance adaptable to a variety of settings, developing a global health education plan, and providing supporting infrastructure including assessment and evaluation mechanisms, such as the recently developed Canadian global health core competencies (Gao *et al.* 2015). Although some experts recommend that schools deliver the global health curriculum through specific time quotas (Houpt *et al.* 2007), we encourage a less prescriptive approach in education plans such as the use of guiding principles (Brewer 2007). Continued assessment and evaluation will ensure that education evolves in response to the needs of all stakeholders. This includes defining and assessing outcomes such as resource stewardship, the impact of hands-on work with marginalised populations, the effectiveness of curricula in preparing students for such work, and the impact on students' training and careers. Mechanisms for assessment include 360 degree feedback by students, faculty, international partners and global health experts. Working together with all stakeholders, faculties of medicine can build a core global health component in their curriculum.

This strategy has worked in the past. Once evidence had been assembled and with advocacy from students and educators, the AFMC developed pre-departure training, released national guidelines, gained approval from all medical schools and had it entrenched in licensing standards in 3 years (Anderson *et al.* 2008, Anderson *et al.* 2012). With coordinated support from the global health community, leading Canadian medical schools, the accreditation council and the licensing body have become interested and motivated to improve medical education by including global health. Such an advocacy-oriented approach provides an optimistic path for rapid advancement in the field with concerted interest and effort.

Across Canada, we have not yet reached an optimal global health education. However, the way forward will be clearer with national, coordinated approaches. By working together, trainees, physicians and our patients will arrive at a healthier and more equitable destination.

Acknowledgements

The authors wish to thank the directors, administrators, teachers of global health and the medical student leadership who participated in the survey and interviews. We would also like to thank the following individuals for reviewing the draft and providing editorial feedback: Kelly Anderson, Lynda Redwood-Campbell, Tim Brewer and Megan Arthur.

Funding/Support: Funding for this research was provided by the Global Health Office, Western University, London, Canada. Dr Cherniak was

Table 7.2 Recommended areas of global health competencies in the literature (Arthur *et al.* 2011, Battat *et al.* 2010, Jogerst *et al.* 2014, Gao *et al.* 2015)

• Global burden of disease	A B J G
• Health implications of travel, migration and displacement	A B G
• Healthcare disparities between countries	B
• Primary care within diverse cultural settings	B G
• Skills to interface better with different populations, cultures and healthcare systems	B G
• Social and economic determinants of health	A G
• Population, resources and the environment	J G
• Healthcare in low resource settings	A G
• Globalisation of health and healthcare	A J G
• Human rights in global health	A G
• Health equity and social justice	J
• Travel medicine	B G
• Immigrant health	B G
• Sociocultural and political awareness	J G
• Collaboration, partnering and communication	J G
• Ethics	J G
• Professional practice	J G
• Capacity strengthening	P
• Programme management	P
• Strategic analysis	P G

A: Arthur *et al.* 2011
B: Battat *et al.* 2010
J: Jogerst *et al.* CUGH 2015 – Global citizen level
P: Jogerst *et al.* CUGH 2015 – Programme-oriented basic operational level
G: Gao *et al.* CFMS/AFMC 2015

supported by the McGill University Department of Global Health while working on this study.

Other disclosures: None.

Ethical approval: The health sciences Research Ethics Board at Western University reviewed the surveys, interview guides and provided ethical approval.

References

Ablah, E., Biberman, D.A., Weist, E.M., Buekens, P., Bently, M.E., Burke, D., Finnegan, J.R., Flahault, A., Frenk, J., Gotsch, A.R., Klag, M.J., Rodriguez, Lopez M.H., Nasca, P., Shortell, S., Spencer, H.C. 2014. "Improving global health education: development of a global health competency model." *American Journal of Tropical Medicine and Hygiene* 90(3):560–565. 10.4269/ajtmh.13–0537.

Anderson KC, Slatnik MA, Pereira I, Cheung E, Xu K, Brewer TF. 2012. "Are we there yet? Preparing Canadian medical students for global health electives." *Academic Medicine* 87:206–209. 10.1097/ACM.0b013e31823e23d4.

Anderson, K., Bocking, N., Slatnik, M., Pattani, R., Breton, J., Saciragic, L., Dhillon, S., Brewer, T.F. 2008. "Preparing Medical Students for Low-Resource Setting

Electives: A Template for National Pre-Departure Training Guidelines. A Report of the Resource Group on Global Health of the Association of Faculties of Medicine of Canada and the Canadian Federation of Medical Students Global Health Program." Ottawa, ON: Association of Faculties of Medicine of Canada (AFMC). Accessed January 19, 2017. www.old.cfms.org/downloads/Pre-Departure%20 Guidelines%20Final.pdf.

Arthur, M.A., Battat, R., Brewer, T.F. 2011. "Teaching the basics: core competencies in global health." *Infectious Disease Clinics of North America* 25:347–358. 10.1016/ j.idc.2011.02.013.

Battat, R., Seidman, G., Chadi, N., Chanda, M.Y., Nehme, J., Hulme, J., Li, A., Faridie, Nazlie, Brewer, T.F. 2010. "Global health competencies and approaches in medical education: a literature review." *BMC Medical Education* 10:94. 10.1186/ 1472-6920-10-94.

Benzian, H., Greenspan, J.S., Barrow, J., Hutter, J.W., Loomer, P.M., Stauf, N., Perry, D.A. 2015. "A competency matrix for global oral health." *Journal of Dental Education* 79(4):353–361.

Busing, N., Rosenfield, J., Rourke, J. 2010. "The future of medical education in Canada: A collective vision for MD education." Ottawa, ON: The Association of Faculties of Medicine of Canada (AFMC). Accessed January 19, 2017. http:// cou.on.ca/wp-content/uploads/2010/01/COU-Future-of-Medical-Education-in-Canada-A-Collective-Vision.pdf.

Brewer, T.F. 2007. Creating Global Health Curricula for Canadian Medical Students. Report of the AFMC Resource Group on Global Health. Ottawa, ON: AFMC. Accessed January 22, 2017. https://afmc.ca/pdf/pdf_2007_global_health_report.pdf.

Brewer T.F., Hall, T. 2010. "Global Health Essential Core Competencies." Ottawa, ON: AFMC Resource Group/Global Health Education Consortium (GHEC).

Brewer, T.F., Clarfield, M., Davies, D., Garg, B., Greensweig, T., Hafler, J., Hou, J. *et al.* 2015. "A Universal Curriculum for Global Health. The Bellagio Global Health Education Initiative. June 2015 Meeting Summary." Bellagio, Italy: The Bellagio Global Health Education Initiative. Accessed January 22, 2017. http://bellagi- oglobalhealth.education/wp-content/uploads/2016/01/Bellagio-GHEI-June-2015- Meeting-Summary.pdf.

Chase, J., Evert, J. 2011. *Global Health Training in Graduate Medical Education: A Guidebook, 2nd Edition.* San Francisco, CA: GHEC/iUniverse.

Cherniak, W., Drain, P.K., Brewer, T.F. 2013. "Educational objectives of interna- tional medical electives – a literature review." *Academic Medicine* 88(11):1778–1781. 10.1097/ACM.0b013e3182a6a7ce.

Dauphinee, W.D., Mandin, H. 2015. "Objectives for the qualifying examination." Version 3.3.14. Ottawa, ON: Medical Council of Canada (MCC).

Drain, P.K., Holmes, K.K., Skeff, K.M., Hall, T.L., Gardner, P. 2009. "Global health training and international clinical rotations during residency: current status, needs, and opportunities." *Academic Medicine* 84:320–325. 10.1097/ACM.0b013e3181970a37.

Evert, J., Mautner, D., Hoffman, I. 2008. *Developing Global health Curricula: A Guidebook for US & Canadian Medical Schools. A Collaboration of AMSA, GHEC, IFMSA- USA, and R4WH.* Ed. Tom Hall. Washington, DC: American Medical Student Association (AMSA), Global Health Education Consortium (GHEC), the International Federation of Medical Students Association-USA, Ride for World Health. Accessed January 23, 2017. www.mcgill.ca/globalhealth/files/globalhealth/ CurriculoumGuidebook2ndedition2008.pdf.

Frank, J.R. (Ed). 2005. "The CanMEDS 2005 Physician Competency Framework. Better Standards. Better Physicians. Better Care." Ottawa, ON: Royal College of Physicians and Surgeons of Canada (RCPSC). Accessed January 20, 2017. www.royalcollege.ca/portal/page/portal/rc/common/documents/canmeds/resources/publications/framework_full_e.pdf.

Frank J.R., Snell, L., Sherbino, J. (Eds). 2015. "The CanMEDS 2015 Physician Competency Framework." Ottawa, ON: RCPSC. Accessed January 20, 2017. www.royalcollege.ca/rcsite/documents/canmeds/canmeds-full-framework-e.pdf.

Gao, G., Kherani, I., Halpine, M., Carpenter, J., Sleeth, J., Mercer, G., Moore, S., Kapoor, V. 2015. "Global Health Core Competencies In Undergraduate Medical Education." Ottawa, ON: CFMS-Global Health Program and AFMC-Global Health Working Group. Accessed January 22, 2017. www.cfms.org/files/position-papers/2015%20Global%20Health%20Core%20Competencies.pdf.

Houpt, E., Pearson, R., Hall, T. 2007. "Three domains of competency in global health education: recommendations for all medical students." *Academic Medicine* 82:222–225. 10.1097/ACM.0b013e3180305c10.

Howard, C.R., Gladding, S.P., Kiguli, S., Andrews, J.S., John, C.C. 2011. "Development of a competency-based curriculum in global child health." *Academic Medicine* 86(4):521–528. 10.1097/ACM.0b013e31820df4c1.

Izadnegahdar, R., Correia, S., Ohata B, Kittler, A., ter Kuile, S., Vaillancourt, S., Saba, N., Brewer, T.F. 2008. "Global health in Canadian medical education: current practices and opportunities." *Academic Medicine* 83(2):192–198. 10.1097/ACM.0b013e31816095cd.

Jogerst, K., Callendar, B., Adams, V., Evert, J., Fields, E., Hall, T., Olsen, J., Rowthorn, V., Rudy, S., Shen, J., Simon, L., Torres, H., Velji, A., Wilson, L. 2015. "Identifying interprofessional global health competencies for 21st-century health professionals." *Annals of Global Health* 81(2):239–247. 10.1016/j.aogh.2015.03.006.

Kittler, A., Ohata, B., Vaillancourt, S., Correia, S., Izadnegahdar, R., Brewer, T.F. 2006. "Towards a Medical Education Relevant to all: the Case for Global Health in Medical Education. A Report of the Resource Group on Global Health of the Association of Faculties of Medicine of Canada." Ottawa, ON: Association of Faculties of Medicine of Canada (AFMC).

Koplan, J.P., Bond, T.C., Merson, M.H., Reddy, K.S., Rodriguez, M.H., Sewankambo, N.K., Wasserheit, J.N. 2009. "Towards a common definition of global health." *Lancet* 373:1993–1995. http://dx.doi.org/10.1016/S0140-6736(09)60332-9.

Lavallee, B., Neville, A., Anderson, M., Shore, B., Diffey, L. 2009. "First Nations, Inuit, Métis Health CORE COMPETENCIES. A Curriculum Framework for Undergraduate Medical Education." Ottawa, ON: Indigenous Physicians Association of Canada and AFMC. Accessed January 22, 2017. https://afmc.ca/sites/default/files/documents/en/Medical-Education/Aboriginal-Health-Needs/CoreCompetenciesEng.pdf.

Liaison Committee on Medical Education (LCME). 2015 "Data collection instrument for full accreditation surveys." Washington, DC: American Medical Association (AMA) and AAMC.

Loh, L.L., Cherniak, W., Dreifuss, B.A., Dacso, M.M., Lin, H.C., Evert, J. 2015. "Short term global health experiences and local partnership models: a framework." *Globalization and Health* 11:50. 10.1186/s12992-015-0135-7.

Maclellan, A.M. 2005. "The Social Accountability Initiative Moves Forward" In AFMC Forum, edited by David Hawkins. Ottawa, ON: AFMC. Accessed January

22, 2017. https://afmc.ca/sites/default/files/documents/en/Publications/AFMC-Newsletter/Gravitas/2005/2005_march_forum.pdf.

Medical Council of Canada (MCC). 2005. "Considerations for Cultural-Communication, Legal, Ethical and Organizational Aspects of the Practice of Medicine." Accessed June 7, 2013. http://mcc.ca/wp-content/uploads/CLEO.pdf.

Moineau, G.M., Rourke, J., Busing, N., Rosenfield, J. 2015. "The Future of Medical Education in Canada (FMEC): A Collective Vision for MD Education – Five Years of Innovations in Canada's Faculties of Medicine." Ottawa, ON: AFMC. Accessed January 20, 2017. https://afmc.ca/pdf/fmec/FMEC-MD-2015.pdf.

RCPSC. 2013. "Indigenous health values and principles statement." Ottawa, ON: RCPSC. The Indigenous Health Advisory Committee and the Office of Health Policy and Communications. Accessed January 22, 2017. www.royalcollege.ca/rcsite/documents/health-policy/indigenous-health-values-principles-report-e.pdf.

Redwood-Campbell, L., Pakes, B., Rouleau, K., MacDonald, C.J., Arya, N., Purkey, E., Schultz, K., Pottie, K. 2011. "Developing a curriculum framework for global health in family medicine: emerging principles, competencies, and educational approaches." *BMC Medical Education* 11:46. 10.1186/1472-6920-11-46.

Schmitz, C. 2013. Hamburg, Germany: LimeSurvey Project. www.limesurvey.org.

Shortell, S., Curran, J. 2006. Master's Degree in Public Health Core Competency Development Project. Washington, DC: Association of Schools of Public Health (ASPH). Accessed January 22, 2017. www.aspph.org/app/uploads/2014/04/Version2.31_FINAL.pdf.

Torjesen, K., Mandalakas, A., Kahn, R., Duncan, B. 1999. "International child health electives for paediatric residents." *Archives of Pediatric Adolescent Medicine* 153(12):1297–1302. 10.1001/archpedi.153.12.1297.

Watterson, R., Matthews, D., Bach, P., Kherani, I., Halpine, M., Meili, R. 2015. "Building a framework for global health learning: an analysis of global health concentrations in Canadian medical schools." *Academic Medicine* 90(4):500–504. 10.1097/ACM.0000000000000648.

Wilson, L., Harper, D.C., Tami-Maury, I., Zarate, R., Salas, S., Farley, J., Warren, N., Mendes, I., Ventura, C. 2012. "Global health competencies for nurses in the Americas." *Journal of Professional Nursing* 28:213–222. 10.1016/j.profnurs.2011.11.021.

World Federation on Medical Education (WFME) Task Force on International Standards in Basic Medical Education. 2015. "Basic Medical Education. WFME Global Standards for Quality Improvement. The 2015 Revision." Ferney-Voltaire, France and Copenhagen, Denmark: WFME. Accessed January 20, 2017. http://wfme.org/standards/bme/78-new-version-2012-quality-improvement-in-basic-medical-education-english/file.

World Federation on Medical Education (WFME) Task Force on International Standards in Basic Medical Education. 2003. "Basic Medical Education. WFME Global Standards for Quality Improvement." Copenhagen, Denmark: WFME. Accessed January 20, 2017. http://wfme.org/standards/bme/3-quality-improvement-in-basic-medical-education-english/file.

Xu, J.J., Pereira, I., Liu, W., Herbert, C. 2011. "Assessing the effectiveness of pre-departure training for professional healthcare students working in resource-limited settings." *University of Toronto Medical Journal* 88(3):199–204. Accessed January 20, 2017. http://utmj.org/index.php/UTMJ/article/view/1350.

8 A profile of international electives programming at Canadian medical schools

Akshaya Neil Arya and Kristin Neudorf

This chapter details a study that describes and categorises international health electives (IHEs) offered at all 14 English-speaking Canadian medical schools in 2012–13. It was completed as part of the study discussed in *Chapter 7*. While there is evidence of benefits of participating in such global health placements, there is a paucity of research or evaluation as to which opportunities or programmes are most effective and appropriate for students, or the medical facilities and communities that host them. This work may assist in the design of studies comparing these opportunities within other nations' medical education systems.

All participating medical schools identified at least one international site where some type of partnership which facilitated student elective experiences existed, most often an informal one. All schools had electives in clinical settings where students either observed or participated, depending on the level of training. Four schools cited opportunities for medical students to participate in research projects, and nine schools included community outreach or development work as part of elective experiences. Six medical schools had at least some sites with on-site faculty supervision from the sending institution. A further six schools indicated that while faculty did not accompany students and supervise them directly, they had previously travelled to the site to ensure appropriateness for student placements. We hope that this project can lay the groundwork for subsequent evaluations of IHEs, and facilitate the sharing of lessons learned and best practices between schools.

Introduction

International health electives in Canadian schools have not been systematically studied. We wanted to understand how IHE initiatives developed at English-speaking medical schools in Canada, what types of international opportunities were available to trainees, and how partnerships were formed between Canadian schools and the international medical facilities that hosted their students.

Methods

This survey was piggybacked on to the study described in *Chapter 7* (see "Methods") and the survey instrument was developed by the authors. Follow-up interviews of administrative faculty were administered in February to March 2013 with verbal consent obtained before each interview. The interviews were conducted by phone or through internet voice software, transcribed word-for-word and thematically analysed by the authors. The survey results and quantifiable interview results were analysed by calculating simple descriptive statistics using Microsoft Excel. Both the survey and interviews were approved for use by the Research Ethics Board at Western University.

Results

International health elective opportunities

All medical schools (14/14) described opportunities offered to students to have "local" experiences within low resource or underserved communities, and international global health electives at both the preclinical and clinical stage of their education. Most schools also offered international opportunities for residents, but because these types of electives were generally organised and coordinated by individual departments rather than the medical schools' global health office or administrator, it was beyond the scope of our research project to collect comprehensive information on postgraduate electives.

All medical schools (14/14) required students to participate in pre-departure training (PDT) prior to doing an international elective in a low resource setting. Many schools expressed concern about liability implications of allowing students to do placements in countries considered unsafe by Canada's Ministry of Foreign Affairs, although it appeared that few restrictions were placed on students who were returning to family or countries with which they had association.

While all schools had students participating in clinical settings during electives, the nature of the students' activities varied considerably between the preclinical and clinical stage of training, as preclinical students are limited in their ability to provide meaningful clinical assistance. Clinical trainees often use IHEs to fulfill their clerkship or elective requirements, and are therefore required to demonstrate clinical skills as part of the elective, as they would if they were doing a placement in Canada at that stage of their training.

The majority of Canadian medical schools developed IHEs that extended beyond clinical work or observation also to include a community development (9/14) or research (4/14) component. Sixty-four per cent (9/14) had established some type of interdisciplinary project that provided international elective opportunities for students from a range of health or science disciplines outside of medicine. This included nursing, dental, physio and occupational therapy, public or community health, epidemiology, pharmacy, veterinary, engineering, or science graduate students.

Seventy-nine per cent (11/14) provided information about the length of time that students spent on international electives. Three schools required students to spend a minimum of 2 to 3 weeks on-site, and eight schools had a minimum somewhere between 4 and 6 weeks. One of those schools required students to be involved in project planning, research and hand-over for a total of 18 months, and within that timeframe students spent approximately a month on site.

International partner sites

While difficult to quantify, a recurring theme during interviews with faculty was the desire to develop long-term, sustainable IHE programmes with partners – many cited the example of Making the Links (*Chapter 31*). All schools (14/14) identified international sites where some type of partnership existed, either through a formal institutional memorandum of understanding or through informal relationships between faculties to facilitate student elective experiences. These connections resulted largely from individual faculty connections with host institutions. No school formalised arrangements with all their partners, which meant there were no standardised principles guiding such relationships within schools, let alone among schools across Canada. The extent to which schools organised the elective experience varied, not just between schools, but also within, making it difficult to quantify such information in absolute terms. Some schools had sites that they recommended to students, but largely left it to the student to organise and coordinate with the local contact person. Other schools had highly organised electives, where much of the coordination and curriculum was arranged between the school and the host institution, directly involving faculty or staff. At some schools students could be involved in faculty-developed longitudinal research or community outreach projects. Most schools had multiple partners – official or unofficial – and the nature of elective opportunities varied from one partner to the other.

The importance of bilaterality including exchange of personnel and capacity building in the form of research, training or community development initiatives came up frequently in interviews, whether or not a school engaged in such activities. Half of the Canadian schools (7/14) provided opportunities for trainees from partner institutions to visit their site, and six schools provided opportunities for faculty exchange while others attempted more capacity building addressing locally identified needs.

Supervision and evaluation

All schools had a process to ensure student supervision during IHEs in place, although it varied within and among schools, depending on the nature of the partnership, the level of faculty involvement and the timing of student elective periods. Forty-three per cent (6/14) indicated that they had at least one elective experience in which their own faculty supervised students on site during their IHE, either accompanying them on the journey, or having faculty physically based in the host community. Eight schools indicated that they had a process for vetting host sites and connecting with local supervisors to ensure adequate monitoring of students.

Fifty-seven per cent (8/14) relied solely on local preceptors to supervise students. In cases in which faculty did not accompany students on elective, students were required to identify a supervisor prior to embarking on the placement. Thirty-six per cent (5/14) of schools indicated that while faculty did not accompany students and supervise them directly, they had previously travelled to a partner site and had vetted it to ensure appropriateness for student placements. At such sites, clear communication with partners about the school's curriculum and the students' level of training might reduce the likelihood that students would be expected to perform tasks beyond their level of training. Twenty-one per cent (3/14) of schools indicated that faculty rarely or never visited a site with or without students.

Of nine schools which were able to provide information about assessment of students' performance during electives, 89 percent (8/9) indicated that students' supervisors were required to provide some form of evaluation in order for students to receive credit and/or funding from the school. Assessment forms were the primary means for obtaining feedback on the students' performance, although this was not necessarily a requirement for preclinical IHEs in which students were not receiving academic credit. Four of these eight schools also required students to submit a reflection paper after their elective as part of the assessment process whether through a global health office or through an undergraduate medical education office.

The students' experience: selection, funding learning objectives, and de-briefing

The process for vetting students prior to international placements varied among schools. Half (7/14) of the schools selected students for electives and/ or elective funding based on a written application, three schools required students to meet with faculty to assess their suitability for an IHE, and two schools had a formal interview process.

Funding was available at 79 percent (11/14) of schools in the form of scholarships or grants that students could apply for to cover some or all of the costs of their elective. Two schools involved students in fund-raising for community outreach projects as part of their placement experience. One school required students to pay a fee for elective participation, which was used for elective operations, such as compensating on-site supervisors and coordinators for their time.

Only three schools required a formal meeting with a designated faculty member, usually through a global health office, prior to embarking on an elective. Such meetings are meant to examine preparation but also risk of infectious disease, HIV prophylaxis, N-95 masks for tuberculosis as well as personal safety and appropriate supervision. These considerations also could have been dealt with at a mandated travel clinic visit and also in PDT.

All schools (14/14) required students to establish learning objectives before going on clinical electives. At 71 percent (10/14) of schools students took responsibility for developing objectives (sometimes with guidance from faculty templates), and at the other 29 percent (4/14) objectives were developed or recommended for the students by faculty.

Faculty learning objectives, determined by interview, varied and were often loosely defined. The majority of the learning objectives were based on standardised CANMEDs (Royal College of Physicians and Surgeons of Canada (RCPSC), 2015) and CANMEDS-FM (College of Family Physicians of Canada (CANMEDS-FM) 2009) family medicine objectives (CFPC). Examples of specific learning objectives include enhancing clinical skills, learning a foreign language, understanding different healthcare systems, understanding clinical ethics, increasing cultural awareness, learning to manage diseases rarely seen at home, understanding differences in medical education, gaining surgical experience and functioning in a low resource setting. These objectives could be achieved by attending lectures, participating in clinical work, and/or engaging in research projects.

Schools provided varied opportunities for students to debrief and reflect on their IHE. Fifty-seven per cent (8/14) required students to write a reflective paper, and 71 percent (10/14) required students to make a presentation about their experience. The majority of schools offered some type of in-person debriefing, with 29 percent (4/14) providing an opportunity for a one-on-one meeting with faculty, and 64 percent (9/14) offering a more informal group debriefing session among students. At three schools debriefing was mandatory, while at ten schools it was optional for students.

Discussion

The types of international elective experiences available to Canadian undergraduate medical trainees vary significantly between, and sometimes within, schools with respect to location, objectives and evaluation, as well as the nature of partnerships, preparation, curricula and faculty supervision. Pedagogical research addressing these variables systematically in terms of outcomes to students, programmes and host sites may be useful.

While a compilation of such opportunities at medical schools did not seem to be done, Herrick and Reades developed a database of relations of the top 100 institutions in the Times Higher Education World University Rankings 2015–16, literally mapping these findings. Of institutions in the Global South, Makerere and Addis Ababa University had the most relations (Herrick and Reades 2016). Top US universities (in particular in the northeast) had relations primarily in southern Africa while western European universities had more in southeast Asia. The study identified fewer relationships with Chinese and Indian universities relative to their population. Herrick unfortunately does not seem to have characterised such relationships further, even by faculty (Herrick and Reades 2016).

PDT, because of presumed positive impact on hosts, is considered by some as a part of social accountability (Wallace and Webb 2014). A movement towards addressing these issues began with efforts to improve PDT, which has now been mandated for accreditation, although not standardised, at medical schools across Canada (and in the USA (Liaison Committee on Medical Education (LCME)) to prepare students better for the realities of working in a vastly different cultural and medical context (Anderson and Bocking 2008). Indeed, all 14 medical schools in our study had implemented faculty-led PDT that was mandatory for any student travelling to low-income countries for an elective. This was a considerable increase from 2005–06, when only four of 17 schools offered faculty-led, mandatory PDT (Izadnegahdar *et al.* 2008). Anderson *et al.* (2012) found compulsory PDT changed from 11/17 (65 percent) to 16/17 (94 percent) between 2008 and 2010 (Anderson *et al.* 2012) and PDT was mandatory in six out of 11 (55 percent) to 11/16 (69 percent), but the majority of these were run with budgets less than $500 and were often student-run with faculty involvement (Anderson *et al.* 2012). Several in our study saw the need for, and sometimes tried to implement, specific training for different groups of trainees (students and sometimes residents): high-income country clinical settings, low and middle-income country non-clinical settings, research and low resource settings within Canada.

Although no study has examined performance in the field, Xu *et al.* (2011) using pre and post-training questionnaires and focus groups found a greater improvement in scores of what they termed objective competencies such as safety and health, than subjective ones such as ethical and cultural issues. There were innovations as several schools explored online options to teach didactic components of PDT. Anderson *et al.* (2012) also found language competency training in only ten of 16 schools, but this was not assessed by us. Our Global Health Office at Western University implemented non-compulsory language training in Spanish, Arabic, Mandarin and Swahili, the language of our partner sites, believing this would assist both in practical terms but also helping with cultural competency and making people more sensitive to host needs.

The pre and post-travel consultation visit has been centralised and standardised at many Canadian schools, with mandating the availability and distribution of post-exposure prophylaxis (PEP) kits and N95 masks for high-risk situations. As Anderson found (Anderson *et al.* 2012), although nine out of 16 schools mandated PEP kits, only one supplied these, assuming they would be available through a students' individual drug plans.

It appears that self-organised electives, wherein the sending institution had no relationship with the host and little knowledge or control, made up a substantial proportion of student electives. The lack of vetting of all sites and/

or accompaniment of students meant that such experiences could not be considered "safe."

This Making the Links programme (University of Saskatchewan, Medical College 2016) is one model addressing many of these deficiencies. While intuitively this seems to be a preferred approach, this also has not been systematically evaluated in terms of student or host outcomes.

Having community development and research components provides a more rounded educational experience, but it can also satisfy students' desire to help, even at the preclinical stage of training when their clinical skills are limited.

The institutional interest, direction and consideration of issues and standardisation around safety for students and the programmes and communities in which they engage was laudable. But such standardisation imposes increased demands, human and financial, on hosts, and downloading can threaten social accountability goals of schools. Furthermore, lack of standardisation of training and the wide variety of experiences offered or allowed at Canadian medical schools would create challenges for implementation and integration, leading to questions about whether pedagogical goals are consistently met. Although there has been much work done at medical schools in Canada to develop ethical IHE opportunities for students, more needs to be done in terms of programme evaluation and sharing lessons learned between schools. As with other aspects of medical education, there is a need to develop and share best practices for IHEs and engage in rigorous and ongoing evaluation of such programmes to ensure quality. The WEIGHT guidelines and WMA statement on ethics (*Chapter 13*), are examples of the development of best practices, to protect the patient, the trainee and the sending programme (Crump *et al.* 2010).

We believe that moving to more reciprocal arrangements, standardising objectives and competencies, sharing experiences among schools, and following the WEIGHT criteria may help lead to better experiences for the students but also for the communities and programmes with which they engage. Paying more attention to the voices of those communities and programmes is also important and may be the subject of further research.

Acknowledgements

The authors wish to thank the directors, administrators and teachers of global health, who took time from busy schedules for interviews and students who provided guidance, especially Bill Cherniak and Mary Halpine who were involved in the design of the online survey. We would also like to thank the following individuals for reviewing the draft and providing editorial feedback: Kelly Anderson, Lynda Redwood-Campbell, Videsh Kapoor, Jill Allison, Shawna O'Hearn.

Funding/Support: Funding for this research was provided by the Global Health Office, Western University, London, Canada.

Other disclosures: None.

Ethical approval: The health sciences Research Ethics Board at Western University reviewed the surveys and interview guides and provided ethical approval.

References

Anderson KC, Slatnik MA, Pereira I, Cheung E, Xu K, Brewer TF. 2012. Are we there yet? Preparing Canadian medical students for global health electives. *Academic Medicine* 87:206–209. www.ncbi.nlm.nih.gov/pubmed/22189881.

Anderson K, Bocking N. 2008. "Preparing Medical Students for Electives in Low-Resource Settings: A Template for National Guidelines for Pre-Departure Training." AFMC Global Health Resource Group and CFMS Global Health Program. www.old.cfms.org/downloads/Pre-Departure%20Guidelines%20Final. pdf.

College of Family Physicians of Canada (CANMEDS-FM). 2009. www.cfpc. ca/uploadedFiles/Education/CanMeds%20FM%20Eng.pdf   or   www.cfpc.ca/ ProjectAssets/Templates/Resource.aspx?id=3031.

Crump JA, Sugarman J, and WEIGHT (Working Group on Ethics Guidelines for Global Health Training). 2010. "Ethics and best practice guidelines for training experiences in global health." *American Journal of Tropical Medicine and Hygiene* 83(6):1178–1182. doi:10.4269/ajtmh.2010.10-0527.

Herrick C, Reades J. 2016. Mapping university global health partnerships. *Lancet Global Health* 4(10):e694   www.thelancet.com/pdfs/journals/langlo/PIIS2214-109X(16)30213-3.pdf.

Izadnegahdar R, Correia S, Ohata B, Kittler A, ter Kuile S, Vaillancourt S, Saba N, Brewer JF. 2008. "Global health in Canadian medical education: current practices and opportunities." *Academic Medicine* 83(2):192–198. doi:10.1097/ACM. 0b013e31816095cd.

Royal College of Physicians and Surgeons of Canada (RCPSC). 2015. Frank JR, Snell L, Sherbino J, editors. Can Meds 2015 Physician Competency Framework. Ottawa: Royal College of Physicians and Surgeons of Canada. www.royalcollege. ca/rcsite/canmeds/canmeds-framework-e or www.cfpc.ca/uploadedFiles/Education/ CanMeds%20FM%20Eng.pdf.

University of Saskatchewan, College of Medicine. 2016. "Certificate in Global Health." Accessed August 11, 2016. http://medicine.usask.ca/programs/making-the-links.php#Courses.

Wallace LJ, Webb A. 2014. "Pre-departure training and the social accountability of international medical electives." *Education in Health* 27:143–147. www.research-gate.net/publication/261180403_Pre-Departure_Training_and_the_Social_ Accountability_of_International_Medical_Electives.

Xu JJ, Pereira IJ, Liu WW, Herbert CP. 2011. "Assessing the effectiveness of pre-departure training for professional healthcare students working in resource-limited settings." *University of Toronto Medical Journal* 88(3):199–204.

9 Pre-departure training

Approaches and best practices

*Tracy L. Rabin, Matthew DeCamp, Alison
Doucet, Mei Elansary, Gabrielle A. Jacquet,
Michael Peluso, Jeremy Sugarman and Tricia Todd*

Introduction

Students planning to travel abroad to study or participate in health-related activities are in distinct need of high quality pre-departure training. Health and medical systems vary tremendously throughout the world and, many of these students, both pre-health and health professions students, will be working in a clinical environment and may be actively engaging in healthcare delivery. As a result, pre-departure training is essential to protect both the students and the communities with whom they will interact. Indeed, pre-departure training is now widely regarded as an essential part of any global health training experience.

The Working Group on Ethics Guidelines for Global Health Training (WEIGHT) (Crump, Sugarman, and Working Group on Ethics Guidelines for Global Health Training (WEIGHT) 2010) and the Forum on Education Abroad (2013) have both identified content areas that should be included in pre-departure training. These include the following: understanding the norms of professionalism, standards of practice, cultural competence, dealing appropriately with conflicts, language capability, personnel safety and implications of differential access to resources. It is also recommended that students develop an understanding of key sociocultural, political and historical aspects of the host community. Finally, students should recognise the need to be adaptable, sensitive to local priorities and be respectful and humble learners.

Although the importance of this pre-departure content is widely recognised, it is not yet clear what the most effective delivery method is. Multiple institutions have independently developed pre-departure training programmes. These are sometimes tailored to a specific institutional need, but they also have the potential to be shared and used by others. In this chapter, we compare and contrast six such programmes. Rather than being an exhaustive list of all existing programmes, they represent a diversity of pedagogical approaches, each with its own advantages and disadvantages. Table 9.1 identifies the key characteristics of each tool. The remainder of the chapter elaborates upon each characteristic before closing with some comments on the current state of pre-departure training and future research needs.

Table 9.1 A comparison of pre-departure tools

Pre-departure tool	Audience	Content	Delivery mode	Completion confirmation	Evaluation of the tool
Ethical Challenges in Short-term Global Health Training (ethicsandglobalhealth.org)	Medical, nursing, public health students, as well as postgraduate learners and trainees	10 cases: 1. Developing cultural understanding 2. Ensuring personal safety 3. Exceeding level of training 4. Ensuring sustainable and appropriate benefits 5. Addressing ancillary benefits 6. Recognising Burdens 7. Shifting resources 8. Telling the "truth" 9. Selecting a research project 10. Understanding informed consent for research	Open access Online Self-guided Case-based Ideally, programme leaders should integrate the cases into small or large group discussions, provide additional didactic sessions tailored to their programme, and/or ask trainees to reflect on their experiences in light of the ethics concepts presented before, during and after trainees' time abroad.	Certificate of completion available for each case	Use: As of this writing, approximately 5 years after launch, the sites continue to receive hundreds of visits per month and are required by several global health programmes (DeCamp *et al.* 2013). Impact: Unpublished data on pre and post-curriculum testing suggest it increases knowledge of ethics and confidence in managing ethical issues. Reach: User demographics suggest that the curriculum is reaching its target audience (i.e., those with little prior global health ethics training relevant to short-term experiences).
Global Ambassadors for Patient Safety (GAPS) (z.umn.edu/hccgaps)	Preclinical, undergraduate students or professional trainees	Six key content areas: 1. Benefits of a global learning experience 2. Finding an appropriate global health experience 3. Choosing a programme that fits your needs 4. Preparing to learn 5. Learning ethically while abroad 6. Applying what you learn	Open access On-line Self-guided	GAPS oath signed in many languages, provides evidence of a commitment to ethical behaviour	There is not a formal evaluation for GAPS. Tracking shows that it has been used in over a dozen countries, with an increasing number of new users every year. The path is acquired by completing a knowledge quiz, and many organisation users – such as the University of MN require the oath as evidence of completion of the programme.

| The Practitioner's Guide to Global Health (www.edx.org/course/practitioners-guide-global-health-bux-globalhealthx#!) | Undergraduate and graduate students, as well as medical trainees and health volunteers | Part 1: The big picture *6–12 months in advance* Why do you want to have a global health learning experience? What kind of experience is right for you and your current level of training? When would be a good time? Where should you do it? How will you fund it? Part 2: Preparation and on the ground *1–3 months in advance* Logistics of planning, security, transportation, communication, personal, health, academic; health: vaccinations and prophylaxis; preparing to learn and to serve: cultural awareness and sensitivity; packing; logistics and cultural awareness on the ground; dealing with unexpected situations on the ground. Part 3: Reflection *2 weeks prior to return* Preparing to return home: unexpected feelings and health issues, as well as for planning for future work and sustainability. | Open access Online course (split into 3 parts) Self-guided Designed to be used according to a specific timeline Incorporates a variety of educational techniques, including an: interactive discussion board, video vignettes, case-based scenarios | Participants take mid-course and post-course exams to measure their progress, which is tracked on the website. Can also pay US$50 to obtain a verified certificate of attendance | Although participants are evaluated via the built-in online exams, the programmes themselves have not been evaluated. |

(continued)

Table 9.1 (cont.)

Pre-departure tool	Audience	Content	Delivery mode	Completion confirmation	Evaluation of the tool
McGill University Pre-departure Orientation Workshop	Mandatory for medical students going abroad and strongly encouraged for residents	Main competencies addressed are cultural safety, language, ethical, personal health and travel safety. Thought-provoking scenarios that touch upon each of these competencies (either alone or in combination) have been developed to illustrate the challenges and explore/solicit possible solutions to common issues. One week prior to the workshop, compulsory reading material is made available online (password-protected) to This includes recent literature on ethical dilemmas (such as medical tourism), setting academic goals for rotations in non-academic centres, cultural paradigms of health, and logistics of safe travel. In addition, a 60-min video created by the university's rector's office on legal issues and travel safety has to be viewed and a quiz answered and submitted before the start of the workshop.	In-person half-day workshop offered semi-annually. Six preceptors. (family physicians, some specialists and student alumni), facilitate each workshop. The format is problem-based learning/case scenarios in small groups (10–12 students). Each group works through approximately 7 scenarios. Facilitators encourage discussion between the groups. Multiple logistics issues are usually raised and answered during the small group sessions.	Proof of attendance and completion of the final quiz sent by email to each student.	Programme has attempted to obtain feedback on the workshop and preceptors using surveys and debriefing sessions, but participation has been low due to long delays between the workshops and the time of travel.

| Yale School of Medicine Global Health Clinical Ethics Curriculum (www.mededportal. org/publication/ 10232) | Health profession students | The curriculum includes both a pre-travel component (including the following case topics: clinical limits, burdens on the host, financial obligations, resource allocation, navigating local culture, and photography ethics), as well as a framework for a post-return debriefing workshop. | Curriculum freely available online via MedEdPORTAL. Six case studies to be used in 90-minute sessions – ideal for groups no larger than 25 students, as the sessions combine both small and large group exercises. Facilitated by faculty and returnee students. | Workshop attendance serves as evidence of completion of the curriculum. | The curriculum includes pre-workshop, post-workshop, and post-travel questionnaires, to be used to assess the impact of the session on the learners. Analysis of the pre-workshop, post-workshop, and post-trip questionnaires has been conducted by the authors and indicates that the students who have engaged in these pre-departure workshops demonstrate improved awareness of the range of ethical dilemmas that they might encounter while engaged in clinical work abroad, and had increased their self-rated ability to identify and negotiate these situations. Importantly, those students who had participated in this workshop prior to travel felt more prepared to manage the ethical dilemmas that they encountered during their clinical rotations, compared to those who did not participate (Kallem et al., 2013). |

(*continued*)

Table 9.1 (cont.)

Pre-departure tool	Audience	Content	Delivery mode	Completion confirmation	Evaluation of the tool
Ethics Simulation in Global Health (*ESIGHT*) – University of California San Francisco	Health profession trainees	Ethical categories: cultural differences, professional issues, limited resources, personal moral development. Ethical issues: informed consent, extent of training of local staff, scope of practice, humility and self-awareness, truth telling, corruption, material shortage, establishing a moral compass, privacy and confidentiality, over-involvement, dealing with moral distress.	Simulation based learning. Since the pilot of *ESIGHT* the simulations have been run twice annually at UCSF, and over 150 trainees have gone through the exercises. The number of scenarios has expanded to eight, including scenarios based in global health settings in the USA.	Workshop attendance serves as evidence of completion of the curriculum.	Initial data showed that the simulations were realistic and effective. Many trainees remarked about the "visceral" feelings in the simulations that are reminiscent of the feelings they had encountered in prior real-world ethical dilemmas. Realism and emotional state – the vast majority of participants believed that the simulations were realistic and put them in a mental or emotional state similar to those felt while encountering an ethical dilemma in a resource-constrained setting. Perceived effectiveness compared to traditional training modalities – 100 percent of the participants agreed that simulation-based training was more effective than traditional approaches to teaching global health ethics. Effectiveness in the field – Participants felt *ESIGHT* prepared them for the ethical dilemmas they may face.

[O1]www.who.int/whr/2000/media_centre/press_release/en/

Audience

Because of the growing interest in study abroad at the undergraduate, graduate, and professional educational level, there are many audiences in need of global health pre-departure training. Undergraduate students, health profession students, postgraduate trainees and even practising health professionals all require pre-departure training. For undergraduate students (or even students in health professional programmes who are preclinical) there is the need to focus on how their limited knowledge and experience shapes what they should or should not be doing in a healthcare setting. By contrast, postgraduate and practising health professionals may need to be less concerned about technical expertise and more aware of the importance of ensuring reciprocity and capacity building in settings abroad. At the same time, some pre-departure training content, such as cultural humility, linguistic capability and attention to the potential unintended consequences of the trainees' presence are arguably common to all audiences.

Although the tools in this chapter can be used for all the audiences identified above, some are more geared towards a specific audience. For example, Global Ambassadors for Patient Safety (GAPS) is specifically geared towards a preclinical audience, while the others are generally focused on clinical trainees (e.g., medical, nursing and other health profession students). The concepts taught will also apply to more advanced professionals (e.g., practising clinicians). However, when case scenarios are structured for less experienced trainees, such as medical or nursing students, the use of that case for practising health professionals may require adaptation and effort to make this application clear.

Delivery mode

There are two modes of delivery used for pre-departure training, online and in-person; each modality has benefits and drawbacks. Online learning can provide both synchronous and asynchronous activities, which may increase access to the content and allows the learner to proceed flexibly at their own pace (Schonfeld 2005). At the same time, for education to be effective, learners using online education tools must be self-motivated and responsible for learning the content. By contrast, interactive, in-person settings demand a high level of engagement; however, participants receive a large amount of real-time feedback and support.

Online

The online tools highlighted in this chapter are open-access, self-guided resources that can be used asynchronously. All of the online tools supply information and resources for users, but they differ in terms of their intended use. For example, *Ethical Challenges in Short-term Global Health*

Training is a self-contained site that can be accessed and utilised at any point in the preparation for a global experience, including by trainees whose programmes may provide little formal pre-departure training. To engage learners, the creators solicited real world scenarios from global health practitioners and developed them into ten interactive, query-based cases with corrective feedback that can be completed at the learner's own pace (DeCamp *et al.* 2013). Although ideally incorporated into a more formal curriculum where, for example, trainees can discuss the ten cases and debrief, this is not strictly necessary (and many programmes are using the cases alone for pre-departure ethics training).

The *Global Ambassadors for Patient Safety* is also available in an online format, and can be used as an independent learning platform, or can be applied in an in-person workshop setting.

The Practitioner's Guide to Global Health has a unique approach and timeline. Part 1 of the guide is recommended to be taken 6–12 months before departure, part 2 to be taken 1–3 months before departure, and part 3 is the culminating reflection exercise upon return home. Any of these three tools could be incorporated into pre-existing, in-person pre-departure training offered by organisations who sponsor global training experiences or used independently by students or organisations planning a global experience. All three provide valuable access and flexibility in application or use.

In-person

The McGill workshop, the Yale *Global Health Clinical Ethics Curriculum*, and the UCSF ethics simulation (*ESIGHT*) are all in-person programmes that require faculty, staff and student participation. In developing the curricula, all three programmes have engaged health professionals, including students, who had previous global health elective experience, and they also encourage involvement of student leaders to facilitate its ongoing use in education. This creates opportunities for students who have returned from training experiences to mentor and teach other students, as well as be mentored by the faculty who administer the programme. Not incidentally, it also offers a chance for the student mentors to debrief their own prior elective experience; of note, the Yale curriculum includes a specific framework for conducting in-person post-return debriefings for students who had participated in the pre-departure workshop.

A common challenge among in-person training is that it requires significant time and support. With growing demand for pre-departure training, for example, McGill had difficulty identifying enough preceptors to facilitate the required small group discussions (leading McGill to consider an online format for future pre-departure training).

The *ESIGHT* simulation programme is unique in taking advantage of recent work on the value of simulation as an education method (Alluri *et al.*

2016, Hawkins and Tredgett 2016, Baptista *et al.* 2016, Couto *et al.* 2015, Muniandy and Nyein 2015). Using focus groups of global health faculty (nurses, pharmacists and physicians), *ESIGHT* creators gathered data on the most commonly faced ethical dilemmas in global health settings. The focus groups informed the development of several simulation scenarios. An ethicist was consulted to develop a rubric for faculty debriefings that highlighted the salient ethical principles from the scenarios. While simulation training is exciting and engaging, it may be the most resource intense and requires the most expertise to be used widely.

Content

The content for all of the pre-departure training tools highlighted in this chapter reflect the WEIGHT and Forum on Education Abroad standards. Important common themes include information on how trainees can ensure their personal safety abroad, the importance of language ability, and awareness of the history, culture and health issues unique to the country they will visit. Any comprehensive pre-departure training should address logistics and provide information about topics related to daily life during the experience, including transportation, food and housing.

Nevertheless, the tools vary in their emphasis. Some tools, for instance, are intended as a more comprehensive overview of pre-departure preparation; *GAPS*, the McGill programme, and *The Practitioner's Guide* are good examples of this. Others, including *Ethical Challenges in Short-term Global Health Training*, *ESIGHT*, and the Yale *Global Health Clinical Ethics Curriculum* (Elansary *et al.* 2015) focus uniquely on the ethical aspects of global health training. These subtle differences in content are important, because individuals who run global health training programmes may find that one or the other best complements their own expertise and existing pre-departure training.

Completion confirmation

Most tools have identified a way of confirming completion, frequently obtained through some type of feedback or final assessment that minimally verifies that an individual has completed the course. Such certificates should not be confused with competency, however. Particularly for online courses, certificates of completion cannot alone reflect how engaged a learner was in the particular course. As an alternative to a traditional certificate, the GAPS programme asks students to sign an oath after successful completion of a post-course quiz. The oath comes in multiple languages and states that the student is aware of the limitations of activities they should be involved in when abroad. The oath can also be used to educate the host as to the scope of training and practice a student should be involved in while participating in the global experience.

Evaluation

Evaluation is a critical component of pre-departure training. Without evaluation, programmes cannot know whether pre-departure training is meeting its stated goals. In general terms, evaluation can take two basic forms: evaluation of the tool itself (i.e., evaluation of users' experiences with the tool, such as how much they enjoyed it or what changes they might like to see) and evaluation of the tool's effectiveness (i.e., evaluation of its use, its effects on knowledge, skills, attitudes and so on).

Although each pre-departure training tool includes some type of evaluation, they vary in what they evaluate and in whether this evaluation is largely for tool developers versus for programme leaders. For example, *Ethical Challenges in Short-term Global Health Training* has evaluated use statistics, collects data on users' experience with the site, and has conducted pre- and post-tests to evaluate its effect on ethics knowledge and attitudes. However, these evaluation methods are not available to global health training programme leaders. Other tools, such as GAPS, *ESIGHT*, and the McGill programme, have conducted similar evaluations. By contrast, Yale's curriculum includes sample pre-workshop, post-workshop, and post-trip questionnaires that the developers used at Yale to assess the impact of the programme on the learners, and which other programmes are able to adapt and use as well.

At present, the evaluation of each tool's effectiveness in changing trainee behaviour while abroad is in an early stage. For instance, both UCSF and Yale have demonstrated that trainees reported that the pre-departure training was helpful during their experience abroad. Nevertheless, this is not the same as demonstrating evidence of specific behaviours while abroad, differences in host community perceptions of trainees who undergo pre-departure training, or improved effectiveness of the global health training programme itself (among other potential outcomes of interest).

Conclusion

The primary driver in any pre-departure training is to provide the students the information they need to be safe and behave professionally and appropriately while also ensuring the safety and welfare of the host community, including patients. The pre-departure tools highlighted in this chapter all share these goals. Notable similarities include a number of overlapping content areas (e.g., personal safety, cultural awareness and humility, and attention to ethical issues). In terms of delivery, most are case-based, and even though some can be used entirely online, most include (or at least recommend) in-person instruction to accompany the online content.

The areas where the tools differ represent an opportunity for transformative learning tailored to particular programme and trainee needs. Any teaching and learning methodology has advantages and disadvantages; relevant factors include learners' preferred learning style, the ability to tailor the tool's content to a specific programme's setting, convenience, cost, efficiency and effectiveness. For example, free online training in isolation may be an efficient way to deliver knowledge-based content but does not afford rich discussion of complex concepts in a group or simulation setting. By contrast, workshops or simulations are engaging educational experiences but may be time and resource intensive beyond the means of some programmes. Fortunately most of the tools include an open access component, allowing users to explore them and decide which best fits their needs.

Several challenges lie ahead. One is that there is often no mechanism to require pre-departure training for students and trainees who participate in experiences abroad through unofficial channels (e.g., arranged with individual faculty members and self-funded, private providers, religious institutions etc.). Another is that, at present, limited information exists to define the best practices for the delivery of pre-departure training for health-related programmes. In particular, there is limited evidence that training improves student or trainee behaviour abroad, improves longer-term programme sustainability and effectiveness, or is positively perceived by the communities where trainees visit. This creates an opportunity and a need for additional research on existing tools, perhaps including their comparative evaluation. Future attention should turn to more rigorously examining the behavioural effects of curricula like ethicsandglobalth.org in real world settings, their comparative effectiveness, and their relative impact on programme sustainability and success (Rahim *et al.* 2016).

Acknowledgements

To the team who put together the *ESIGHT* simulations: Tina Brock, Tea Logar, James Harrison, Stacy James-Ryan, Marcia Glass and Phuoc Le. The project was funded by a UCSF Academy of Medical Educators Innovations Funding grant.

To the Yale Global Health Clinical Ethics Curriculum team: Mei Elansary, Stacey Kallem, Oluwatosin Onibokun, Michael Peluso, John Thomas and Tracy Rabin.

References

Alluri, R.K., P. Tsing, E. Lee, and J. Napolitano. 2016. "A randomized controlled trial of high-fidelity simulation versus lecture-based education in preclinical medical students." *Medical Teacher* 38(4). doi:10.3109/0142159X.2015.1031734.

Baptista, R.C., L.A. Paiva, R.F. Gonçalves, L.M. Oliveira, M.F. Pereira, and J.C. Martins. 2016. "Satisfaction and gains perceived by nursing students with medium and high-fidelity simulation: A randomized controlled trial." Nurse Education Today 46:127–132. doi:10.1016/j.nedt.2016.08.027. Epub 2016 Aug 30.

Couto, T.B., S.C. Farhat, G.L. Geis, O. Olsen, and C. Schvartsman. 2015. "High-fidelity simulation versus case-based discussion for teaching medical students in

Brazil about pediatric emergencies." Clinics (Sao Paulo) 70(6):393–399. doi:10.6061/
clinics/2015(06)02. Epub 2015 Jun 1.

Crump, J., J. Sugarman, and Working Group on Ethics Guidelines for Global Health
Training (WEIGHT). 2010. "Ethics and Best practice guidelines for training experiences in global health." *American Journal of Tropical Medicine and Hygiene*
83(6):1178–1182.

DeCamp, M., J. Rodriguez, S. Hecht, M. Barry, and J. Sugarman. 2013. "An ethics curriculum for short-term global health trainees." *Globalization and Health*
doi:10.1186/1744-8603-9-5.

Elansary M., S. Kallem, M. Peluso, J. Thomas, and T. Rabin. 2015. Global Health
Clinical Ethics. MedEdPORTAL Publication; 2015. Available from: www.meded-
portal.org/publication/10232   (http://dx.doi.org/10.15766/mep_2374-8265.10232#
sthash.n4WYJanM.dpuf).

Forum on Education Abroad. 2013. "Standards Guidelines Undergraduate Health-
Related Programs Abroad." last modified March. accessed November 15, 2016.
https://forumea.org/resources/standards-of-good-practice/standards-guidelines/
undergraduate-health-related-programs-abroad/.

Hawkins, A., and K. Tredgett. 2016. "Use of high-fidelity simulation to improve communication skills regarding death and dying: a qualitative study." *BMJ Palliative
Care* doi:10.1136/bmjspcare-2015-001081.

Kallem, S., M. Peluso, and T. Rabin. 2013. "Identification and management of ethical dilemmas during global health clinical rotations: Evaluating the impact of pre-
departure training on student knowledge, skills, and attitudes." Poster presented at
CUGH Annual Meeting: Washington, DC.

Muniandy, R.K., K.K. Nyein, and M. Felly. 2015. "Improving the self-confidence
level of medical undergraduates during emergencies using high fidelity simulation."
Medical Journal of Malaysia 70(5):300–302.

Rahim, A., F. Knights Née Jones, M. Fyfe, J. Alagarajah, and P. Baraitser. 2016.
"Preparing students for the ethical challenges on international health electives: a
systematic review of the literature on educational interventions." *Medical Teacher*
38(9): October 1-911-20. doi:10.3109/0142159X.2015.1132832.

Schonfeld, TL. 2005. "Reflections on teaching healthcare ethics on the web." *Science
and Engineering Ethics* 11(3):481–494.

10 Understanding service-learning basics and best practices

Richard Kiely, Jeanne Moseley and Rebecca Stoltzfus

Introduction

The term service-learning is becoming more familiar to faculty and administrators as an experiential approach to pedagogy, research and community development. This chapter will provide definitions and key concepts, and describe the main components of high quality service-learning programmes, illustrated through current global health service-learning programmes that Cornell University's Global Health Program has established in Tanzania, Zambia and the Dominican Republic.

Addressing global health problems requires the knowledge and expertise of diverse social organisations and institutions, including higher education (Seifer 1998). Service-learning connects the resources amassed in universities with local and international communities and serves as a nexus for reforming education, transforming students into responsible citizens and addressing societal needs (Jacoby 2015).

Global health employers and service-learning educators cite numerous reasons for engaging students in understanding and addressing problems in local and international communities (Cashman and Seifer 2008). Global service-learning can help students develop cultural knowledge, humility and empathy in addition to technical and interdisciplinary skills (Kiely 2004). First-hand exposure to health disparities challenges students to explore their role as global citizens acting on beliefs and values that support common human dignity (Cene *et al.* 2009, Hartman and Kiely 2014a).

Service-learning in the global and health education context can have a transformative impact on students, faculty, institutions and communities (Kiely 2004). However, incorporating service-learning into global health education programmes is a complex, challenging and counter-normative approach to teaching, research and capacity building in communities and university leaders, faculty and administrators may be hesitant, citing pedagogical challenges, resource constraints or risk management concerns (Grusky 2000). Thus, it is critical for campus and community stakeholders involved in the design and delivery of service-learning courses or programmes to consider thoughtfully the purposes of the endeavour and establish criteria for maintaining quality.

Fortunately, the field of service-learning has developed a strong evidence base and a set of quality models and practices (Cashman and Seifer 2008, Jacoby 2015).

The following sections provide an introduction to evolving definitions, key concepts, components and resources to guide the design, delivery and evaluation of global health service-learning programmes.

Definition of service-learning

The language and definitions that describe domestic and international service-learning have evolved over the past few decades and depend on the institution, purpose and context of the service. Jacoby defines service-learning as "a form of experiential education in which students engage in activities that address human and community needs, together with structured opportunities for reflection designed to achieve desired learning outcomes." (Jacoby 2015, pp. 1–2). A distinguishing characteristic of service-learning is the intention to balance benefits to the student and to the recipient of the service, as well as balanced attention to the quality of the service provided and the learning that ensues.

When service-learning crosses borders of nation, class, or culture, the opportunities for learning become more rich and complex, encompassing cross-cultural, linguistic, disorienting and (potentially) immersive dimensions of service-learning (Hartman and Kiely 2014b). For example, Hartman and Kiely (2014b) define global service-learning in both domestic and international contexts as:

> ...a community-driven service experience that employs: structured, critically reflective practice to better understand: common human dignity; self; culture; positionality; socio-economic, political, and environmental issues; power relations; and social responsibility, all in global contexts.
>
> (p. 60)

Global service-learning is therefore well suited for the emerging field of global health, which emphasises equity, transnationality and the translation of knowledge into action.

Community-driven service outcomes

The element of service and its outcomes in global health education programmes can take many forms (Seifer 1998), as can the definition of community. We define community broadly, as "a group of people with diverse characteristics who are linked by social ties, share common perspectives, and engaged in joint action in geographical locations or settings" (MacQueen *et al.* 2001). An exciting element of service-learning in global health is the development of new and innovative models of service which aim to meet the needs of diverse community stakeholders while educating students. By co-designing programmes with partners, each service-learning programme provides unique opportunities for cross-cultural collaboration, learning, and service. The following are several examples of service outcomes of undergraduate non-clinical service-learning programmes in global health.

Collaborative policy case studies

In the bi-institutional course Global Health and Development in Tanzania, Cornell University undergraduate global health students and Kilimanjaro Christian Medical University College (KCMUCo) students work together in teams to research an important public health issue affecting the local community. Each team of two Cornell and two KCMUCo students chooses a topic of interest, collects data on its prevalence and impact, and conducts stakeholder interviews to understand diverse perspectives on the issue, its causes and consequences. Ultimately, each group is responsible for writing and presenting a policy case study that outlines sustainable policy options for their topic. The teamwork involved in this process provides important opportunities for all participants to expand their perspectives on global and public health issues and to strengthen critical thinking, research, communication and interpersonal skills. These policy case studies are used in teaching second and third-year medical students at KCMU College, and several have been published.

Cornell students also develop policy papers in the service-learning programme in Lusaka, Zambia under the direction and guidance of the Southern African Institute for Policy and Research (SAIPAR). The health policy issues are defined by partner and community stakeholder needs. Students conduct literature reviews and interview stakeholders to develop a written policy paper, and also present their findings for SAIPAR, partner organisations and relevant community stakeholders. The students' combined work contributes directly to the mission of SAIPAR to improve policy making, research capacity and governance in Zambia. This model of service-learning demonstrates a responsiveness to the needs of partnering organisations and serves as an important catalyst for bringing together diverse stakeholders for the generation of new ideas on complex global health, development and governance issues.

Community-engaged research

In the Dominican Republic, Cornell's global health students and faculty have partnered with students and faculty of the Autonomous University of Santo Domingo (UASD) to create a Dominican global health programme, RenaSer. Together the Cornell and UASD global health students conduct research projects in collaboration with Fundación Centro ANDA, a community-based natural healing centre in a low income *barrio* of the city founded by a local physician. From year to year, student teams are developing action research projects on themes of urban gardens, living with diabetes, urban sport and physical fitness, and gender norms of young adults.

Relationships and partnerships as an outcome

Students are important actors in the building of relationships and partnerships. For service-learning programmes to be meaningful and sustainable, the development of relationships and trust with partners is a foundational process and outcome. Partnerships have taught us that relational work itself is a form of service to individuals and communities when relationships bridge disparities of power, culture, and access to healthy environments. For example, by placing students in family homestays with woman-headed households in the Dominican *barrio*, and by including homestay family members in the programme's reflective discussions, we have observed increased neighbourhood engagement with health issues and with the Fundación Centro ANDA. The cultivation of relationships between partners, students, community members and educators takes time and demands open communication. This means creating space to listen to the complex needs and concerns of diverse stakeholders and then being responsive to the challenges and changes that inevitably emerge in the partnerships.

Student learning outcomes

Service-learning in global health can be designed to meet a wide variety of student learning outcomes; however, we have found it useful to think in terms of four broad categories of outcomes. These categories are relevant at any level of education, although the specific outcomes and competencies will differ substantially depending upon the (multi)disciplinary scope of the programme and also for clinical versus preclinical versus non-clinical programmes.

Technical or disciplinary learning outcomes

These learning outcomes relate to the content area of the service engagement; for example, early child development in the context of India's Integrated Child Development Scheme, or pain and pain management in the context of palliative care, or monitoring and evaluation in the context of a donor-funded programme. High quality service-learning programmes provide academic support to these learning outcomes through a variety of means: a reading list with assigned questions, in-person or web-based lectures, structured journaling assignments for participant observation and discussion platforms with peers or mentors. Academic content may be delivered concurrently to the service, or may be delivered before the service activity as a pre-departure course or seminar. In the latter case, it is important to structure learning prompts and reflections that help students integrate their experiential learning with theories and readings on the topic.

Professional skills

Service-learning provides opportunities for students to practise and hone skills that will be necessary for a successful career. For clinical level professional students in supervised clinical settings, these may include clinical skills. However, service-learning can also facilitate growth in valuable non-clinical professional skills. In a recent survey of 49 global health project directors (USAID 2016), these skills were deemed most valuable: programme management, monitoring and evaluation, communication, strategy and project design, and teamwork. Service-learning can be designed to provide students mentored work opportunities that build these skills. Students value opportunities to contribute to project outputs and deadlines, as do their future employers.

Personal growth

To thrive in global health, practitioners need to develop particular sets of personal attributes that may be included as explicit learning outcomes of service-learning programmes. The realities of global health present unexpected and sometimes harsh challenges to students' assumptions and values. Other students may discover that they do not want to work long term in the circumstances in which they find themselves, or they may make significant lifestyle changes to fit a new world view. Service-learning is usually a humbling experience, a good thing for students coming from positions of privilege. Students often grow dramatically in the personal domain, clarifying their own values and world view, gaining empathy and insight into inequalities and injustice, and gaining grit and confidence. In USAID's survey of project directors (USAID 2016), the following attributes were cited as most salient for success: understanding context and realities of global health; flexibility, adaptability and creativity; and cultural sensitivity.

Intercultural competence

Students learn to function in another environment, develop an understanding of another culture, and gain an appreciation of perspectives and belief systems that are different from their own. Immersive programmes of significant duration can provide intensive language learning experiences. Excellent service-learning programmes also teach students how to assess and manage risks for themselves and their peers in diverse environments. Managing personal health risks and social and emotional challenges is a necessary aspect of intercultural competence in low resource settings.

These four categories above offer a starting point for specifying the learning outcomes for students. In our experience, it is best to work with the community partner to specify three to five student learning outcomes and strive to deliver them at high quality, rather than to proliferate many learning outcomes. The choice of learning outcomes guides the design of academic supports, mentorship, assignments, reflection prompts, and assessment of the service-learning programme.

Components of service-learning programmes

We refer to service-learning *programmes* because they are more than academic courses with a service component. The nature of service-learning programmes requires that programme leaders plan for student preparation, health and safety, planning and communication with diverse institutional and community stakeholders and cultural adjustment issues as well as academic learning components and service project design and sustainability. In addition, it is important to consider the sequence and alignment of activities that prepare students before, during and after the service-learning experience (Evert *et al.* 2014). Effective service-learning programmes often include the key components below.

Pre-service training or coursework

Thorough orientation and preparatory coursework or programming is a critical part of an effective service-learning programme. Given the complex nature of health-related issues and disparities in resource-poor global community settings, participants need to be well prepared with the skills, knowledge and attitudes necessary for engaging in health-related service-learning activities (Cene *et al.* 2009). Pre-service coursework provides essential training, cultural and area studies, and practical suggestions to assist students in engaging in high quality service work (Cashman and Seifer 2008).This may be done through seminars or workshops that utilise simulations, readings, role-plays and discussions with past student participants. In addition, it is helpful to provide students thorough orientation materials in writing, preferably in one handbook or website. However, nothing can totally prepare students for what they will experience in an unfamiliar cross-cultural context. Therefore, ongoing on-site orientation, supervision and mentorship by appropriate staff or health professionals is also critical (Evert *et al.* 2014).

Local community partnerships

Service-learning programmes cannot function without well-developed community partnerships that emphasise the importance of reciprocity and significant community involvement (Jacoby 2015, Kiely and Nielsen 2002). Those who have a stake in the service component should have significant involvement and control in the design, implementation, evaluation and ongoing maintenance of service-learning activities. This may or may not include a formal agreement (i.e., memoranda of understanding) describing roles, responsibilities, procedures for communication and evaluation and budgetary commitments. Effective partnerships make explicit short and long-term commitments to the programme. A community advisory board may be helpful to ensure relevance of the service work and provide a formal structure and process for communication and community voice.

Clear and useful understandings of service

While service may take a wide variety of forms, there is agreement among service-learning scholars and practitioners (Grusky 2000, Siefer 1998) that the service component must meet the following criteria:

- Students participate in a set of organised and supervised community-based service and learning activities in order better to serve a constituency.
- The service is useful and addresses needs, concerns and issues identified by community stakeholders.
- The service draws from community knowledge and assets and builds capacity.
- All stakeholders involved must have a well-defined, mutually constructed set of expectations and develop long and short-term goals to achieve sustainable service work.

Structured critical reflection

Collier and Williams (2005) have described reflection in service-learning as "a person's intentional and systematic consideration of an experience, along with how that person and others are connected to that experience, framed in terms of particular course content and learning objectives" (p. 84). Ideally students will have multiple structured opportunities to reflect critically before, during and after on their service-learning experience. Critical reflection represents the hyphen that connects the service with learning (Eyler and Giles 1999), and should be a central component of all service-learning programmes (Hatcher *et al.* 2004). Reflection may be structured in a variety of ways, including dialogue, discussion, journals, or other writing assignments (Cashman and Seifer 2008). Critical reflection that is enriched through readings or individualised feedback also helps to prevent reinforcement of prejudice and development of incorrect assumptions about those in the community being served (Eyler and Giles 1999).

Supervision and mentorship

Service-learning offers students a unique opportunity to observe how faculty, peers and community health practitioners and professionals respond to a variety of practical situations (Evert *et al.* 2014). Given the cross-cultural immersion experience that service-learning and global health programmes entail, faculty, students and community members tend to spend a significant amount of time travelling, living, eating and working together. Ideally students have opportunities to question probe this aspect of the experience and benefit from the active reflection of their mentors. Faculty and health professionals in service-learning settings actively engage with students and can provide immediate on-site demonstrations and feedback on student work (Kiely and Nielsen 2002). In contexts that are complex and unpredictable, faculty members often re-think their teaching styles and are required to maintain flexibility regarding their instructional role and course activities. The lived curriculum is not entirely under the control of the faculty member or programme leaders. Thus, faculty need to be prepared for uncertainty and variation in their relationships with students and be intentional about modelling professionalism and mentoring students to understand better appropriate health practices, cultural norms and expectations (Kiely and Nielsen 2002).

Ethical practice

Delivery of healthcare is governed by local and host country policies, and students must not provide healthcare that they are not qualified or legally permitted to undertake (Evert *et al.* 2014). It is important to educate students to recognise host-country policies and guidelines regarding what they are permitted to do and to observe (Parsi and List 2008). All programme staff, faculty and community partners should be aware of these guidelines and provide consistent preparatory training and on-site supervision to ensure that students do not engage in activities that might cause harm or discomfort to patients and others receiving healthcare services (Cene *et al.* 2009, Logar *et al.* 2015). We have found it useful to work with scenarios and role-plays to equip students to recognise and respond appropriately in moments when social dynamics might entice them to overstep bounds.

Evaluation and assessment

Evaluation provides important empirical data for determining programme impact and identifying programme areas that need improvement (Evert *et al.* 2014). While traditional classroom evaluations tend to focus on student learning outcomes and the quality of instruction, service-learning evaluations also focus on the quality of social interaction, the usefulness of service work and the application of learning in practical situations. A comprehensive evaluation should draw from methods that document the quality of the relationships among students, faculty, institutional and community partners (Jacoby 2015). Ongoing evaluation of learning processes, service activities and relationships is key to sustaining high quality global service-learning experiences. Students should also participate in the evaluative process during and after participation in the programme. An electronic portfolio can be an effective way to ensure students document and apply their learning before, during and after completion of the service-learning and global health programme. Before completing the programme, it may be helpful for students to create an action plan for transferring and applying their learning in meaningful ways in new contexts (Kiely 2004).

The dynamic nature of service-learning programmes: challenge and opportunity

Integrating service-learning into global health education programmes is a dynamic process that brings rich opportunities and also significant challenges. It is not uncommon for faculty, staff and student leaders to become over-whelmed or stretched too thin as they strive to create and sustain programmes on scant budgets or without sufficient effort allocation. Websites, gatherings and online communities for service-learning practitioners offer substantial resources. See for example: Campus Compact (www.campuscompact.org), Community–Campus Partnerships for Health (www.ccph.org), and Global Service Learning (www.GlobalSL.org).

In spite of challenges, however, global service-learning programmes provide unparalleled opportunities for the mutual growth of everyone involved – faculty, staff, students and partners alike. Indeed, it is the vitality of learning for all participants that is often the most critical sustaining force behind this approach to global health education.

Acknowledgements

The authors wish to thank Allison Lapehn for her editorial support.

References

Cashman, S. and S. Seifer. 2008. "Service-Learning: An integral part of undergraduate public health." *American Journal of Preventative Medicine* 35(3):273–278.

Cené, C., M. Peek, E. Jacobs and C. Horowitz. 2009. "Community-based teaching about health disparities: combining education, scholarship, and community service." *Journal of General Internal Medicine* 25(2):130–135.

Collier, P. and D. Williams. 2005. "Reflection in action: the learning–doing relationship." In: *Learning through serving: A student guidebook for service-learning across the disciplines*, edited by C. Cress, P. Collier and V. Reitenauer, 83–97. Sterling, VA: Stylus.

Eyler, J. and D. Giles. 1999. "*Where's the learning in service-learning?*" San Francisco: Jossey-Bass.

Evert, J., P. Drain and T. Hall. 2014. *Developing global health programming: a guidebook for medical and professional schools.* 2nd ed. San Francisco, CA: Global Health Education Collaborations Press.

Grusky, S. 2000. "International service learning." *The American Behavioral Scientist* 43(5):858–867.

Hartman, E. and R. Kiely. 2014a. "A critical global citizenship." In: *Crossing boundaries: Tension and transformation in international service-learning*, edited by P. Green and M. Johnson, 215–242. Sterling, VA: Stylus.

Hartman, E. and R. Kiely. 2014b. "Pushing boundaries: Introduction to the global service- learning special section." *Michigan Journal of Community Service Learning* 21(1):55–63.

Hatcher, J.A., R.G. Bringle and R. Muthiah. 2004. "Designing effective reflection: what matters to service-learning." *Michigan Journal of Community Service Learning* 11(1):38–46.

Jacoby, B. 2015. "*Service-learning essentials: Questions, answers and lessons learned.*" San Francisco: Jossey-Bass.

Kiely, R. and D. Nielsen. 2002. "International service-learning: the importance of partnerships." *Community College Journal* 39–41.

Kiely, R. 2004. "A chameleon with a complex: searching for transformation in international service-learning." *Michigan Journal of Community Service Learning* 10(2):5–20.

Logar, T., P. Le, J. Harrison and M. Glass. 2015. ""First do no harm": teaching global health ethics to medical trainees through experiential learning." *Bioethical Inquiry* 12:69–78.

MacQueen, K.M., E. McLellan, D.S. Metzger, S. Kegeles, R.P. Strauss, R. Scotti, L. Blanchard and R.T. Trotter II. 2001. "What is community? An evidence-based definition for participatory public health." *Am J Public Health* 91(12):1929–1938.

Parsi, K. and J. List. 2008. "Preparing medical students for the world: service learning and global health justice." *Medscape Journal of Medicine* 10:268.

Seifer, S. 1998. "Service-learning: community–campus partnerships for health professions education. *Academic Medicine* 73(3):273–277.

USAID. 2016. Infographic on Closing Gaps in Global Health Professionals' Education. www.ghfp.net/content/infographic-closing-gaps-gh-professionals-education. Accessed on April 16, 2016.

11 Fair trade learning

Janice McMillan, Cody Morris Paris,
Becky L. Spritz and Cynthia Toms-Smedley

Introduction to fair trade learning

Global educational programmes and partnerships come in many forms and iterations and with varying levels of success in bringing about positive outcomes for all stakeholders. While programme outcomes begin with good intentions and have documented contributions, critics have also acknowledged issues of power, positionality and neocolonialism (Grusky 2000, Stoeker and Tryon 2009, Reynolds 2014, Vrasti 2013). Ideally, global partnerships prioritise reciprocity in relationships and are built on cooperative, cross-cultural participation. Ethical community partnerships require participants and institutions to examine their potential impacts on vulnerable communities (Wood *et al.* 2011) and evaluate the effectiveness of service learning (Bringle and Hatcher 2002).

Recently, there has been a call for more clear guidance: "service-learning must be grounded in a network, or web, of authentic, democratic, reciprocal partnerships and … as a way to incorporate mutuality and reciprocity, resulting in more appropriate, inclusive, and sustainable development" (Jacoby 2003, p. 11). Crabtree (2008) also notes that "we need more than an ethos of reciprocity as a guide; we need the … on-the-ground strategies that are more likely to produce mutuality" (p. 26). As a result, the first iteration of fair trade learning (FTL) principles emerged in 2013, to help advance just global partnerships through specific ethical standards.

FTL is a global educational partnership exchange that prioritises reciprocity in relationships through cooperative, cross-cultural participation in learning, service and civil society efforts. It foregrounds the goals of economic equity, equal partnership, mutual learning, cooperative and positive social change, transparency and sustainability. FTL explicitly engages the global civil society role of educational exchange in fostering a more just, equitable and sustainable world.

The first iteration of the FTL standards was catalysed by the best thinking from host communities, academics working in service learning and applied lessons from community developed organisations and volunteer sending agencies. Principles of best practice have been evident in university service learning since its inception (Dorado and Giles 2004, Porter and Monard 2001, Wood *et al.* 2011). In an attempt to address this disconnect Slimbach gathered years of insights by probing the curricula and central assumptions of international education and service learning with the following question: "What kind of program, for what kind of student, for what kind of world?" He summarised his insights in a document entitled, "Program Design for the Common Good" (Slimbach 2013), which played a formative role in the first draft iteration of FTL standards (Hartman *et al.* 2014).

The FTL construct also emerged through the efforts of the Association of Clubs (AOC) in Petersfield, Jamaica through a model of community tourism that prioritised participatory budgeting and community-driven development with their partner organisation, Amizade Global Service Learning (Hartman 2015). The construct that emerged from their lived experience of reciprocity has helped the organisations "stay honest" with one another as they, "uphold ethical, community-centered principles despite market pressures to do otherwise" (Hartman *et al.* 2014, p. 110).

These conversations between Amizade and multiple academic and volunteer programme design experts have led to FTL. However, the intention of FTL is not to limit and prescribe – and therefore present discomfort – with the language or best practices. In fact, the purpose of the rubric is not to present a settled understanding of the "service," "development," "community" or even "partnership" – as these terms have led to fragmented conversations concerned with delineation rather than collaboration. Instead, the intention of the FTL standards is to create spaces for dialogue, transparency and mutual benefit between global educational partners.

The FTL standards adhere to the following nine principles (Hartman 2015, p. 225):

1. Explicit dual purposes in our work, serving community and students simultaneously, and explicitly not privileging students over community.
2. Community voice and direction – at every step in the process.
3. Institutional commitment and partnership sustainability – and supporting multidirectional exchange.
4. Transparency, specifically in respect to economic relationships and transactions.
5. Environmental sustainability and footprint reduction.
6. Economic sustainability in terms of effort to manage funding incursions in the receiving community and fund development at the university in a manner that takes a long view of the relationships involved.
7. Deliberate diversity, intercultural contact and reflection systematically to encourage intercultural learning and development among participants and community partners.
8. Global community building – in the sense that we keep one eye always on the question of how this work pushes us into better relationships around

the world; how our civil society networks grow into community; how our efforts abroad should inform our actions at home.

9. Proactive protection of the most vulnerable populations.

The importance of FTL for ethical global partnerships

One student reflected that one of the most important lessons she learnt was that even if students want to help, this does not necessarily mean that they can or should help.

Importance of context: rethinking practice

FTL offers us one way to begin thinking about the importance of grounding service learning practice in the realities of the local context and community. In particular, thinking about the practice of service learning in the context of FTL principles begins to move us in useful and important ways towards more just and ethical partnership-based practice. For many, global service learning (GSL) offers students the opportunity to gain an understanding of and "bear witness to" a range of global concerns, e.g., poverty and inequality, in contexts very different from their own. These experiences can lead to a range of civic outcomes, enabling students to become engaged and caring "global citizens" (Cermak *et al.* 2011) and to experience some degree of personal or social transformation (Kiely 2004, King 2004).

However GSL is not viewed by all as inherently transformative, particularly from communities in theGlobal South. It is often argued to be a kind of "tourism" (Salazar 2004, Prins and Webster 2010), with confusion as to "who" the community is (Link *et al.* 2011). Service relationships can reinforce problematic, internal divisions within host communities (Cermak *et al.* 2011, Camacho 2004 in McMillan and Stanton 2014) and many programmes do not actually achieve the reciprocity they strive for (Grusky 2000).

Such programmes would do well to focus on some of the FTL practice principles – in particular those linked to student-centredness. These principles, following Hartman *et al.* (2014) have as their focus, an aim of "maximizing students' learning and experiences before, during and after their participation in programmes" (p. 114). In terms of thinking about them from a Global South perspective, the most important among them include:

- instilling "an ethical vision of human flourishing" (principle 1.9)
- using reflection to connect the students' experiences with goals on global civic engagement and intercultural learning (principle 1.11)
- providing a learning environment that both supports and challenges students (principle 1.12)
- mentoring, especially from host communities (principle 1.15)

Emphasis on these principles can generate deeply reflective students who understand the complexity and interconnectedness of a practice like GSL.

Co-creation and transformation

Simonelli *et al.* (2004) have developed an approach to community collaboration that is "producing a refined theory and practice of service" (p. 43). Such an approach, they argue, begins with making sense of the community's own way of understanding and defining service. Drawing from this understanding, service continues through a commitment to acompañar (accompany) the community before, during, and after the service experience, producing what the authors believe is "a program and relationship based on symmetry and sustainability".

This approach reflected in the FTL standards (Hartman *et al.* 2014) principles of actively seeking to include "the voices of the marginalised" (p. 112) and the importance of engaging in ongoing dialogue with community partners to ensure that the partnership can "contribute to community-driven efforts that advance human flourishing" (p. 112). Simonelli et al (2004) argue that we need an "understanding [of] how the community or neighborhood fits into the larger power environment or political landscape" (p. 55). In other words, we need to pay critical attention to the context in which the partnership is located. In particular, they state as one of their programme goals to "[p]rovide long-term accompaniment to communities *in their process of autonomous … development*" (p. 44; emphasis added).

This notion of "accompaniment" is reflected in the concept of "generativity reciprocity" whereby the collaboration between university and community becomes a space of "co-creation" and where the partnership "produce[s] something new together that would not otherwise exist" (Hartman *et al.* 2014). In looking at this through a lens from the Global South, what is crucially important is that it could contribute to

> transformation of individual ways of knowing and being or of the systems of which the relationship is a part. The collaboration may extend beyond the initial focus as outcomes, as ways of knowing, and as systems of belonging evolve.
>
> (Hartman *et al.* 2014)

This is complex work, however, often requiring not only new sets of skills and knowledge but perhaps more importantly, new sensitivities and ways of viewing the world. This in turn asks how we, as educators and facilitators of possible social change, are ourselves "present" in the work (McMillan and Stanton 2014). We need, in other words, to include an ontological project in our work: both ourselves and our students must surface and consider critically our views and feelings about service (McMillan and Stanton 2014).

FTL in health education

The implementation of FTL principles within global volunteer health initiatives supports and extends recommendations for global health training within the public health sector (Crump, Sugarman and the Working Group on Ethics Guidelines for Global Health Training (WEIGHT) 2010, Evert *et al.* 2011). FTL promotes sustainable, reciprocal learning partnerships to the mutual benefit of the community and to the volunteers. This requires didactic training to ensure a minimal level of competency in relevant content areas, and an understanding of the cultural and sociopolitical contexts of a community that impact health and health access. It also requires a continuous dialogue with partners to plan and evaluate projects, and reflection before, during and after the experience to ensure ethical delivery of services.

The desire of students and trainees in the health professions to gain global field experience has led to a proliferation of global volunteer health programmes. As practitioners, educators and global citizens, we each bear the responsibility to ensure these programmes are delivered ethically and are not repeating history by exploiting countries and cultures for the sake of the experiential learning of students.

FTL's emphasis on mutually beneficial, reciprocal community partnerships helps to address these challenges. By ensuring community input in the planning and evaluation stages of a programme, FTL allows the programme leader to discuss what is needed, and to negotiate with community leaders the parameters of what the programme can provide. Transparent and frank communications with community leaders help to revise expectations for the programme and to ensure the programme addresses the community's needs, while taking care that students are not practising beyond the bounds of their education and training. Pre-trip planning to tailor the students' learning outcomes to the community's needs and the design of a corresponding curriculum that complements and enhances community goals for the programme is essential. Pedagogically, it also builds accountability into the service experience by holding us – as teachers and practitioners – accountable for our students' learning and competency.

Preparing students to deliver a global health intervention involves far more than the completion of training models on the signs and symptoms of various conditions and disorders, however. It requires a shift in our conceptualisation of physical and psychological health away from a western medical model and toward a cultural world view (Crump, Sugarman and the Working Group on Ethics Guidelines for Global Health Training (WEIGHT) 2010). Attitudes and beliefs about the causes and consequences of health and wellbeing are embedded within community and culture, as are perceptions of disability and health-related behaviours such as when to seek treatment and care (Ravindran and Myers 2012). Moreover, even when medical beliefs and practices change, the lives of individuals reside within the communities and cultures that frame their experiences of everyday life (Mills 2014).

How, then, can we prepare our students for working as health providers in a global context? As programme leaders and instructors, we can use FTL to promote students' cultural world views through continuous discussions of responsible engagement (Hartman *et al.* 2014). By deconstructing traditional service models involving a service provider as the "expert," FTL prompts critical reflection about what we think we know, and how knowledge is defined by our cultural context (Ravindran and Myers 2012). As instructors, we can use this approach to teach students to question and critically examine their own cultural frame of reference. In so doing, students develop the skills for engaging responsibly and respectfully across diverse cultures.

An FTL approach also offers unique opportunities for exploring the "need" for international service organisations. What historical, political and economic forces have contributed to a particular community need? A systematic analysis of the interconnections between health, education, government and politics moves students beyond simple service delivery models to consider the ways in which global health overlaps with other critical dimensions of global human rights such as equity, justice and peace (O'Donnell 2012). To be effective, however, instructors must take care to explore students' intellectual and emotional responses to these issues thoroughly. Ideally, these opportunities for reflection are offered in multiple ways – through reflective journaling, small group discussions and one-on-one conversations – before, during, and after the experience to allow each student an individualised path and pace for self-discovery.

The continued development of FTL and most recent conversations, publications, standards, and tools are available at www.globalsl.org/ftl.

References

Bringle, R. and Hatcher, J. 2002. "Campus–community partnerships: the terms of engagement." *Journal of Social Issues* 58(3):503–516.

Camacho, M. 2004. "Power and privilege: community service learning in Tijuana." *Michigan Journal of Community Service Learning* 10(3):31–42.

Cermak, J., Christiansen, J.A., Finnegan, A., Gleeson, A. and White, S. 2011. "Displacing activism? The impact of international service trips on understandings of social change." *Education, Citizenship and Social Change* 6(5):5–19.

Crabtree, R. 2008. "Theoretical foundations for international service-learning." Michigan Journal of Community Service-Learning 15(1):18–36.

Crump, J.A., Sugarman, J. and the Working Group on Ethics Guidelines for Global Health Training (WEIGHT). 2010. "Ethics and best practice guidelines for training experiences in global health." *American Journal of Tropical Medical Hygiene* 83(6):178–182. doi: 10.4269/ajtmh.2010.10-0527.

Dorado, S. and Giles, D. 2004. "Service-learning partnerships: paths of engagement." *Michigan Journal of Community Service Learning* 11(1):25–37.

Evert, J., Huish, R., Heit, G., Jones, E., Loeliger, S. and Schmidbauer, S. 2011. "Global health ethics." In: *Oxford Handbook of Neuroethics*, edited by J. Illes and B. J. Sahakian. Oxford: Oxford University Press.

Grusky, S. 2000. International service learning: a critical guide from an impassioned advocate." *American Behavioral Scientist* 43(5):858–867.

Hartman, E. (2015) "Fair trade learning: a framework for ethical global partnerships." In: *International Service Learning: Engaging Host Communities*, edited by M. A. Larsen, 215–234. New York: Routledge.

Hartman, E., Paris, C.M. and Blache-Cohen, B. 2014. "Fair trade learning: ethical standards for community-engaged international volunteer tourism." *Tourism and Hospitality Research* 14(1/2):108–116.

Jacoby, B. and Associates. 2003. *Building Partnerships for Service Learning*. San Francisco: Jossey-Bass.

Kiely, R. 2004. "A Chameleon with a complex: searching for transformation in international service learning." *Michigan Journal of Community Service Learning* 10(2):5–20.

King, J. 2004. "Service-learning as a site for critical pedagogy: a case of collaboration, caring, and defamiliarization across borders." *Journal of Experiential Education* 26(3):121–137.

Link, H., McNally, T., Sayre, A., Schmidt, R. and Swap, R. 2011. "The definition of community: a student perspective." *Partnerships: A Journal of Service Learning and Civic Engagement* 2(2):1–9.

McMillan, J. and Stanton, T. 2014. "'Learning service' in international contexts: partnership-based service-learning and research in Cape Town, South Africa." *Michigan Journal of Community Service Learning* 21(1):64–78.

Mills, C. 2014. *Decolonizing Mental Health: The Psychiatrization of the Majority World*. New York: Routledge.

O'Donnell, K.S. 2012. "Global mental health: a resource primer for exploring the domain." *International Perspectives in Psychology Research, Practice, Consultation* 1(3):191–205. doi: 10.1037/a0029290.

Porter, M. and Monard, K. 2001. "Ayni in the global village: building relationships of reciprocity through international service learning." *Michigan Journal of Community Service Learning* 8(1):5–17.

Prins, E. and Webster, N. 2010. "Student identities and the tourist gaze in international service-learning: a university project in Belize." *Journal of Higher Education Outreach and Engagement* 14(1):5–32.

Ravindran, N. and Myers, B.J. 2012. "Cultural influences on perceptions of health, illness, and disability: a review and focus on autism." *Journal of Child and Family Studies* 21(2):311–319. doi: 10.1007/s10826-011-9477-9.

Reynolds, N. 2014. "What counts as outcomes? Community perspectives of an engineering partnership." *Michigan Journal of Community Service Learning* 20(1):79–90.

Salazar, N. 2004. "Developmental tourists vs. development tourism: a case study." In: *Tourist Behavior: a Psychological Perspective*, edited by A. Raj, 85–107. New Dehli: Kanishka Publishers.

Simonelli, J., Earle, D. and Story, E. 2004. "Acompanar obediciendo: learning to help in collaboration with Zapatista communities." *Michigan Journal of Community Service Learning* 10(3):43–56.

Slimbach, R. 2013. "International Education Program Design for the Common Good." Globalsl.org. http://globalsl.org/international-education-program-design-for-the-common-good/.

Stoecker, R. and Tryon, E. 2009. *The unheard voices: Community organizations and service-learning*. Philadelphia: Temple University Press.

Vrasti, W. 2013. *Volunteer Tourism in the Global South: Giving Back in Neoliberal Times*. Oxon, UK: Routledge.

Wood, C., Banks, S., Galiardi, S., Koehn, J. and Schroeder, K. 2011. "Community impacts of international service learning and study abroad: an analysis of focus groups with program leaders." *Partnerships: A Journal of Service Learning and Civic Engagement* 2(1):1–23.

Part II
Ethics

12 Clear as mud

Power dynamics in global health volunteerism

Alyssa Smaldino, Judith N. Lasker and Catherine Myser

Introduction

Throughout the colonial periods in much of Africa, Asia and the Americas, a message of improving health through the application of western bio-medical interventions became part of the colonial system, with the goal of protecting European settlers from unknown illnesses and enhancing the African population as needed for labour in extractive industries (Lasker 1977). Western medical practices also acted as a protective shield for other activities and practices that elevated the status of European colonists while segregating and marginalising local populations. For example, in 1899 the Liverpool School of Tropical Medicine published information stating that if Europeans sought to prevent malarial infection among their communities in West Africa, they must segregate from Indigenous dwellings by at least 0.5 miles. This enabled European populations to access the services necessary for maintaining good health while marginalising Indigenous populations and mainstreaming the idea of "unsanitary natives," which resurfaced during the HIV/AIDS epidemic in the late 20th century (Barron 2008).

More people are now travelling to Africa, Asia and Latin America (herein referred to as the "Global South") than ever before. The global volunteering industry, which provides students, professionals, church members and others with short-term volunteer opportunities, generates several billion dollars in revenue annually. One segment of this enterprise is referred to as "voluntourism," because the emphasis is on tourists having volunteer opportunities; "volunteering" can be used to apply to the broader population of people who travel primarily to provide services rather than primarily for tourism (Hartman *et al.* 2014). The focus of this analysis is on short-term health-related volunteering.

Given the historical context in which these programmes exist, power dynamics play out in many ways between western volunteers (individuals from high-income countries (HICs)) and their Global South counterparts. There are at least five main groups of actors in most volunteer activities; hence, the power relationships can easily become complex. These groups are: (1) the sponsoring organisation in HICs (also known as the "Global North"), which could be a non-governmental organisation (NGO), a religious institution, a university, a voluntourism company, or a corporation; (2) donors who contribute to the sponsoring organisations; (3) the people who travel and volunteer; (4) organisations in the host country that partner with the sponsor; and (5) the patients/community members in the host country.

In this chapter we will focus on the power relations between the sponsoring organisations and host organisations, but we recognise that this is but one dimension of the situation and that the relative standing and goals of all five groups must be considered. The power dynamics between organisations also represent a much larger picture that includes the power of the sponsor or volunteer's country relative to the host's country, particularly given that most volunteers are of European descent while most patients are of non-European descent or represent Indigenous people. The racial stereotypes that were formalised under colonial rule continue to influence who has power on both a macro and micro scale.

Some sponsoring organisations from the Global North exacerbate power dynamics by simply appearing in a poor community without any local connections (Lasker 2016a). Those that do partner with local organisations often ask for no more than logistical (housing, transportation) and translation services, rather than engaging with local organisations to define a project collaboratively to address the needs of the community (Catholic Health Association 2015). In this model, the sponsor organisation decides what a volunteer group should do and how they should do it. This ignores the host community's own sense of what it needs and suggests that volunteers and sponsor organisations have the power to determine what services are accessible in the host community regardless of individuals' reality in that place.

It is also important to note that in many cases, centuries of colonial rule, medical missions and global health volunteering have created "attractive" global health activities that are popular with volunteers but are not entirely relevant to communities. Because volunteers bring resources with them to host communities, many host organisations will pitch what they know "sells" with volunteers instead of pitching what they actually need, for fear that they will be rejected and the resources will disappear in turn.

A number of sponsoring organisations will equip their volunteers with medical scrubs, white coats and stethoscopes, giving the perception that they are trained medical doctors. Misperceptions about the role, training and expertise of volunteers is possible (DeCamp *et al.* 2014). In reality, many volunteers are not trained medical professionals. Regardless of their actual training, it is common for students to believe that direct experience with patient care in a "developing" medical setting can help improve their chances of getting accepted into medical school, and this belief is not unfounded. A number of medical schools list "medical experience" as an expectation for applicants (Princeton Review 2017), setting students up to demand or expect direct patient interaction in clinical settings that are often highly sensitive and complex. Not only does this exacerbate power dynamics, it can lead to harmful clinical outcomes that host organisations and clinics are then responsible for addressing. Not only students, but university administrators and faculty are implicated in these dynamics and therefore have a responsibility to understand and prevent unethical medical activities from occurring as best they can.

At a hospital in Tanzania untrained high school and undergraduate students commonly volunteer while wearing white coats. Sometimes the organisations sending volunteers insist they wear white coats, and some companies even provide them as part of the package. Untrained volunteers regularly deliver babies, often unsupervised by trained Tanzanian health professionals. The white coats give both patients and local health professionals the impression that volunteers possess medical training, which is at once potentially harmful and highly unethical (Sullivan 2016).

> Case Study: An organisation in Central Africa hosts health professional students who offer annual "health education" classes over a 4–6 week period on topics requested by the host organisation. There are a number of power dynamics that play out and diminish the impacts of the programme.

- Qualifications: The students wear medical scrubs throughout their time on site, even though they are not medical students. This creates a false perception that they have been trained in the knowledge they are sharing, even though they have not been.
- Language: As the classes are offered for adult refugees from many African countries, the lectures are simultaneously translated from English into as many as three additional languages. The translators have no science or health backgrounds, leading to mistranslations such as "uncircumcised men have a greater chance of transmitting HIV/AIDS than circumcised men" translated from English to French as "only uncircumcised men transmit HIV/AIDS, whereas circumcised men cannot."
- Insufficient Context: Students had a lack of relevant historical, cultural and political knowledge to question why certain questions are asked and how to respond appropriately. For example, questions about "how to identify a virgin" are answered only as physiology questions, without any reference to their cultural basis.
- Thus, volunteers who are ill-equipped to navigate their experiences upon arrival in a host community can easily create unanticipated risks and harms, despite intending benefits.

Making a difference: perspectives from the frontlines

When seeking to understand and address the global power dynamics that have developed throughout history in order to improve global health, it is essential to listen to the voices of those who have been most affected by short-term volunteer programmes. However, data and stories that take host communities' perspectives into consideration are hard to come by. Most of the literature on this topic looks at the value of volunteering for the volunteers themselves, but if existing power dynamics themselves can lead to poorer health outcomes (Krieger 2001), the global health community has a responsibility to begin systematically collecting data and stories from the Global South related to perceptions of power. In doing so, global health practitioners and trainees can be given the tools and information to listen to communities and invest in their existing solutions so that power can more readily be shifted and host communities and organisations can achieve their missions.

The Catholic Health Association surveyed 49 hospital and clinic faculty from 14 countries, all of whom had hosted medical volunteers, to understand what aspects of these experiences worked most and least for their communities. Nearly 70 percent of respondents reported that volunteers need to improve in their ability to train local staff to provide better patient care. About 65 percent said that volunteers need a better understanding of local customs and culture, and 50 percent reported that volunteers' willingness to learn from the local community should improve (Catholic Health Association 2015). All three of the most important qualities for volunteers to improve in, therefore, relate in some way to the human dynamics between volunteers, staff and community members. At the core of volunteer experiences, perceptions of who has power to treat patients, who has greater knowledge, and whose customs are "normal" can make or break the experience for the host community. These findings are entirely consistent with the results of the few studies that ask host community staff about their experiences with volunteers from wealthier countries (Kraeker and Chandler 2013, Laleman *et al.* 2007).

Similarly, researchers at the University of Toronto conducted a survey with one of their partner organisations in Kenya that sought to determine what the host organisation perceives to be the three most challenging aspects of managing volunteer programmes. Kenyan staff reported that establishing a culture of mutual respect, host organisations' involvement in selecting the volunteers, and designing a programme that benefits both the host community and volunteer are the three most challenging, but important, factors in establishing mutually beneficial volunteer opportunities (Ouma and Dimaras 2013). Once again, the perspective of host organisation staff members is focused primarily on the human elements of the relationships between sponsoring organisations and host organisations. Respect between all individuals and equal involvement of all stakeholders in determining programme objectives can occur if sponsoring organisations and volunteers approach the experiences with an understanding of the power dynamics at play and a clear objective to manage them.

An example of the deleterious effects of power differentials emerged from the Catholic Health Association study: While 75 percent of host organisation representatives said that there is an opportunity to provide feedback to visiting organisations, a number of them also said that the fear of losing the partnership is a major obstacle to providing real feedback. Even when they do offer feedback, they note that it is rarely incorporated into future planning efforts (Catholic Health Association 2015a). Sponsoring organisations must be particularly concerned about these dynamics if they aspire to have a real and effective partnership.

Managing power in the pursuit of health

Sponsoring organisations should help volunteers understand the symbols of power that they may be travelling with. In doing so, sponsoring organisations can help prepare volunteers to prevent flaunting these symbols.

Symbols of power: resources

> [Foreign] surgical teams only work on the tip of the iceberg when it comes to addressing the medical problems of this country. The problems of Guatemala – corruption, lack of resources, lack of education – all come from poverty. So poverty is the root of the problem, and surgery does not address poverty.
>
> (Guatemalan surgeon from Green *et al.*)

At the root of the global health crisis is not sickness; according to many, it is poverty. Yet, it is not poverty of ability or capacity. Host communities understand that volunteers commit enormous amounts of resources to participate in medical missions and volunteer activities. Not only do volunteers spend large sums of money to participate in these activities, they bring with them passports, visas, vaccination cards and other forms of identity and protection that are often difficult to come by for an individual living in a country in the Global South. Volunteers should make efforts to avoid ostentatious displays of these material items and be sensitive to the power they hold by nature of owning these possessions.

There are also many medicine-specific forms of technology and equipment that can exacerbate problematic dynamics and technical challenges if they are not considered in advance of a volunteering experience. Volunteers are keen to carry medical equipment and medications with them on volunteer trips, many of which can be helpful to the host community, but not all. If a clinic does not have stable electricity, a high-voltage refrigerator will simply become a waste of space. If a laboratory already has a centrifuge, another may not be useful.

Furthermore, many host organisations have expressed frustrations with the large quantities of expired medications donated by volunteers. In Green and colleagues' interviews with staff of Guatemalan host organisations, many individuals reported that their staff spent vast amounts of valuable time sorting through and disposing of expired medicine that was brought by volunteers from the USA. "If the medications aren't fit for human consumption in the US, why should they be fit for human consumption in a poor country?" one person questioned (Green *et al.* 2009). Sponsoring organisations should prepare volunteers to consider which technologies and materials are necessary to meet their trip objectives, and encourage them to leave all non-essential objects at home.

Symbols of power: race and language

> The world conference [against racism, racial discrimination, xenophobia, and related intolerance] recognises that these historical [racial] injustices have undeniably contributed to poverty, underdevelopment, marginalisation, social exclusion, economic disparities, instability and insecurity that affect many people in different parts of the world, in particular in developing countries (Farmer 2004). Declaration of the World Conference against Racism, Racial Discrimination, Xenophobia, and Related Intolerance, signed by representatives of 150 countries.

There are also non-materials symbols that carry power, such as Caucasian ethnicity and the English language. As previously mentioned, migration patterns of volunteers in the global health arena have often focused on individuals from the Global North travelling to "help" countries in the Global South. Because people of European descent have greater access to the wealth needed to travel internationally, volunteers are often light-skinned, and host community members are often dark-skinned. These racial factors have been at play for centuries and are often deeply ingrained in the subconscious of both volunteers and host community members. In fact, in the 19th century when Europeans first began providing medical care to Indigenous African and Asian populations, disease transmission was assumed to be a racial characteristic, leading to extreme segregationist policies and the racism underlying the origination of phrenology and eugenics (Barron 2008). Volunteers must understand the historical factors at play that may create unconscious bias in their interactions; they must understand that being called "mzungu," or "gringo," both of which are slang for "white person," is not an insult, but a cultural code that has deeply personal meaning to communities that have been historically oppressed and controlled by "white" people. Volunteers should be given space to reflect upon these symbols of power before, during, and after volunteer experiences.

Symbols of power: photography

> Photography has become almost as widely practiced an amusement as sex and dancing – which means that ... it is mainly a social rite, a defense against anxiety, and a tool of power.
>
> (Susan Sontag 2001)

Volunteers should carefully consider whether and how to travel with materials that reflect or symbolise power, such as a camera. When considering the documentation of volunteer experiences, one must be thoughtful about how photographs are taken, what they represent, and where they are ultimately shared. If a photograph represents a false reality, or the camera creates a barrier between volunteer and community, the necessity of the image should be reconsidered. Volunteers should also be sure to gain permission to take pictures, post them, or circulate them for any reason. Often it will be necessary to plan this in advance in order to develop media releases and waivers in local languages that can be read to those who are not able to read. (See also *Chapter 27.*)

Conclusion: is mutuality in global health volunteerism possible?

There are enormous historical and cultural challenges faced by volunteers seeking to alleviate or reduce power dynamics between themselves and their host organisation and community. Organisations that sponsor volunteer trips also have goals that might conflict with the aim of reducing power differentials. For example, organisers of overseas health trips may have demands for recruitment and retention of students, employees, or church members as a primary concern. Activities may also be driven by sponsoring organisations seeking enhanced reputation or increased income (whether for profit or for services), even if the volunteering itself does not help communities (Lasker 2016b). Yet, it is possible, with the appropriate preparation and training, to enhance mutuality in global health volunteer programmes. Three key guidelines should be followed.

1. Cultivate long-term mutual relationships with well-evaluated host organisations.
   There are examples of global health programmes that form long-term relationships between unique volunteer groups and host organisations. For example, GlobeMed, an organisation founded by a group of students in 2007, is a network of 60 long-term partnerships between university-based chapters and grassroots organisations. While individual students transition between leadership positions each year, there is continuity in the relationship between the university and organisation, allowing students' fund-raising, advocacy and volunteering efforts to evolve alongside the community's needs each year. Many of the principles and values applied in GlobeMed partnerships are similar to the fair trade learning model, which was pioneered by Amizade-Global Service Learning (Hartman *et al.* 2014) and detailed in *Chapter 11.* Fair trade learning is grounded in the recognition that the individuals and communities that host volunteers are uniquely impacted by visitors and should be offered fair working conditions and compensation, hold significant voice in the orchestration of programming, and be offered proper professional development opportunities. These principles can be applied by other sponsoring organisations hoping to cultivate long-term relationships that value respect, trust and mutual learning between volunteers and host organisations.

2. Ground experiences in a sustained learning process about the historical and sociocultural dynamics of global health.

    A few hours, or even a few weeks, of preparation is not enough for volunteer experiences. Volunteers who want to make a meaningful, long-lasting impact should take the time to learn about the historical and sociocultural dynamics of global health through formal and/or informal education. All student volunteers from GlobeMed, for example, engage in weekly dialogue about global health dynamics and systems for at least one year before they travel abroad, in addition to 10 weeks of learning specifically about the host community prior to departure. Other sponsoring organisations can help volunteers gain essential contextual knowledge by facilitating a learning process focused on understanding the history of the host community.

3. Develop tangible skills that can add unique value to host organisations and communities.

    Sponsoring organisations should develop an understanding of which assets and skills the host organisation and community already possess in order to avoid duplication of efforts or undermining of local talent. Host organisations can value from a unique skill set that is not locally identifiable or accessible, such as advanced surgical techniques or documentary film production. Sponsoring organisations should either review asset maps and needs assessments that have been developed in the community or produce them with the leaders of host organisations. This will help sponsoring organisations know how their volunteers can add the most value and recruit accordingly.

Managing power in volunteer experiences requires a significant amount of intention, but those who are willing to spend the resources and time to travel and volunteer abroad should be held to high standards in their preparation. Ultimately, if the deeply entrenched power dynamics of global health cannot shift, health goals cannot be met; therefore, it is all of our responsibilities to understand the context in which we seek to do good, and to act accordingly.

References

Barron, Daniel. 2008. "Tropical medicine's contribution to colonial racism." *Crossroads* 3:1.

Catholic Health Association. 2015. *Short-Term Medical Mission Trips Survey Results.* St Louis, MO.

DeCamp, Michael, Enumah S, O'Neill D, Sugarman J. 2014. "Perceptions of a short-term medical programme in the Dominican Republic: voices of care recipients." *Global Public Health* 9(4):411–425. doi: 10.1080/17441692.2014.893368.

Farmer, Paul (2004). "An anthropology of structural violence." *Current Anthropology* 45: 305–325.

Green, Tyler, Green, Heidi, Scandlyn, Jean, and Andrew Kestler. 2009. "Perceptions of short-term medical volunteer work: a qualitative study in Guatemala." *Globalization and Health* 5:4.

Hartman, Eric, Paris, Cody, and Brandon Blache-Cohen. 2014. "Fair trade learning: ethical standards for community-engaged international volunteer tourism." *Tourism and Hospitality Research* 14:108–116.

Kraeker, Christian and Clare Chandler. 2013. "'We learn from them, they learn from us': global health experiences and host perceptions of visiting health care professionals." *Academic Medicine* 88:483–487.

Krieger, Nancy. 2001. "Theories for social epidemiology in the 21st century: an ecosocial perspective" *International Journal of Epidemiology* 30:668–677.

Laleman, Geert, Kegels, Guy, Bruno Marchal *et al.* 2007. "The contribution of international health volunteers to the health workforce in sub-Saharan Africa." *Human Resources for Health* 5. doi: 10.1186/1478-4491-5-19.

Lasker, Judith. 1977. "The role of health services in colonial rule: the case of the Ivory Coast." *Culture, Medicine, and Psychiatry* 1:277–297.

Lasker, Judith. 2016a. "*Hoping to Help; the Promises and Pitfalls of Global Health Volunteering.*" Ithaca, NY: Cornell University Press.

Lasker, Judith. 2016b. "International Health Volunteering; Understanding Organizational Goals." *Voluntas: International Journal of Voluntary and Nonprofit Organizations* 27:574–594.

Ouma, Brian and Helen Dimaras. 2013. "Views from the global south: exploring how student volunteers from the global north can achieve sustainable impact in global health." *Globalization and Health* 9:32.

Princeton Review. 2017. "How to Make Your Medical School Application Stand Out." www.princetonreview.com/med-school-advice/make-your-medical-school-application-stand-out.

Sontag, Susan. 2001. *On Photography*. New York: Picador.

Sullivan, Noelle. 2016. "Global poor's medical care would be unethical in US." *Orlando Sentinel* Feb. 25. www.orlandosentinel.com/opinion/os-ed-health-care-third-world-022616-20160225-story.html.

13 Existing and emerging ethical standards in global health education

Matthew DeCamp, John A. Crump,
Jeremy Sugarman, Tricia Todd,
Xaviour Walker and Ahmed Ali

With increasing interest in global health has come a variety of standards and guidelines designed to help health professionals and trainees understand the best practices associated with participating in a global health-related experience (Ahn *et al.* 2015). The history of standards and guidelines for global health research is far more extensive than for global health practice. It is only recently that organisations responsible for training and education programmes abroad have begun talking about and developing standards and guidelines (AmeriCares Medical Outreach 2013). These programmes often overlap with those focusing on volunteering and service. The volunteer, service and mission sector has also engaged in evolving efforts to set standards and best practices (Stone and Olson 2016, International Medical Corps 2016, Medical Teams International 2016). This chapter will highlight a few of the guidelines and policies that have been developed in the past decade, including the WEIGHT guidelines, the World Medical Association (WMA) policy statement, and the Forum on Education Abroad Guidelines.

Working Group on Ethics Guidelines for Global Health Training (WEIGHT)

In the early 2000s, burgeoning interest and demand for global health training among students and trainees led universities in high income countries increasingly to offer short-term experiences in many low resource settings (Crump and Sugarman 2008). From these training opportunities arose ethics concerns for: patients and other potential beneficiaries, such as community members, trainees, local staff and host institutions and sending institutions (Crump, Sugarman and Working Group on Ethics Guidelines for Global Health Training (WEIGHT) 2010). While considerable scholarly and policy attention had been given to ethical issues surrounding research conducted across international borders and under circumstances of unequal wealth or power (Singer and Benatar 2001), at the time less had been given to the ethical issues associated with education, training and service initiatives of global health programmes, and no formal ethical guidelines were available for global health training experiences.

To develop ethics and best practice guidelines, WEIGHT was formed in 2009 with the support of funding from the Wellcome Trust. WEIGHT members were selected through a process of consultation with leaders in global health and ethics. Recognising the importance of an inclusive process, explicit attention was given to ensuring members represented a diverse range of perspectives (including funders, short-term programmes organisers, host communities and ethicists) and geographical locations (including high and low income countries). Of 13 initial membership invitations, ten (77 percent) accepted. Those who declined were replaced by persons with similar expertise and experience to create a balanced membership (Crump, Sugarman and Working Group on Ethics Guidelines for Global Health Training (WEIGHT) 2010). A literature review was conducted for publications relevant to ethics concerns for global health training. Following distribution of the findings of the literature review, WEIGHT met in person in March 2010 to draft a preliminary set of ethics and good practice guidelines through group discussion around ethical issues that have arisen for individuals and institutions that send or receive trainees in global health. The guidelines were developed through a moderated workshop format. All members were given the opportunity to raise and discuss dissenting views for each recommendation. Agreement was reached by consensus. Drafts of the guidelines were circulated to the group for final revisions until consensus was obtained. The primary goal of the guidelines is to facilitate the structuring of an ethically responsible global health training programme and to discourage the implementation and perpetuation of imbalanced and inequitable global health training experiences and programmes (Crump, Sugarman and Working Group on Ethics Guidelines for Global Health Training (WEIGHT) 2010).

The WEIGHT guidelines were published in December 2010 (Crump, Sugarman and Working Group on Ethics Guidelines for Global Health Training (WEIGHT) 2010). The guidelines address the need for structured programmes between partners, the importance of a comprehensive accounting for costs associated with programmes, the goal of mutual and reciprocal benefit, the value of long-term partnerships for mitigating some adverse consequences of short-term experiences, characteristics of suitable trainees, the need to have adequate mentorship and supervision for trainees, preparation of trainees, trainee attitudes and behaviour, trainee safety and characteristics of programmes that merit support by sponsors.

Box 13.1 WEIGHT guidelines

Sending and host institutions

Well-structured programmes seem to be the optimal means of ensuring optimal training programmes in global health. Developing and maintaining well-structured programmes generally involves a sustained series of communications and seems to have a common set of attributes as listed below, and may include clear delineation of roles and responsibilities of all parties, budgets, duration of attachments, participation in and distribution of written reports and other products. We recommend that sending and host institutions should do the following.

1. Develop well-structured programmes so that host and sender as well as other stakeholders derive mutual, equitable benefit including:

a.   Discuss expectations and responsibilities of both host and sending institutions and agree on terms before programme implementation; the terms may be outlined within a memorandum of understanding. Revisit the expectations and responsibilities on a periodic basis.
b.   Consider local needs and priorities regarding the optimal structure of programmes.
c.   Recognise the true cost to all institutions (e.g., costs of orientation, insurance, translation, supervision and mentoring, transportation, lodging, healthcare, administration) and ensure that they are appropriately reimbursed.
d.   Aspire to maintain long-term partnerships so that short-term experiences may be nested within them.
e.   Promote transparency regarding the motivations for establishing and maintaining programmes (e.g., to meet an educational mission, to establish a relationship that might be used to support research, to meet student need) and identifying and addressing any conflicts of interests and conflicts of obligations (e.g., to local patients, communities, or local trainees compared with the global health trainees) that may result from such a programme.

2. Clarify goals, expectations, and responsibilities through explicit agreements and periodic review by:

a.   Senders and hosts.
b.   Trainees and mentors.
c.   Sponsors and recipients.

3. Develop, implement, regularly update, and improve formal training for trainees and mentors, both local and foreign regarding material that includes:

a.   Norms of professionalism (local and sending);
b.   Standards of practice (local and sending);

c. Cultural competence, e.g., behaviour (local and sending) and dealing effectively with cultural differences;

d. Dealing appropriately with conflicts (i.e., professionalism, culture, scientific and clinical differences of approach);

e. Language capability;

f. Personal safety; and

g. Implications of differential access to resources for foreign and local trainees.

4. Encourage non-threatening communication to resolve ethical conflicts as they arise in real time and identify a mechanism to involve the host and sending institutions when issues are not readily resolved.

5. Clarify the trainees' level of training and experience for the host institution so that appropriate activities are assigned and patient care and community wellbeing is not compromised.

6. Select trainees who are adaptable, motivated to address global health issues, sensitive to local priorities, willing to listen and learn, whose abilities and experience matches the expectations of the position, and who will be good representatives of their home institution and country.

7. Promote safety of trainees to the extent possible (e.g., vaccinations, personal behaviours, medications, physical barriers, security awareness, road safety, sexual harassment, psychological support, insurance and knowledge of relevant local laws).

8. Monitor costs and benefits to host institutions, local trainees, patients, communities and sponsoring institutions to ensure equity.

9. Establish effective supervision and mentorship of trainees by the host and sending institution, including the selection of appropriate mentors and supervisors and facilitating communication among them.

10. Establish methods to solicit feedback from the trainees both during and on completion of the programme, including exit interviews, and track the participants post-training to evaluate the impact of the experience.

Trainees

Trainees themselves play an important role in the quality of global health experiences. It is essential that trainees understand their responsibility in this regard, not only to ensure their personal experience is a good one, but that their actions and behaviours can have far-reaching and important implications. To help meet such responsibilities, we recommend that trainees should do the following:

1. Recognise that the primary purpose of the experience is global health learning and appropriately supervised service. The duration of the training experience should be tailored so that the burden to the host is minimised.
2. Communicate with their local mentor through official channels regarding goals and expectations for the experience before the training, and maintain communication with mentors throughout the experience.
3. Learn appropriate language skills relevant to the host's locale as well as sociocultural, political and historical aspects of the host community.
4. Seek to acquire knowledge and learn new skills with appropriate training and supervision, but be cognisant and respectful of their current capability and level of training.
5. Participate in the process of communicating to patients and the community about their level of training and experience so that appropriate activities are assigned and patient care and community wellbeing is not compromised.
6. Recognise and respect divergent diagnostic and treatment paradigms.
7. Demonstrate cultural competency (e.g., personal dress, patient privacy, culturally appropriate and inappropriate gestures, gender issues, traditional beliefs about health, truth telling, social media) and engage in appropriate discussions about different perspectives and approaches.
8. Take measures to ensure personal safety and health.
9. Meet licensing standards, visa policies, research ethics review, training on privacy and security of patient information, and other host and sending country requirements.
10. Follow accepted international guidelines regarding the donation of medications, technology, and supplies (World Health Organization 2000) (World Health Organization 1999).
11. If research is planned as part of the training experience, develop the research plan early and in consultation with mentors, focus on research themes of interest and relevance to the host, understand and follow all research procedures of the host and sending institution, obtain ethics committee approval for the research before initiation of research, and receive appropriate training in research ethics.
12. Follow international standards for authorship of publications emanating from the global health experiences and discuss these issues and plans for presentations early in collaborations.
13. When requested, be willing to share feedback on the training experience and follow up information on career progression.

14. When seeking global health training outside of a well-structured pro-gramme, potential trainees should follow the guidelines for institutions (above) so as to maximise the benefits and minimise potential harms of such training experiences.

Sponsors

Sponsors of global health training programmes understandably desire high quality experiences for trainees as well as minimising any potential adverse consequences related to programmes they support. By requiring recipients to be involved with high quality global health training programmes as a condition of receiving funds, sponsors can play an important role in creating and maintaining such programmes. Where practicable, we recommend that sponsors should do the following:

1. Promote the implementation of these guidelines.
2. Consider local needs and priorities, reciprocity and sustainability of programmes.
3. Ensure that the true costs are recognised and supported (e.g., costs of orientation, insurance, translation, supervision and mentoring, transportation, lodging, healthcare, administration, monitoring and evaluation).
4. Execute explicit agreements with recipients, with periodic review, to help clarify goals, expectations and responsibilities.
5. Aim to select trainees who are adaptable, motivated to address global health issues, sensitive to local priorities, willing to listen and learn, whose abilities and experience match the expectation of the position, and who will be a good representative of their home institution and country.
6. Promote safety of trainees to the extent possible (e.g., vaccinations, personal behaviours, medications, physical barriers, security awareness, road safety, sexual harassment, psychological support, insurance, and knowledge of relevant local laws).
7. Encourage effective supervision and mentorship by the host and sending institution.
8. Require that sponsored programmes comply with licensing standards, visa policies, research ethics review, training on privacy and security of patient information, and other host and sending country requirements.
9. Encourage the collection and evaluation of data on the impact of the training experiences.

(reprinted with permission from American Journal of
Tropical Medicine and Hygiene)

Although formal evaluation of uptake has not been undertaken, it appears that tertiary institutions have used the WEIGHT guidelines to design and modify global health training programmes. The guidelines have also been used by global health students to prepare for and improve training experiences. Furthermore, they have been adapted into a free online course on ethics challenges in short-term global health training oriented particularly towards pre-departure training for global health students (http://ethicsandglobal-health.org) (DeCamp *et al.* 2013).

As one of the first sets of formal ethics and best practice guidelines specific to global health training, WEIGHT laid the foundation for future research in this area. For instance, WEIGHT identified a number of data gaps in ethics and global health training such as benefits and burdens to patients, host communities, local trainees and host institutions. Filling these data gaps could lead to future improvements to the guidelines, which in turn should translate into better programmes in which at least some of the ethical challenges could be mitigated or properly addressed.

World Medical Association statement on international electives

The World Medical Association (WMA) was founded in 1947 and is an international organisation representing 111 national medical associations. The WMA has a long history of addressing the ethical challenges that face physicians across the globe. They are responsible for the cornerstone documents in medical ethics including the Declaration of Geneva (World Medical Association 1948), known as the modern Hippocratic Oath, and the Declaration of Helsinki (World Medical Association 2013) regarding the use of humans in medical research. Through the Junior Doctors Network, the WMA identified the need for a credible consensus among the international community of physicians for the growing practice of global health electives.

A working group composed of members from all continents, many who themselves had a first-hand experience in global health electives placements, developed the initial recommendation for the policies following a literature review. The WMA policy statement on the ethical considerations of global medical electives was designed as a resource for use by national medical associations, sponsor institutions such as universities, local host communities and others involved in the global medical elective process. The WMA policy on the ethical considerations of global medical electives should augment the current available global health electives' policies and guidelines. It is understood that no single approach will be perfect for all countries and the WMA hopes by introducing the policy and through its members and partners to start a series of nationwide debates and policies that can be tailored and implemented locally.

Box 13.2 WMA statement on ethical considerations in global medical electives

Adopted by the 67th General Assembly of the World Medical Association, Taipei, Taiwan, October 2016

Preamble

• Medical trainees are increasingly participating in global educational and service experiences, commonly referred to as 'international medical electives' (IMEs). These experiences are normally short term, i.e., less than 12 months, and are often undertaken in resource limited settings in low and middle income countries.

• Although IMEs can provide valuable learning experience, this must be weighed against the potential risks to the host community, the sponsor organisation and the visiting trainee. Successful placements help to ensure that there are mutual benefits for all parties and are built upon an agreed understanding of concepts including non-maleficence and justice.

• Published ethical guidelines, such as the Ethics and Best Practice Guidelines for Training Experiences in Global Health by the Working Group on Ethics Guidelines for Global Health Training (WEIGHT), call on sponsor institutions (i.e., universities and organisations facilitating electives) to commit to sustainable partnerships with host institutions and local communities. All parties are also called upon to work collaboratively in creating professional guidelines and standards for medical electives.

• In turn, trainees undertaking IMEs must adhere to relevant ethical principles outlined in WMA ethical documents, including the WMA's Declaration of Geneva, the WMA International Code of Medical Ethics (World Medical Association 2016b) and the WMA Statement on the Professional and Ethical Use of Social Media (World Medical Association 2016c).

Recommendations

Therefore the WMA recommends that:

• Sponsor institutions work closely with host institutions and local communities to create professional and ethical guidelines on best practices for IMEs. Both institutions should be actively engaged in guideline development. The sponsor organisation should evaluate the proposed elective using such standards prior to approval.

- Guidelines should be appropriate to local context and endorse the development of sustainable, mutually beneficial and just partnerships between institutions and the patients and the local community, with their health as the first consideration. These must take account of best practice guidelines, already available in many countries.
- Guidelines must hold patient and community safety as paramount, and outline processes to ensure informed consent, patient confidentiality, privacy and continuity of care as outlined in the WMA International Code of Medical Ethics (World Medical Association 2016b).
- Guidelines should also outline processes to protect the safety and health of the trainee, and highlight the obligations of the sponsor and host institutions to ensure adequate supervision of the trainee at all times. Institutions should consider means of addressing possible natural disasters, political instability and exposure to disease. Emergency care should be available.
- Sponsor and host institutions have a responsibility to ensure that IMEs are well planned, including, at a minimum, appropriate pre-departure briefings, which should include training in culture and language competency and explicit avoidance of any activity which could be exploitative, provision of language services as required, and sufficient introduction and guidance at the host institution. Post-departure debriefing should be planned on return of the trainee, including reviewing ethical situations encountered and providing appropriate emotional and medical support needed.
- It is expected that the trainee will receive feedback and assessment for the experience so that he/she can receive academic credit. The trainee should have the opportunity to evaluate the quality and utility of the experience.
- Trainees must be fully informed of their responsibility to follow instructions given by local supervisors, and to treat local host staff and patients with respect.
- These guidelines and processes should be reviewed and updated on a regular basis as sponsor and host institutions develop more experience with one another.
- National medical associations should develop best practices for IMEs, and encourage their adoption as standards by national or regional accrediting bodies, as feasible, and their implementation by sponsor and host institutions.

(reproduced with permission from the World Medical Association)

Forum on Education Abroad guidelines for undergraduate health-related programmes abroad

The University of Minnesota approached the Forum on Education Abroad in 2009 asking for a set of standards for sending and host institutions to use to guide programmes serving pre-health students. The Forum on Education Abroad is a 501(c)(3) non-profit membership association recognised by the US Department of Justice and the Federal Trade Commission as the standards Development Organisation for the field of education abroad (The Forum on Education Abroad 2016).

The forum agreed on the development of the standards and an international committee of both health professionals and education abroad professionals was created in 2011 to begin work. A primary literature review identified a few existing guidelines and standards, and from the literature review an initial set of standards was developed. Once developed, The Forum on Education Abroad invited discussions and input from other international members. The final standards were presented to the forum in March 2012. After review by the executive board, the recommendation was made to refer to them as guidelines for undergraduate health-related programmes abroad (The Forum on Education Abroad 2013).

The guidelines are relevant for a wide range of programme types including: academic, for-credit, direct enrollment, hybrid, centre-based, field research and non-credit-bearing internship and volunteer programmes. They are applicable to: semester, year-long, summer, and short-term programmes; and programmes organised by domestic and international universities and education abroad providers. The guidelines are specific to programmes serving students registered at a US undergraduate institution and participating in volunteer, experiential, observation, internship, or other learning activity in a clinic, hospital or community health setting.

The guidelines address all aspects of a global experience from programme development through evaluation. There are ten categories: purpose, programme planning and development, student learning and development, academic framework, clinical or community health experiences, preparing for the learning abroad environment, student selection and code of conduct, organisational and programme resources, health safety and security and ethics and integrity.

The guidelines are used by forum member organisations to assess the quality of their own programmes. The forum provides a variety of trainings to assist organisations understand the guidelines and how to apply them. While the guidelines are valuable, they have not been broadly applied, partly because tools are needed to help the vast array of organisations involved in providing global health-related experiences operationalise them.

Box 13.3 Forum guidelines for undergraduate health-related programmes abroad

Updated March 2013

Can be accessed at: https://forumea.org/resources/standards-of-good-practice/standards-guidelines/undergraduate-health-related-programs-abroad/

There is a growing interest in global health among college students in the USA. Some are interested because of a passion to "help people;" others see pursuing a health-related activity as a way to gain experiences that will help them be successful when applying to medical school or another health profession. With the increase in interest in global health has come an increase in organisations trying to serve these students and give them experiential learning opportunities in health settings. The concern that has been raised by many focuses on the safety and ethical nature of the types of experiences these students are having when abroad. These standards have been created to support sending institutions and hosts that serve students who are involved in experiential learning in health-related settings outside the United States.

These guidelines should be used to augment the forum's standards of good practice for education abroad.

These guidelines are designed for a wide range of programme types including: academic, for-credit, direct enrollment, hybrid, centre-based, field research and non-credit-bearing internship and volunteer programmes. They are applicable to: semester, year-long, summer and short-term programmes; and programmes organised by domestic and international universities and education abroad providers.

These guidelines are specific to programmes serving students registered at a US undergraduate institution and participating in volunteer, experiential, observation, internship or other learning activity in a clinic, hospital or community health setting. Such experiences provide an excellent learning opportunity for students but also present unique challenges not typically encountered in other education abroad programmes. While any experiential-based learning activity can involve interfacing with individuals or communities, public health or patient care activities involve interactions that affect health and wellbeing, and therefore have the potential of putting individuals', communities' and the students' health at risk.

In addition, students who travel abroad for health-related programmes will frequently find themselves in under resourced communities. This is particularly true for students who have an interest in public health and healthcare, because they have a strong desire to serve others. While there may be some validity to this assumption, there are also some serious challenges faced by both students and programmes when students confuse service with learning. When students go abroad and participate in service-learning programmes (e.g. volunteer, internship, etc.) in under resourced communities where there may be health workforce shortages and overburdened health professionals, students may be viewed as being there to help fill the human resources needs in a healthcare or public health setting. This can put students, patients and communities at risk. If health professionals in other countries are not fully aware of the students' present level of education, they may assume students are prepared to provide services for which they have not yet been trained. In addition, students from resource rich countries, like the United States, may have an inflated opinion of their own skills and talents. When given the opportunity to participate in direct patient care, these untrained students may not recognise the risk they pose to themselves and to patients.

Purpose: All programmes (including sending institutions, hosts and experiential settings) that arrange and provide experiential opportunities for students in hospitals, other clinical settings, or community/public health settings should provide appropriate and relevant learning and observation experiences for the students. By doing so, they will ensure the safety of the patients and communities with whom the student interacts.

Programme Planning and Development: Programmes serving undergraduate students should ensure experiences that take into consideration the needs of the community and patients in coordination with the students' learning needs. Therefore, all programmes should:

1. Respect the public health and healthcare needs of the community when developing learning opportunities for students.
2. Match student capacity including knowledge, skills and competencies with the capacity necessary for the experiences they are engaged in so patient and community wellbeing are not compromised.
3. Ensure students receive training that articulates and limits their patient interaction to the same level of patient/community interaction that they would have in a volunteer position in the United States.
4. Ensure that students understand and comply with all applicable licensing policies, visa policies, research ethics, data privacy and security and any other health policy related to their experiential position.

5. Ensure all experiential sites are legitimate and adhere to international, national and local laws with regard to providing patient and community care (e.g., patient privacy training, immunisations, etc.).
6. Ensure students meet language competency or that language services are available for students in all settings. Programmes should consider compensating translators when they are required to assist in student interactions.
7. Ensure pre-departure training, on-site orientation and re-entry assessment and feedback are available for all students. These should address ethics and impart an understanding of the students' responsibility for their actions while abroad.

Student Learning and Development: Programmes should identify appropriate student learning and development outcomes specific to the experience:

1. Ensure learning and development outcomes are appropriate for undergraduate students.
2. Ensure learning outcomes focus broadly on professionalism, standards of practice, ethics, cultural competency, language proficiency, community health, patient safety and personal safety.

Academic Framework: Programmes should clearly articulate the academic requirements of students prior to placing them in an experiential setting.

1. Ensure undergraduate students have adequate academic education that matches expectations in the experiential setting, including but not limited to medical language skills.
2. When students are involved in research, ensure all projects are reviewed by the appropriate oversight body for every entity involved.

Clinical or Community Health Experiences: Experiential opportunities should be offered in collaboration with established, licensed healthcare and public health organisations located in the host communities. Prior to students participating in an experience, host programmes should negotiate and come to agreement with the experiential institutions to ensure student learning and safety objectives will be met. Through negotiation, host programmes and experiential institutions will:

1. Establish that the primary purpose of the experience is learning about healthcare and public health and provide an opportunity for students to learn through observation, as well as relevant and appropriate activities that do not exceed the students' education and training level.
2. Clearly distinguish between the learning role and the service role of students and ensure any student service is within their scope of training and education.
3. Ensure that the sending institution, the host and the experiential setting staff understand students' current capability and level of education, and provide a learning experience that is relevant.
4. Ensure that students are educated to understand the local culture that influences the healthcare and public health of the community and that students are prepared to function professionally and interact appropriately with local practitioners and community members.
5. Engage with existing healthcare and public health organisations and avoid ignoring, displacing, disregarding or circumventing those organisations and professionals by providing experiences outside of those systems.
6. Negotiate and clearly articulate supervision responsibilities by all involved organisations. Ensure the safety of the students and those whom the students interact with and that the students remain in the observer and learner role.
7. Provide support for clear and efficient communication between the host, experiential setting and the students.
8. Ensure students have a safe place to report activities they are asked to perform that are out of scope of their education, training, knowledge and skills.
9. Ensure that any research results, project reports audio/visual products are submitted to and reviewed by the local institutions prior to submission for publication. Provide credit and acknowledgement for local authors and contributors.

Prepare for the Learning Abroad Environment: Both sending institution and host ensure that students are appropriately prepared for their learning abroad experience in a public health or patient care setting and that students are aware of and can articulate appropriate and inappropriate activities.

1. Sending institutions and hosts provide orientation information that puts health in a social-cultural context and provides sufficient comparative information about health systems, health status and public health

allowing students to adjust their perceptions and expectations prior to participating in experiential settings.

2. Hosts and experiential settings provide ongoing orientation and teaching of relevant and appropriate skills to ensure the health and wellbeing of both students and those they are interacting with.
3. Sending institutions and hosts clearly articulate that the experience is intended as an observation and learning experience only.
4. Students are made aware of their obligation to act appropriately and not engage in activities beyond their education level.

Student Selection and Code of Conduct: Programmes provide a fair and transparent policy for student selection and conduct.

1. Programmes clearly articulate the expected knowledge and competencies needed to be successful in the experiential setting. These will include language, cultural, interpersonal and academic knowledge.
2. Students are selected based on the expected knowledge and competencies required for the programme.
3. Programmes have clearly articulated code of conduct that is provided in writing to students.
4. Students agree to abide by the code of conduct while participating in the programme.

Organisational and Programme Resources: Programmes and experiential settings have adequate financial, human and facility resources to provide health services and a learning environment for students.

1. Programmes are sufficiently staffed to train and oversee the students while in an experiential setting.
2. Students are made aware of the limits of an organisation's resources and to be respectful of the resources they are using in the interest of meeting their educational objectives.

Health, Safety, and Security: Sending institutions will articulate clear expectations for hosts and their partnering experiential sites regarding health, safety and security of the students. Sending institutions will explain that if expectations are not met, partnerships may be dissolved and students removed from the site. Sending institutions should:

1. Select host partners and experiential settings with comprehensive health, safety, security and risk management policies to protect students, patients and the community's health and wellbeing.
2. Provide students with information about infectious diseases endemic to the host community and any potentials health risks that students might be exposed to during their programme.
3. Arrange for students to have appropriate supervision at the experiential site and compensate supervisors or other persons supporting students in a mutually agreed upon fashion.
4. Include in pre-departure and/or on-site orientation information about safety protocols when working in patient care settings and training on what to do in the case of an incident of exposure.
5. Clearly articulate policies to protect the health and safety of students in patient care or community health settings in the event of an outbreak or other health risks.
6. Ensure that students are made aware that they are responsible for recognising their own limitations, educate and empower them to decline when asked to perform activities outside their scope of training to protect themselves, the patients and the community.
7. Have policies in place to address students who work outside their scope of practice and clearly articulate those policies to students during orientation.

Ethics and Integrity

8. Sending institutions or organisations have an ethical obligation to ensure that supervisors/host sites understand the level of education and qualifications (or lack thereof) of the students, as well as the appropriate nature, scope and limitations of the students' activities.
9. Sending institutions and organisations should recognise the implicit power differential that exists in educational partnerships that involve partners with disparate levels of resources and influence.
10. Sending institutions and organisations should recognise the risk of paternalism, exploitation, and neocolonial behaviour on behalf of institutions from resource rich environments when engaging with partners in low resource settings.
11. Sending institutions or organisations as well as host institutions and local supervisors should be familiar with and utilise relevant ethical guidelines and best practices.

12. Human dignity and patient autonomy should be prioritised such that educational agendas of the student or the sending organisation should not be prioritised over patient safety, autonomy, dignity and the provision of health services.
13. If culturally acceptable, host sites and onsite supervisors should make patients aware of the students' learner status and ask patient permission for student presence during and involvement in clinical encounters.
14. Meet World Health Organization quality and process standards for donation of equipment, pharmaceuticals and other medical supplies.

(reproduced with permission from
The Forum on Education Abroad)

Conclusion

While the guidelines identified in this chapter are not the only guidelines in existence, they are important contributions to the field. One concern is the growing number of standards and guidelines, potentially adding confusion for those working or being educated in global health. A recent article in *Academic Medicine* addresses the short-term global health programmes that are proliferating and providing opportunities for students and trainees to participate in a short-term global health experience (Melby *et al.* 2016). The article sets out four principles that if followed will benefit both the trainee and the community. The principles are not dissimilar to those found in the WEIGHT guidelines or the forum guidelines. As more and more standards, codes of conduct, guidelines, best practices and principles are developed it poses the potential to create confusion and distract from mechanisms to monitor adherence to existing guidelines. In addition, with no one single organisation responsible for global health or global health ethics, it creates both a vacuum and an opportunity for collaboration in both the development of standards and best practices, and the assurance that the standards are being met.

References

Ahn, R., K. Tester, Z. Altawi and T.F. Burke. 2015. "The need for professional standards in global health." *AMA Journal of Ethics* 17(5):456.

AmeriCares Medical Outreach. 2013. "AmeriCares Medical Outreach: Best Practices Study A Literature Review." accessed October 1, 2016, http://medicaloutreach.americares.org/wp-content/uploads/Americares-MedOutreachPracticesStudy-Lit-Review-Final.pdf.

Crump, J., J. Sugarman and Working Group on Ethics Guidelines for Global Health Training (WEIGHT). 2010. "Ethics and best practice guidelines for training experiences in global health." *American Journal of Tropical Medicine and Hygiene* 83(6):1178–1182.

Crump, J. and J. Sugarman. 2008. "Ethical considerations for short-term experiences by trainees in global health." *Journal of the American Medical Association* 300(12):1456–1458.

DeCamp, M., J. Rodriguez, S. Hecht, M. Barry and J. Sugarman. 2013. "An ethics curriculum for short-term global health trainees." *Globalization and Health* doi: 10.1186/1744-8603-9-5.

International Medical Corp. 2016. "International Medical Corp Code of Conduct." accessed October 1, 2016. https://secure.ethicspoint.com/domain/media/en/gui/29929/code.pdf.

Medical Teams International. 2016. "Medical Teams International Team Code of Ethics and Conduct." accessed October 1, 2016. www.medicalteams.org/docs/default-source/Volunteer-Materials/team_code_of_ethics_and_conduct.pdf?sfvrsn=2.

Melby, M., L. Loh, J. Evert, C. Prater, H. Lin and O. Khan. 2016. "Beyond medical 'missions' to impact short-term experiences in global health (STEGHs): ethical principles to optimize community benefit and learner experience." *Academic Medicine* 91(5):633–638.

Singer, P. and S. Benatar. 2001. "Beyond Helsinki: a vision for global health ethics improving ethical behaviour depends on strengthening capacity." *BMJ* 322:747–748.

Stone, G.S. and K.R. Olson. 2016. "The ethics of medical volunteerism." *The Medical Clinics of North America* 100(2):237.

The Forum on Education Abroad. 2016. "Standards Guidelines: Undergraduate Health Related Programs Abroad." accessed October 1, 2016. https://forumea.org/resources/standards-of-good-practice/standards-guidelines/undergraduate-health-related-programs-abroad/.

World Medical Association. 1948. "WMA Declaration of Geneva (2006 edition)." World Medical Association, last modified May, accessed April 28, 2017. October 1, 2016. www.wma.net/policies-post/wma-declaration-of-geneva/. www.wma.net/en/30publications/10policies/g1/.

World Medical Association. 2013. "World Medical Association Declaration of Helsinki." *Journal of the American Medical Association* 310(20):2191–2194.

World Health Organization, 1999. Guidelines for Drug Donations. World Health Organization, Geneva.

World Health Organization, 2000. Guidelines for Health Care Equipment Donations. World Health Organization, Geneva.

14 Ethical challenges in student experiences of global health research

Kate Standish and Kaveh Khoshnood

Student involvement in global health is expanding beyond clinical activities and students in disciplines beyond medicine are participating in greater numbers (Ablah *et al.* 2014, Hill *et al.* 2012). More high income country (HIC) students now participate in research in low and middle income countries (LMICs) (Mckinley *et al.* 2008), ranging from small student-initiated research projects, to year-long research internships with international organisations and assistantships on large faculty-led studies. Such variety is reflected in the landscape of global health, which is increasingly interdisciplinary and partnership driven, with a focus on prevention, social justice and capacity building (Costello and Zumla 2000, Fried *et al.* 2010, Merson 2014, Frenk *et al.* 2010). This contrasts, however, with a more limited view of global health ethics for trainees. Ethical discussions under the guise of "global health" often focuses narrowly on clinical healthcare delivery by medical students (Rahim *et al.* 2016) and institutional review board protocols for student researchers. As more students participate in collaborative, interdisciplinary and community-based research, they require greater exposure to emerging paradigms of global health research ethics and better preparation and support for common ethical challenges.

Paradigms of ethical practices in global health research have quickly evolved. Most students are taught western biomedical research ethics, which stands on the principles of autonomy, beneficence, non-maleficence and justice (as described in the Belmont Report, the Declaration of Helsinki and CIOMS guidelines). However, this individualistic framework is not well matched for global health research, which often involves communities, populations and partnerships (Pinto and Upshur 2009).

The inadequacy of western biomedical ethics in global health research surfaced in part from the debate regarding standards of care for research subjects in LMICs, from which emerged the imperative to understand the context in which research is conducted, and to interpret ethical guidelines through community engagement (Benatar and Singer 2000). The very inequities that global health practitioners seek to address are recognised as a source of ethical challenges when HIC researchers work in LMICs (Jentsch 2004, Oleksiyenko and Sá 2009, Tan-Torres Edejer 1999).

New paradigms of global health research ethics specifically confront these inequities in power and resources between individual researchers, institutions and countries at both the micro-level – protection of individuals and communities – and at the macro-level – requirements of fair distribution of research benefits and burdens and other considerations of social justice. Proposed ethical frameworks for global health research address process (e.g., research design, participants' rights, partnership, capacity building) and outcomes (e.g., benefit sharing, social value, solidarity, innovation) (Pinto and Upshur 2009, Ijsselmuiden *et al.* 2010, Emanuel *et al.* 2004, Tan-Torres Edejer 1999). HIC researchers are now challenged to collaborate with LMIC researchers to maximise benefits to communities (rather than to HIC researchers' careers), and to help ensure that LMIC researchers acquire the tools and experience to address local research needs independently (Benatar and Singer 2010).

HIC students, as naturally self-interested learners, may have the most trouble complying with such ethical benchmarks. Trainees' limited experience, resources and time make it difficult to establish successful research projects in low resource settings, and their priority on learning may interfere with other outcomes such as local benefit (Jentsch and Pilley 2003, Hunt and Godard 2013). The ethical challenges health professional students face in low income settings have been discussed in medical literature over the past two decades (Banatvala and Doyal 1998, Roberts 2006, Shah and Wu 2008, Pinto and Upshur 2009, Bishop and Litch 2000). Across different disciplines and fieldwork activities ranging from education to research and clinical care, common ethical dilemmas surface: students question whether their activities benefit the local community, recognise their own cultural biases and privileged status as HIC outsiders, work within resource differentials, and navigate different ethical frameworks (Table 14.1) (Elit *et al.* 2011, Abedini *et al.* 2012, Durham 2014, Harrison *et al.* 2016, Crabtree 2013, Hatfield *et al.* 2009, Provenanzo *et al.* 2010, Standish 2016).

These publications, by HIC authors, are beginning to define the role of ethics in student global health research, but a full accounting should be guided by the perspectives of their LMIC counterparts. Host faculty, staff, students and research participants may have different definitions or interpretations of ethical priorities and challenges, although a dearth of those perspectives in global health literature reflects the very inequities that plague the field (Sanchez and Lopez 2013, Crane 2011). Recent qualitative studies have explored host perceptions of ethical issues in short-term global health electives (STEGHs), including the mismatch between visitors' expectations and local needs, a lack of cultural competency, and burdens on local staff and students of hosting visitors (Kumwenda *et al.* 2015, Kraeker and Chandler 2013, Bozinoff *et al.* 2014, see also literature review *Chapter 19*). Fewer studies have looked at host perspectives of visiting student researchers, although many challenges caused by inequities in international research partnerships have been identified (Murphy *et al.* 2015, Costello and Zumla 2000). Discussion of

Table 14.1 Common ethical challenges and relevant training and support for students

Ethical challenges and examples	Training and support
Differences in ethical frameworks and standards • Variations in informed consent expectations and applicability of autonomy (Harrison, Standish, Durham) • Confidentiality in a collective culture (Durham) • Culturally specific vulnerabilities of participants (Standish)	• Competencies: knowledge of global health ethical frameworks and local systems and culture (Hatfield) • Host country IRB review and ethics training (WEIGHT) • Mentorship by faculty with host country experience and ongoing faculty support as ethical challenges arise (Shah) • Opportunity for reflection throughout experience (Crabtree)
Scope of practice • Practising beyond training level (Abedini, Harrison, Standish)	• Competencies/attitudes: humility (Pinto) • Set clear expectations with hosts of student role (WEIGHT) • Discussions with recently returned students about their experiences (Bender)
Resource differentials and working in limited resource settings • Corruption (Standish, Harrison) • Recognising privilege as foreigner, burdens on hosts (Abedini, Elit) • Participant and staff compensation (Standish, Durham)	• Competencies: social justice, historical inequities (Hunt) • Pre-departure case-based learning (DeCamp, Provenzano, Hunt) • Post-fieldwork debriefing and reflection (Bender) • Funding for hosts and equitable institutional partnerships (WEIGHT)
Research benefits • Questioning if research benefits participants/community (Abedini, Standish, Durham) • Unilateral capacity building that leaves out hosts (Elit)	• Competencies: capacity building, translational research (Hatfield), solidarity (Pinto) • Develop research questions and protocol in collaboration with hosts (WEIGHT)

ethical challenges from both HICs and LMICs will be better prepared when they face similar experiences in their fieldwork.

Recognition of the range of ethical challenges student researchers face should be accompanied by renewed attention to ethical frameworks, relevant pre-departure preparation, and strategies for ongoing support during and after fieldwork (Anderson *et al.* 2012). The broader ethical frameworks described for global health are rightfully reflected in ethics guidelines for clinical electives, but those for student research have been less thoroughly addressed. Pinto and Ross (2009) highlight the potential for power imbalance between HIC and LMIC research partners, and encourage students to be critical of such dynamics. They present a framework that focuses student attention on internal concepts of humility and introspection, and external concepts of solidarity and social justice.

The Working Group on Ethics Guidelines for Global Health Training (WEIGHT), an expert group of global health practitioners and ethicists (these are presented in their entirety in *Chapter 13*), has provided a far-reaching set of best practices aimed at students, host and sending institutions, as well as funders for STEGHs, much of which applies to research (Crump, Sugarman, and WEIGHT 2010). With regard to research, their specific recommendations are as follows:

> If research is planned as part of the training experience, develop the research plan early and in consultation with mentors, focus on research themes of interest and relevance to the host, understand and follow all research procedures of the host and sending institution, obtain ethics committee approval for the research before initiation of research, and receive appropriate training in research ethics.
>
> (Crump, Sugarman, and WEIGHT, p. 1180)

The WEIGHT guidelines call on institutions to provide pre-departure training and ensure research is ethically conducted and beneficial to host communities, but the practicalities of how to implement such recommendations are left to individual students, faculty and universities to develop. In some institutions a single training incorporating travel safety and other logistics is combined with a limited discussion of "ethics," while others provide semester-long programmes to prepare students for the work and challenges they will face. Such guidelines are included in *Chapter 13*. Hunt and Goddard (2013) describe the content and methods they used in training programmes for student researchers, including discussion of historical and socioeconomic inequities, ethical challenges in the conduct of research, and where students can find support when such challenges arise. Others propose students receive ongoing mentorship before, during and after fieldwork. In such a model experienced faculty or postgraduates may help students foresee and address challenges when they arise, and as they later process and reflect on them (Shah *et al.* 2011, Bender and Walker 2013, Abedini *et al.* 2012).

Furthermore, pre-departure ethics trainings are often designed and implemented without empirical evidence regarding content or pedagogical method, and they are usually not rigorously evaluated (Hamadani *et al.* 2009, Wallace and Webb 2015). In their review of published ethics trainings for global health clinical electives, Rahim et al (2016) found only two that evaluated outcomes among students. In those that have done rigorous evaluation of training methods, case-based learning, both in person and online, was found to be an effective modality for ethics training (DeCamp *et al.* 2013, Dharamsi *et al.* 2011). Exploring ethical challenges in global health research through cases in pre-departure trainings may help prepare students to recognise and address such challenges when they arise.

Global health research is carried out along historical lines of inequity and exploitation, which often continue to plague our individual and institutional relationships (Crane 2010). Partnerships in research are beginning to address these challenges (Murphy *et al.* 2015), but in the meantime, students entering such strained collaborations should be cognisant of these histories, and be prepared with the ethical frameworks to question and resist their modern manifestations (Wallace and Webb 2015). New models of student global health experiences should address these inequities, and indeed turn them on their heads such that HIC students and researchers no longer dominate the field (MacFarlane *et al.* 2008). This may be accomplished by designing programmes to optimise benefit to the community, such as the more equitable and future-oriented STEGHs described by Melby et al (2015), and through institutional partnerships in which HIC and LMIC students work and live together (Fyfe 2012, Wheat *et al.* 2016). Introspection and reflection may be as important as ethics training in helping students to avoid and respond to ethical challenges (Ventres and Wilson 2015, Sharma and Anderson 2013). Such models fit within the new paradigms of health education, as recently laid out by the Commission on Education of Health Professionals for the 21st century, which aims to change health education globally so that students can adapt to an increasingly interdependent global health environment (Frenk *et al.* 2010). Specifically they lay out a rubric for moving health education from a formative, expert-producing education, to one that transforms, "produc[ing] enlightened change agents." (Frenk *et al.* 2010).

For many learners, practical research experience in the field may be the most transformative moment of their education. There are a number of steps that may help us guide and empower students through these experiences. First, we must identify the ethical challenges students face in global health research, which will require further exploration of students' experiences, through qualitative studies and programme evaluation. For a complete picture, the perspectives of LMIC preceptors and researchers should be prioritised, as they may have different perceptions of ethical challenges and important insights into how to avoid such challenges and support HIC students. Guidelines specific to student researchers should be based on HIC and LMIC expert opinion and research, as well as student and programme experiences. Evaluation and publication of outcomes of rigorous training and structured global health fieldwork programmes will help more institutions to integrate global health ethics into curricula and implement thorough support structures for students. The promotion of health equity will require many actors, and within each actor is the discomfort with inequity that drives them to become agents of change and is often experienced as an ethical dilemma – how to treat a patient with no access to health insurance, how to compensate research subjects who live in extreme poverty. By guiding student researchers through such challenges, we will help create those agents of change.

References

Abedini, N.C., L.D. Gruppen, J.C. Kolars and A.K. Kumagai. 2012. "Understanding the effects of short-term international service-learning trips on medical students." *Academic Medicine: Journal of the Association of American Medical Colleges* 87(6):820–828. doi: 10.1097/ACM.0b013e31825396d8.

Ablah, E., D.A. Biberman, E.M. Weist, P. Buekens, M.E. Bentley, D. Burke, J.R. Finnegan, *et al.* 2014. "Improving global health education: development of a global health competency model." *American Journal of Tropical Medicine and Hygiene* 90(3):560–565. doi: 10.4269/ajtmh.13–0537.

Anderson, K.C., M.A. Slatnik, I. Pereira, E. Cheung, K. Xu and T.F. Brewer. 2012. "Are we there yet? Preparing Canadian medical students for global health electives." *Academic Medicine: Journal of the Association of American Medical Colleges* 87(2):206–209. doi: 10.1097/ACM.0b013e31823e23d4.

Benatar, S.R. and P.A. Singer. 2000. "A new look at international research ethics." *BMJ (Clinical Research Ed.)* 321(7264):824–826.

Benatar, S.R. and P.A. Singer. 2010. "Responsibilities in international research: a new look revisited." *Journal of Medical Ethics* 36(4):194–197. doi: 10.1136/jme.2009.032672.

Banatvala, N. and L. Doyal. 1998. "When to say no." *BMJ* 316:1404–1405.

Bender, A. and P. Walker. 2013. "The obligation of debriefing in global health education." *Medical Teacher* 35(3):e1027–e1034. doi: 10.3109/0142159X.2012.733449.

Bishop, R.A. and J.A. Litch. 2000. "Medical tourism can do harm." *BMJ* 320(7240):1017. doi: 10.1136/bmj.320.7240.1017.

Bozinoff, N., K.P. Dorman, D. Kerr, E. Roebbelen, E. Rogers, A. Hunter, T. O'Shea and C. Kraeker. 2014. "Toward reciprocity: host supervisor perspectives on international medical electives." *Medical Education* 48(4):397–404. doi: 10.1111/medu.12386.

Costello, A. and A. Zumla. 2000. "Moving to research partnerships in developing countries." *BMJ* 321(7264):827–829.

Crabtree, R.D. 2013. "The intended and unintended consequences of international service-learning." *Journal of Higher Education Outreach* 17(2):43–66.

Crane, J. 2010. "Unequal 'partners'. AIDS, academia, and the rise of global health." *Behemoth* (3):78–97. doi: 10.1524/behe.2010.0021.

Crane, J. 2011. "Scrambling for Africa? Universities and global health." *Lancet* 377(9775):1388–1390.

Crump, J.A., J. Sugarman, and Working Group on Ethics Guidelines for Global Health Training (WEIGHT). 2010. "Ethics and best practice guidelines for training experiences in global health." *American Journal of Tropical Medicine and Hygiene* 83(6):1178–1182. doi: 10.4269/ajtmh.2010.10-0527.

DeCamp, M., J. Rodriguez, S. Hecht, M. Barry and J. Sugarman. 2013. "An ethics curriculum for short-term global health trainees." *Globalization and Health* 9:5. doi:10.1186/1744-8603-9-5.

Dharamsi, S., J.-A. Osei-Twum and M. Whiteman. 2011. "Socially responsible approaches to international electives and global health outreach." *Medical Education* 45(5):530–531. doi: 10.1111/j.1365-2923.2011.03961.x.

Durham, J. 2014. "Ethical challenges in cross-cultural research: a student researcher's perspective." *Australian and New Zealand Journal of Public Health* 38(6):509–512. doi: 10.1111/1753–6405.12286.

Elit, L., M. Hunt, L. Redwood-Campbell, J. Ranford, N. Adelson and L. Schwartz. 2011. "Ethical issues encountered by medical students during international health electives." *Medical Education* 45(7):704–711. doi: 10.1111/j.1365-2923.2011.03936.x.

Emanuel, E.J., D. Wendler, J. Killen and C. Grady. 2004. "What makes clinical research in developing countries ethical? The benchmarks of ethical research." *Journal of Infectious Diseases* 189(5):930–937.

Frenk, J., L. Chen, Z.A. Bhutta, J. Cohen, N. Crisp, T. Evans, H. Fineberg, *et al.* 2010. "Health professionals for a new century: transforming education to strengthen health systems in an interdependent world." *Lancet* 376(9756):1923–1958. doi: 10.1016/S0140-6736(10)61854–5.

Fried, L.P., M.E. Bentley, P. Buekens, D.S. Burke, J.J. Frenk, M.J. Klag and H.C. Spencer. 2010. "Global health is public health." *Lancet* 535–537. doi: 10.1016/S0140-6736(10)60203–6.

Fyfe, M.V. 2012. "Education projects: an opportunity for student fieldwork in global health academic programs." *Journal of Public Health Policy* 33(Suppl 1) (January): S216–223. doi: 10.1057/jphp.2012.42.

Hamadani, F., L. Sacirgic and A. McCarthy. 2009. "Ethics in global health: the need for evidence-based curricula." *McGill Journal of Medicine : MJM : An International Forum for the Advancement of Medical Sciences by Students* 12(2) (January):120.

Harrison, J., T. Logar, P. Le and M. Glass. 2016. "What are the ethical issues facing global-health trainees working overseas? A multi-professional qualitative study." *Healthcare* 4(3):43. doi: 10.3390/healthcare4030043.

Hatfield, J.M., K.G. Hecker and A.E Jensen. 2009. "Building global health research competencies at the undergraduate level." *Journal of Studies in International Education* 13(4):509–521. doi: 10.1177/1028315308329806.

Hill, D.R., R.M. Ainsworth and U. Partap. 2012. "Teaching global public health in the undergraduate liberal arts: a survey of 50 colleges." *American Journal of Tropical Medicine and Hygiene* 87(1):11–15. doi: 10.4269/ajtmh.2012.11-0571.

Hunt, M.R. and B. Godard. 2013. "Beyond procedural ethics: foregrounding questions of justice in global health research ethics training for students." *Global Public Health* 8(6):713–724. doi: 10.1080/17441692.2013.796400.

Ijsselmuiden, C.B., N.E. Kass, N.K. Sewankambo and J.V.Lavery. 2010. "Evolving values in ethics and global health research." *Global Public Health* 5(2):154–163. doi: 10.1080/17441690903436599.

Jentsch, B. 2004. "Making Southern realities count: research agendas and design in North–South collaborations." *International Journal of Social Research Methodology* 7(3):259–269. doi: 10.1080/1364557021000024776.

Jentsch, B. and C. Pilley. 2003. "Research relationships between the South and the North: Cinderella and the ugly sisters?" *Social Science and Medicine* 57(10):1957–1967. doi: 10.1016/s0277-9536(03)00060-1.

Kraeker, C. and C. Chandler. 2013. "'We learn from them, they learn from us': Global health experiences and host perceptions of visiting health care professionals." *Academic Medicine: Journal of the Association of American Medical Colleges* 88(4):483–487. doi: 10.1097/ACM.0b013e3182857b8a.

Kumwenda, B., J. Dowell, K. Daniels and N. Merrylees. 2015. "Medical electives in sub-Saharan Africa: a host perspective." *Medical Education* 49(6):623–633. doi: 10.1111/medu.12727.

MacFarlane, S.B., M. Jacobs and E.E. Kaaya. 2008. "In the name of global health: trends in academic institutions." *Journal of Public Health Policy* 29(4):383–401.

McKinley, D.W., S.R. Williams, J.J. Norcini and M.B. Anderson. 2008. "International exchange programs and U.S. medical schools." *Academic Medicine* 83(10):53–57.

Melby, M.K., L.C. Loh, J. Evert, C. Prater, H. Lin and O.A. Khan. 2015. "Beyond medical 'missions' to impact-driven short-term experiences in global health (STEGHs)." *Academic Medicine* 91(5):633–638. doi: 10.1097/ACM.0000000000001009.

Merson, M.H. 2014. "University engagement in global health." *New England Journal of Medicine* 370(18):1676–1678. doi: 10.1056/NEJMp1400276.

Murphy, J., J. Hatfield, K. Afsana and V.ic Neufeld. 2015. "Making a commitment to ethics in global health research partnerships: a practical tool to support ethical practice." *Journal of Bioethical Inquiry* 12(1): 37–146. doi: 10.1007/s11673-014-9604-6.

Oleksiyenko, A. and C.M. Sá. 2009. "Resource asymmetries and cumulative advantages: Canadian and US research universities and the field of global health." *Higher Education* 59(3):367–385. doi: 10.1007/s10734-009-9254-5.

Pinto, A.D. and R.E.G. Upshur. 2009. "Global health ethics for students." *Developing World Bioethics* 9(1):1–10. doi: 10.1111/j.1471-8847.2007.00209.x.

Provenzano, A.M., L.K. Graber, M. Elansary, K. Khoshnood, A. Rastegar and M. Barry. 2010. "Short-term global health research projects by US medical students: ethical challenges for partnerships." *American Journal of Tropical Medicine and Hygiene* 83(2):211–214. doi: 10.4269/ajtmh.2010.09-0692.

Rahim, A., F. Knights (Née Jones), M. Fyfe, J. Alagarajah and P. Baraitser. 2016. "Preparing students for the ethical challenges on international health electives: a systematic review of the literature on educational interventions." *Medical Teacher*: 1–10. doi: 10.3109/0142159X.2015.1132832.

Roberts, M. 2006. "A piece of my mind. duffle bag medicine." *JAMA : The Journal of the American Medical Association* 295(13):1491–1492.

Sanchez, A. and V.A. Lopez. 2013. "Perspectives on global health from the South." In: *An Introduction to Global Health Ethics*, edited by A.D. Pinto and R.E.G. Upshur. New York, NY: Routledge.

Shah, S. and T. Wu. 2008. "The medical student global health experience: professionalism and ethical implications." *Journal of Medical Ethics* 34(5):375–378. doi: 10.1136/jme.2006.019265.

Shah, S.K., B. Nodell, S.M. Montano, C. Behrens and J.R. Zunt. 2011. "Clinical research and global health: mentoring the next generation of health care students." *Global Public Health* 6(3):234–246. doi: 10.1080/17441692.2010.494248.

Sharma, M. and K.C. Anderson. 2013. "Approaching global health as a learner." In: *An Introduction to Global Health Ethics*, edited by A.D. Pinto and R.E.G. Upshur, 36–46. New York, NY: Routledge.

Standish, K. 2016. "Ethical Challenges in Student Global Health Research Projects." MD Thesis, Yale University School of Medicine.

Tan-Torres Edejer, T. 1999. "North–South research partnerships: the ethics of carrying out research in developing countries." *BMJ* 319(7207):438–441.

Ventres, W.B. and C.L. Wilson. 2015. "Beyond ethical and curricular guidelines in global health: attitudinal development on international service-learning trips." *BMC Medical Education* 15(1):68. doi: 10.1186/s12909-015-0357-7.

Wallace, L.J. and A. Webb. 2015. "Pre-departure training and the social accountability of international medical electives." *Education for Health* 27(2):143–147. doi: 10.4103/1357–6283.143745.

Wheat, S., R. Mendez, R. Musselman, F. Mugadza, S. Shumbairerwa, C. Ndhlovu, P. Wetherill, M. Sadigh and S. Winter. 2016. "Beyond the homestay model: peer mentorship and early exposure in global health education." *Medical Science Educator*. 26:409. doi: 10.1007/s40670-016-0249-4.

15 Why matters

Motivations in global health training

Mary White and Kelly Anderson

Motivations explain, in part, why we hunger to do something or why we engage in certain actions and thoughts. Our motives are often buried in our unconscious such that most of the time we only express those that are rational and socially acceptable. Should motivations matter in global health?

Every year, thousands of individuals from high income countries (HICs) spend weeks or months in low and middle income countries (LMICs) in order to learn, conduct research, or provide service in underserved communities, most seeking to contribute in some way to promoting global health. For similar reasons, some choose to serve in low income communities in their own countries. Given the cost, uncertainty and sometimes discomfort that service in low resource communities involves, what motivates people to seek out these opportunities? Do their motivations make a difference in what they do? We generally assume a coherent correspondence between motivations and anticipated or desired consequences. If a fundamental goal of global health activities is to improve human health worldwide, we would think that that the motivations of these thousands of travellers would parallel this goal. But such congruence between intentions and outcomes is not always what we find.

Medical trainees and other aspiring health professionals comprise a sizeable portion of those who travel in the name of global health. Most are participants in short-term, credit-bearing electives or non-credit-bearing internships, fieldwork, or volunteer activities. The motivations voiced by these individuals largely include desires to learn about tropical medicine and infectious disease, develop cultural sensitivity, learn a foreign language, learn about healthcare in low income countries, provide meaningful service, and conduct research (Holmes *et al.* 2012, Perry 2012). Other, perhaps unvoiced, motivations may include the desire to see the world, to better understand the experiences of those less privileged, to be transformed by immersion in poverty, to fulfill a faith-based commitment, to gain easy academic credit, to practise procedures in ways that are not possible at home, to be seen as a hero, and to have a distinguishing line on a curriculum vitae. What is noteworthy about almost all of these voiced and unvoiced motivations is the degree to which the anticipated benefits are to be gained by the learner, and not necessarily by the host community.

Personnel in low-income clinical settings and communities also have self- or community-serving motives for welcoming foreign visitors. When medical trainees are accompanied by their own medical faculty, these individuals can provide clinical service and teaching that is greatly appreciated by host site personnel and patients (Kumwenda *et al.* 2015). Trainees may also provide useful service appropriate to their level of skill. Other publicly voiced motivations for hosting visitors include the desire to share what medical practice in a low resource setting entails; opportunities for staff development and training; compensation for services as hosts and preceptors, and the hope that linkages with higher income institutions or countries may lead to future training opportunities and other capacity-strengthening benefits (Kumwenda *et al.* 2015). What receiving communities rarely mention is the cost of hosting learners and novice physicians. These include the drain on time due to trainees' additional teaching and supervisory needs, visiting physicians' need for training in local clinical practices, and the fact that unless compensation is pre-arranged, visitors may not be aware that their presence is burdening their hosts at all.

Visiting researchers, an increasing presence in the southern hemisphere, are similarly driven by the desire for meaningful findings but also for outcomes that will lead to further grant support and professional advancement. Needless to say, well-designed research is critical to advances in health and healthcare. But much global health research may also be perceived as ethically fraught (Klitzman 2012, Emanuel *et al.* 2004), benefitting researchers and their sponsors far more than the communities they study and rely on for support (Benatar 2000). This may include studies of no local relevance, that disregard local culture or context, that are logistically infeasible, or that violate local and international research ethics. Pinto and Upshur observe, "Within research, such a questioning of motives is becoming ever more important. Will the research actually address the gap between knowledge and practice, the 'know-do gap', or is it just for the sake of publishing?" (Pintur and Upshur 2009, p. 8).

For partner institutions in low income countries, research collaboration with a foreign university can include benefits of medical and/or technological resources, research training, future partnership opportunities, and (limited) provision of healthcare services. But these benefits, while substantial, may come at a price. Sponsoring researchers' needs for staff support can result in disruption to clinical services, drawing local clinical and administrative personnel away from their usual duties to the higher salaries offered by foreign research partners. By importing drugs and medical supplies and distributing them without regard for the local providers of such goods, visiting researchers may drive local pharmacies out of business or force them to relocate, leaving a void when the researchers eventually depart. In these and other ways, research initiatives can be significantly disruptive of to their host communities.

This may not be the intent, but if the motivation for research is squarely on improving the welfare of the hosting community, one would expect many of these consequences to be anticipated and avoided. Moreover, given the quantities of funding necessary for most international research partnerships, coupled with the indirect grant support received by home institutions, one might expect a portion of those funds to be dedicated to strengthening the partner institution in return for hosting and supporting the project. But international research ethics guidelines have not yet addressed this form of benefit sharing, tacitly suggesting that the health of the surrounding community need not be a priority for researchers (World Medical Association 2002, Council for International Organizations of Medical Sciences (CIOMS) 2002).

The travellers whose motives are most likely to be congruent with the goals of global health are the experienced professionals who commit to working in low-resource settings for substantial periods of time, from months to years. These visitors are most effective when joining an existing health system. They are usually appreciated by their local colleagues and patients, especially when they are clearly committed repeat visitors, familiar to facility personnel, and make an effort to integrate clinical practices with local capacity building. Similarly, those who engage in global health through advocacy and professional work within their home country that impacts domestic policies, practices, research, and markets in the rest of the world, can be seen to have outcomes congruent with intentions.

By contrast, short-term medical missions and brigades can have notable downsides. As mentioned above, visitors who believe they are working where there is little or no healthcare may simply fail to recognise the resources and healers in the local health system. By providing services and medications for free, visitors can disrupt or undermine local healthcare providers and businesses (Bishop and Litch 2000). For patients, continuity of care, including follow-up of surgical procedures, may not be possible once a short-term mission leaves. While some healthcare is usually better than no care, if visitors fail to anticipate what happens when they leave, they can do real harm. In these (and other) ways, even with the best of intentions, the impact of visiting healthcare professionals, whether short or long term, is not always unambiguously positive.

There are also some physicians working in global health whose motives could be said to be chiefly self-serving. These include some who lack the necessary qualifications to practise medicine in their home countries, and others who are working out personal feelings of guilt over their comparative privilege, or possessed of compulsive "rescuer" identities or desires for self-sacrifice. Importantly, while their motives may not be entirely altruistic, many of these individuals may nonetheless provide valuable medical service and care. Clear conjunction between motive and outcome is therefore not always necessary for a positive impact. But if well-intentioned, altruistic professionals can be disruptive, and self-serving visitors can provide valuable benefits, do motives matter at all? If so, why, and how?

For trainees, self-interest, which at least in part underlies most of their daily choices at this stage in their training, should be acknowledged. It is a good thing for a young person to be curious, to want to learn tropical medicine, to want to see the world and how others live, to aspire to a global state of mind (Philpott 2010). For some who primarily seek adventure, if they do so with an open mind, global health experiences may nonetheless be professionally transformative. It would be unreasonable to argue that only a narrow range of motives is acceptable for those who aspire to work in global health. But while some acts done for the wrong reasons may sometimes produce benefits, it is more often the case that acts done for the wrong reasons produce harm. Anecdotal stories abound of medical students who arrive unprepared, knowing nothing of their host country and its culture, who wear offensive clothing, take pictures without permission, engage in practices for which they have no qualifications, shirk their responsibilities in favour of tourism or recreation, fail to take antimalarial medications, get themselves sick with infectious or gastrointestinal diseases, overindulge in drugs and alcohol, or simply convey arrogance in their demeanour. One may wonder at the motives of these students – do they really not care who they offend? Have they no idea what they are getting into? Do they truly feel they have no time to do any pre-departure preparation? Even if their poor showing is the result of ignorance, is that excusable?

Perhaps in some cases ignorance may indeed be a valid defence against charges of flawed motivation. But, because visiting global health workers represent not just themselves but their home institutions and perhaps even broader communities of identity, they and their sending and host institutions must accept certain ethical responsibilities. As described by an international working group on the ethics of global health training, regardless of their personal motives and goals, individuals aspiring to work in global health should be committed to: (1) learning as much as possible about their responsibilities and the anticipated setting in advance; (2) being up to date on required credentialing and licensing; (3) once on site, demonstrating respect for their hosts and the desire to learn from them; and (4) remaining constantly vigilant of their personal safety. Sending and host institutions should also make every effort to: (1) structure partnerships to be mutually beneficial, with clearly articulated expectations and frequent evaluation; (2) recognise the real cost to all individuals and institutions and ensure that they are paid for; (3) invest in developing and maintaining long-term relationships between partner organisations; and (4) be clear and transparent about motivations for partnerships (e.g., teaching, research, or capacity strengthening) (Crump, Sugarman, and the Working Group on Ethics Guidelines for Global Health Training 2010). If these individual and ethical responsibilities are upheld, even without grasping the reasons why they are necessary, it is likely that elective, research and service experiences will be on balance successful – beneficial to both parties in expected and unexpected ways. In short, having the right motivation is an important dimension of ethical behaviour. But even if an individual's motives are unclear, misguided, or misplaced, if he or she is committed to upholding ethical principles of respect, responsibility and accountability, much effective service in the interests of global health may sometimes be achieved.

Finally, let it be noted that there are no more astute observers of human character than one's hosts. How one behaves – how one is seen to engage in a workplace or community – will be watched and judged. Determinations will impact both the success of short-term initiatives and long-term relationships. Host-community personnel that believe they are being used by students, clinicians or researchers for their own self-serving purposes may prove poor partners; more importantly, poor impressions can limit future opportunities, including those for learners and researchers who wish to return in subsequent years. Motivations thus matter for individuals, for host communities, and for the future of global health. No one can travel to a low resource setting without making a difference. The question for each of us is, what kind of difference that will be?

References

Benatar, S.R. 2000. "Avoiding exploitation in clinical research." *Cambridge Quarterly of Healthcare Ethics* 9:562–565.

Bishop, R.A. and Litch, J.A. 2000. "Medical tourism can do harm." *BMJ* 320:1017.

Council for International Organizations of Medical Sciences (CIOMS). 2002. International Ethical Guidelines for Biomedical Research Involving Human Subjects. Accessed October 26, 2016. http://cioms.ch/publications/layout_guide2002.

Crump, J.A., Sugarman, J., and the Working Group on Ethics Guidelines for Global Health Training (WEIGHT). 2010. "Ethics and best practice guidelines for training experiences in global health." *American Journal of Tropical Medicine and Hygiene* 83(6):1178–1182.

Emanuel, E.J., Wendler, D., Killen, J. and Grady, C. 2004. "What makes clinical research in developing countries ethical? The benchmarks of ethical research." *Journal of Infectious Disease* 189:930–937.

Holmes, D., Zayas, L. and Koyfman, A. 2012. "Student objectives and learning experiences in a global health elective." *Journal of Community Health* 37:927–934.

Klitzman, R.L. 2012. "US IRBs confronting research in the developing world." *Developing World Bioethics* 12(2):63–73.

Kumwenda, B., Dowell, J., Daniels, K. and Merrylees, N. 2015. "Medical electives in sub-Saharan Africa: a host perspective." *Medical Education* 49:623–633.

Perry, D.J. 2012. "Effective purpose in transnational humanitarian healthcare providers." *American Journal of Disaster Medicine* 8(3):159–168.

Philpott, J. 2010. "Training for a global state of mind." *Virtual Mentor* 12(3):231–236.

Pinto, A.D. and Upshur, R.E.G. 2009. "Global health ethics for students." *Developing World Bioethics* 9(1):1–10.

World Medical Association (WMA). 2002. "Declaration of Helsinki." (1964, 2002) Accessed October 26, 2016. www.fda.gov/ohrms/dockets/dockets/06d0331/06D-0331-EC20-Attach-1.pdf.

16 From hubris to humility

Towards an appreciation of the philosophy of life in the host country

Dan Hayhoe and Jill Allison

> At the very heart of efforts to instill professionalism, humanism, and cultural openness and humility in medical students is the notion of justice: to treat all patients as individuals – with all the emotional, experiential, and cultural richness and depth that comprise an individual's identity – with fairness and compassion.
>
> (Kumagai and Lypson 2009, p. 782)

Cultural responsiveness, as the epigraph above highlights, is about fairness. The work of global health affords people an opportunity to engage in new and exciting life experiences, but the depth, richness and understanding of what fairness and justice mean in relation to experience can only be fully appreciated with reflection and humility. For many of us, it is only in contemplation on return that we recognise the hubris with which we have sometimes approached the work of engaging culture. In global health programmes, the challenge is to give people the tools to recognise and critically examine their own cultural context and the influence this has on their lives. It is also important to give them the skills to be honest about their lack of familiarity and the need to be open, reflexive and receptive to the importance culture plays in shaping people's experiences in illness, wellness and healing. This takes a measure of courage. As Jack Coulehan notes "[c]ountercultural though it is, humility need not suggest weakness or self-abnegation. Quite the contrary, humility requires toughness and emotional resilience" (Coulehan 2010, p. 201). We use examples from Malawi, Nigeria and Southern Africa to provide illustrations of cultural constructs essential to investigate before engaging with new communities.

Culture is a complex network of social practices, functions, relationships, world view, political influences, belief, and values all of which exist in "layers of meaning" (Faulkner *et al.* 2006, p. 27). It shapes the day-to-day lives of people everywhere but is neither static nor stable, even as its influence may be an obstacle to change. Culture is a paradox: it is both blatantly obvious in its performance and deceptively obscure in its experience. We are often unaware of the impact of culture in our own day-to-day lives. For those of us who work in health sciences faculties and supervise intercultural experiences for students, teaching what is often called cultural competency or cultural responsiveness is perhaps the hardest concept to address. Some scholars have used the image of the iceberg to explain how much of culture actually resides unseen but is still influential.

What we are really aiming to cultivate is a sense of humility and respect for deeply held values and world view – both our own and others. At the same time, we want people to be critically conscious of the fact that there is no neat package in which all of this will be revealed; nor is it likely that any two people from the same community and cultural background will experience and share completely a singular set of ideas, behaviours or interpretations. Thus while we must understand the overarching impact of cultural values, we cannot reduce people to the exotic "other." Addressing the fundamental tension that exists in the epigraph above – between treating individuals and acknowledging collective influences that shape their notions of health and illness – lies in the art of cultural sensitivity as practice.

Another important element in providing tools for critical cultural awareness and humility is to ensure that culture is not represented as an excuse or a reason for an outcome that is not expected or is not positive. For example, it might seem easy to explain a lack of uptake of women's health service as rooted in cultural non-acceptance when, in fact, on deeper analysis, it is poverty that is the obstacle. Global health practitioners and scholars must be prepared to deepen their insights into and understanding of explanatory frameworks used by patients, families, communities and colleagues as they give meaning and importance to an illness or healing event in their lives (Kleinman and Benson 2006). However, the explanatory framework cannot become a way to end a conversation, a mere checklist that provides a way to develop the treatment plan. In the same way, culture should not be confused with poverty and lack of power (Farmer 1999). An ethical and responsive approach will seek to understand the complex reasons why people, for example, may not take up treatments or respond to suggestions or advice. It may not be culture, but rather economics and resource constraints that govern people's priorities and responsiveness to our work.

One of the most important tools that educators and learners have available to them for addressing the challenges of understanding a cross-cultural experience is reflection. As an educator John Dewey noted, the "reconstruction or reorganization of experience" was at the heart of any educational endeavor (Dewey 1916, p. 82). Encouraging a deep reflection on the meaning and transformative potential of any cross-cultural experience must guide the pre-departure and post-return debriefing process.

In fact, what we are suggesting is that the totality of pre-departure training (which includes statistics on morbidities, ratios of healthcare personnel to population, local facilities, personal health and safety, etc.) is only a matter of technical significance without at least some understanding of host country views of selfhood, community, life and death, ethics and morality, and humankind's connection to the spiritual world. Many, if not all, philosophies of life include a spiritual component which speaks to the very essence of the individual's place in human society as well as their interconnectedness to all of their world, both animate and inanimate, from a time prior to their birth to their existence in some form of spirit world after death. Clearly this impacts the understanding of the life–death continuum and shapes the meaning of health, illness and healing. Experiences that challenge and expose our own world view are often most profound when it comes to spiritual values. We provide some concrete examples below as a way of illustrating the importance of a reflective and reflexive approach to cultural competency. A reflexive perspective encourages a deeper sense of self-awareness and the impact our own presence in shaping an encounter or experience.

Ubuntu, Sangomas, Nigerian Juju and Yoruba spiritual beliefs

> This life's dim windows of the soul distort the heavens from pole to pole and lead us to believe a lie, when we see with, not through, the eye.
>
> (William Blake 1757–1827)

The epigraph above and the ensuing segment posit that one's understanding of reality must of necessity be formed by a composite of each person's unique life experience and culture. Consequently truly mutual respect and collaboration must begin with an openness to see through another's eyes.

Ubuntu

Ubuntu is an example of a concept which shapes the values and perspectives on wellness and healing in southern Africa. Ubuntu was first mentioned in the literature in 1846 (Gade 2012). It is discussed in this chapter as both an individual quality and as a philosophy or world view. Ubuntu is not "I think, therefore I am" as Rene Descartes declared, but rather, "I am because you are." The Zulus would say "Umuntu ngumuntu ngabantu," which means that "A person is a person through other persons" (Samkange 1980, p. 2). This strikes an affirmation of one's humanity through recognition of the uniqueness of another. Desmond Tutu describes Ubuntu as "... the essence of being human ... my humanity is caught up and is inextricably bound up in yours. I am human because I belong. It speaks about wholeness, about compassion. You cannot exist as a human being in isolation. It speaks about our interconnectedness. You cannot be a human all by yourself. What you do affects the whole world" (Tutu 1999, pp. 34–5). Similar concepts of the connectedness of human spirit are evident in the Qur'an and Judeo-Christian texts. In order to understand fully the world view of people in different cultural contexts, we must try to grasp their understanding of both self and social relationships.

In Malawi, the Ubuntu philosophy is called Umunthu. According to Bishop Msusa of Zomba this describes a world view that embraces the idea of a single unified family that belongs to God thus including a spiritual component (Mbiti 1990). The western natural-supernatural dualism is somewhat antithetical to this perspective. In many non-western world views, the spiritual or supernatural world lives in contiguity with the natural or material world; they interact with one another and intercede among us. God, humankind and extra-humans are all regarded as integral parts of a single totality of existence. Thus, one's life is fundamentally related to higher and lower levels of life, to other humans, and to one's own interior life. Consequently, a human being is always viewed holistically. When someone is sick, the whole person is sick, both physically and spiritually (Berglund 1976). When someone dies, the Zulu saying is "udlulile emhlabeni" meaning that a person has passed on to another stage of life. This clearly implies that a person does not lose their personhood at death. The whole of society, in the view of those African societies that embrace this view, comprises the living and those who have died but continue to be present among the living in a complex and organic whole (Mcuna 2004). This sense of continuous presence has an impact on both death and end-of-life care as the place of a deceased individual remains important and connected to ongoing social life. The dignity afforded the life-to-death continuum is an essential component of this world view.

No culture is homogeneous and indeed manifests remarkable variance at any given time from rural to urban and within exponentially shortening timeframes in the same geographical locale. The African continent has absorbed waves of people and groups each with their own culture, religion and world view impacting and intermingling with the existing culture. Witness the advent of a labour force from India in East Africa in the 19th century, which profoundly altered the culture of the region, and more recently by the influx of people from China across the entire continent, again with a different religion, spiritual world view and cultural ethos (Moyo 2012). The same pattern of overlapping cultures over time is true of every society. When DH arrived in Malawi in 1989 he was asked by a chief of the Tumbuka people "Have you come planting palm trees?" The reference was to the fact that palm trees were not Indigenous to the area but had been introduced by a different culture to mark the entrances to their places of worship, that is: "Have you come to superimpose a new culture or religion over our own?"

Sangomas

The Sangomas of southern Africa, historically viewed by missionaries and colonialists as "witchdoctors," are essentially diviners while Inyangas are herbalists, although there is frequently the incorporation of both aspects in a given practitioner. Clearly, their world view, as well as that of the significant demographic which seeks out their advice, is inclusive of, and inextricably connected to, a spiritual dimension.

"Traditional healers often outnumber medical doctors by 100/1 or more in most African countries. They provide a large, accessible, available, afford-able human resource pool. They are highly respected, widely distributed and highly consulted since 80 percent of Africans rely on traditional medicine for the majority of their healthcare needs" (King 2000, p. 7).

The UNAIDS review of 2010 states "collaborating with traditional healers in HIV/AIDS prevention and care [demonstrates that] modern and traditional belief systems are not incompatible but complementary" (King 2000, p. 10). Their role is deeply embedded in many cultures in sub-Saharan Africa, and as we collaborate in healthcare it is essential that we remain open to respectfully listening and engendering inclusivity in any dialogue.

Juju in Nigeria

In many parts of west Africa, there is still a pervasive belief in the potency of Juju, which frequently coexists with a belief in western biomedicine without apparent cognitive dissonance. One does well to understand that this belief in the efficacy of Juju existed long before the arrival of Christianity or Islam (Talbot 2007) and indeed may continue as a component of the lives and prac-tices of the adherents of those religions. In the Juju world view, individuals are exact copies of the divine, making their problems both essentially spiritual and embedded within a holistic spiritual framework. As a result there is an intrinsic dimension of meaning and ultimately purpose to their crisis, whether it is physical, spiritual or social. The western mindset conflates the historical timeline of "progression" over thousands of years from magic to religion to science with the ultimate emergence of science as the arbiter of biomedical practice. Juju would posit that all three continue to exist and reinforce each other for our health and social wellbeing (Iroegbu 2010).

Yoruba spiritual beliefs / medicine in Nigeria

"From the earliest beginnings of medicine, mankind has associated the act of curing disease with gods, goddesses and other forms of divine forces. Sickness was recognised as a consequence of disobedience to or sin against these super-natural agents and their moral rules. Magical-empirical approaches to health and disease characterized all archaic civilizations" (Awojoodu and Baran 2009, p. 1). Among the Yoruba of Nigeria (comprising a population of over 30 million in West Africa), as in many African cultures, health and religion are tightly interrelated. In the Yoruba mindset, all healing, including that of the western medical doctor, comes from God.

The tension between western biomedicine and other systems of healing rooted in spirituality and folk traditions is often located in the dichotomy between scientific reason and proof versus the notion of belief which is less rational (Good 1994). Without a full understanding of the meaningful links between healing and world view, we risk diminishing the importance of a community's explanatory model and supplanting it with our own. Again, reflecting on how "belief" in western biomedicine shapes our own world view is crucial to an engaged and respectful partnership in a global health context.

Seduction, hubris and humility

What are the practical implications of understanding this philosophy for a visiting healthcare professional? Some implications are obvious in the contrast between the "individualistic" mindset so prevalent in the west and the more communal identity base in Ubuntu. This influence on a world view will shape ideas on life, death, misfortune and illness as well as ideas about what needs to be done to address illness or bad luck. This should have a profoundly humbling effect on us and engender at least a rudimentary insight into our national partners' thinking. A willingness to accept that such views are different to our own is essential to being able to work in tandem with colleagues and patients in other cultural contexts, regardless of the nature of the project or experience. Many in the Global North function daily in a learned and unquestioned dualistic context of thought in which our world is "automatically" sorted into right and wrong, black and white, good and bad, natural and supernatural. Perhaps this is one of the greatest barriers to humble reflection with respect to understanding many world views which function outside this paradigm with significantly more cognitive dissonance from a western perspective. Without a willingness to suspend our own set of beliefs and ideas, to question or challenge our values, we will be unable to engage fully with the meaning of healing, wellness or illness among others.

"The Reductive Seduction of Other People's Problems" as posited by Courtney Martin is an essential component of our thinking with respect to humility as we engage in North–South dialogue. To attempt to understand our own problem with the "ego of the Global North," she supposes a young boy in Uganda sees the San Bernardino, California shootings on CNN and thinks "I want to help with all that violence and killing of innocent people." So, he forms a charity, raises money and travels to California to offer assistance. He has no knowledge of the National Rifle Association, Second Amendment rights, the gun lobby, social, ethnic and religious stratification, American ethics or issues around immigration, mental illness or family life and values. He knows nothing of North American history and culture … he is just appalled at the level of gun violence in the USA and feels compelled to help out (Martin 2016).

The pervasive hubris of the Global North is evident to any thoughtful person as we read the above narrative and apply it to ourselves. In essence, we don't know what we don't know. Global health projects, learning or teaching are often framed as problem solving, helping or capacity building. Many students will begin with essentially altruistic objectives, but it is crucial to acknowledge local partners, local knowledge and local solutions.

Conclusion

Humility and the capacity to reflect on the meaning of cross-cultural experiences are key elements for developing global citizenship. Much of this begins with a willingness to acknowledge the spiritual realm or world view that shapes our work, both at home and abroad. But that work continues with critical reflection that transforms experience into understanding and enriches respect and partnership. Knowledge may mean a grasp of facts and statistics related to a particular demographic. Wisdom, however, entails the application of that knowledge with humility in collaboration with our colleagues who know more than we ever will about the culture, world view, beliefs and struggles in lived realities far different than our own.

References

Awojoodu, O. and D. Baran. 2009. "Traditional Yoruba medicine In Nigeria: a comparative approach." *Bulletin of The Transilvania University of Brasov* 6(51):129–136.

Berglund, A.-I. 1976. *Zulu Thought Patterns and Symbolism*. Capetown: David Philip.

Coulihan, J. 2010. On Humility. *Annals of Internal Medicine* 153(3): 200–201. doi: 10.7326/0003-4819-153-3-201008030-00011.

Dewey, J. 1916. *Democracy in Education: An Introduction to the Philosophy of Education*. New York: The Free Press.

Farmer, P. 1999. *Infections and Inequalities: The Modern Plagues*. Berkeley: University of California Press.

Faulkner, S.L., J.R. Baldwin, S.L. Lindsley and M.L. Hecht. 2006. "Layers of meaning: an analysis of definitions of culture." In: *Redefining Culture: Perspectives Across the Disciplines*, edited by J.R. Baldwin, S.L. Faulkner, M.L. Hecht and S.L. Lindsley, 27–52. London: Lawrence Ehrlbaum Associates.

Gade, C.B.N. 2012. "What is Ubuntu? Different interpretations among South Africans of African descent." *South African Journal of Philosophy* 31(3):484–503.

Good, B.J. 1994. *Medicine, Rationality and Experience: An Anthropological Perspective*. Cambridge: Cambridge University Press.

Iroegbu, P. 2010. *Introduction to Igbo Medicine and Culture in Nigeria*. USA & Canada: Lulu.com Publishing.

Kleinman, A. and P. Benson. 2006. *Anthropology in the clinic: the problem of cultural competency and how to fix it. PLoS Medicine* 3(10):e294. doi: 10.1371/journal.pmed.0030294.

King, R. 2000. Collaboration with Traditional Healers in HIV-AIDS Prevention and Care in Sub-Saharan Africa – a Literature Review. UNAIDS. www.hst.org.za/uploads/files/Collab_Lit_Rev.pdf.

Kumagai, A.K. and Lypson, M.L. 2009. "Beyond Cultural Competence: Critical Consciousness, Social Justice, Multicultural Education." *Academic Medicine* 84(6):782–787.

Martin, C. 2016. "Reductive Seduction of Other People's Problems." Accessed January 20, 2017. https://medium.com/the-development-set/the-reductive-seduction-of-other-people-s-problems-3c07b307732d#.o8nud7ngb.

Mbiti, J.S. 1969. *African Religions and Philosophy*. Oxford: Heinemann Editorial Publishers.

Mcuna, T.N. 2004. "The Dignity of the Human Person: A Contribution of the Theology of Ubuntu to Theology and Anthropology." Unpublished Master's Thesis, Pretoria, UNISA.

Moyo, D. 2012. *Winner Take All: China's Race for Resources and What It Means for the Rest of the World*. Toronto: HarperCollins.

Samkange, S.J.T. 1980. *Hunhuism or Ubuntuism: A Zimbabwe Indigenous Political Philosophy*. Salisbury: Graham Pub.

Talbot, P.A. 1923, digital 2007. *Life in Southern Nigeria: The Magic, Beliefs and Customs of the Ibibio Tribe*. Abingdon, UK: Routledge.

Tutu, D. 1999. *No Future Without Forgiveness*. London: Rider,Random House.

17 How social accountability in medical education can contribute to global health

Ryan Meili, Shawna O'Hearn, Jan De Maeseneer and Roger Strasser

Achieving the ambitious improvements in health and wellbeing set out in the Sustainable Development Goals (World Health Organization 2016) will require the participation of and leadership from health professionals. The way in which those service providers are trained will play a significant role in whether and how they engage in addressing the world's most pressing health challenges. In this chapter we present the increasing focus on social accountability of medical schools and how this relates to global health. We then describe case examples from three Canadian and one Belgian medical school, and examine what future directions may emerge from what these examples demonstrate.

Social accountability in medical education

In 1995, the World Health Organization (WHO) defined the "social accountability of medical schools" as "the obligation to direct their education, research, and service activities towards addressing the priority health concerns of the community, region and the nation that they have a mandate to serve" (Boelen *et al.* 1995). This followed several decades in which innovative schools had focused on connecting with and responding to community needs (Strasser *et al.* 2015). The Network: Towards Unity for Health began in 1979 with inspiration from the WHO with a group of 19 medical schools – including McMaster University in Canada – that implemented community oriented medical education (Schmidt *et al.* 1991).

In 2001, Health Canada and all Canadian medical schools made a joint commitment to social accountability in the publication, Social Accountability: A Vision for Canadian Medical Schools (Health Canada 2001). This commitment was reaffirmed with the Future of Medical Education in Canada Visions for MD Education (Association of Faculties of Medicine of Canada (AFMC) 2010) and Postgraduate Medical Education (Association of Faculties of Medicine of Canada (AFMC) 2012). Also the College of Family Physicians of Canada (CFPC) has committed to achieving social accountability in family medicine (Buchman *et al.* 2016).

At the international level, the Training for Health Equity network (THEnet) is a group of health profession schools that are guided by a social accountability mandate. Although these schools operate in very different contexts and employ somewhat different strategies, they share nine core principles, including targeting education and research to the health and social needs of the community, and recruiting students from and educating students in underserved communities (Palsdottir *et al.* 2008).

THEnet developed, piloted and published an evaluation framework for socially accountable health professional education (THEnet 2011, Larkins *et al.* 2013) which provided the core content for the Global Consensus on Socially Accountable Education in 2010 (Global Consensus for Social Accountability of Medical Schools 2010). Subsequently, THEnet has been successful in researching, reporting and advocating for socially accountable education (Strasser and Neusy 2010, Larkins *et al.* 2013, Ross *et al.* 2014, Larkins *et al.* 2015). Following the global consensus, the Association for Medical Education in Europe (AMEE) adopted social accountability as one of the elements of the ASPIRE: International Recognition of Excellence in Medical Education programme (www.amee.org).

Global health through a social accountability lens

Socially accountable education prepares future health professionals to address the priority health concerns of society, often with a focus on vulnerable and marginalised populations. Preparing competent graduates requires a broad integration of international and intercultural perspectives throughout the curriculum (Stutz *et al.* 2015).

When considering internationalising the curriculum, the focus has frequently been on international student mobility. These programmes in the health field grew to become known as global health. The research identified benefits for students, such as: gaining knowledge of diseases foreign to the home country; improvement of clinical skills (Drain *et al.* 2007); acquisition of communication and language skills; recognition of cultural, social and economic influences on healthcare (Haq *et al.* 2000); influence on career objectives (Drain *et al.* 2007, Haq *et al.* 2000); and building confidence (Niemantsverdriet *et al.* 2004).

However, the research also identified concerns about student motives to engage in these international health experiences. Questions were raised about how community needs and priorities were taken into consideration while developing and evaluating the programmes (Hanson *et al.* 2011). Through the advocacy of global health leaders, ethics became a component of the pre-departure training in Canadian medical schools. This training extends beyond the classic ethical frameworks to include values such as humility, introspection, solidarity and social justice (Pinto and Upshur 2009). This training also ensures self-reflection of motivations, power-relationships, ethical issues, and impacts on the community (Hanson *et al.* 2011).

Over the past decade, the scholarly focus on ethical dilemmas including risk management, student and patient safety, working beyond competency levels, and burden on partner institutions has challenged faculty, students and partners to rethink the emphasis on international global health (Holland and Holland 2011). This debate created space for the emergence of local global health programmes focusing on refugee health, student-run clinics, service learning opportunities, and engaging with Indigenous communities both in urban and remote areas of Canada.

While the training in ethical frameworks for global health has shaped some of this focus towards local global health. This has been assisted by the Sustainable Development Goals, which apply to all countries. This shift to acknowledge everyone as pivotal to creating equitable and healthy societies is already a visible change within the rethinking of global health.

The emphasis on social accountability within our medical and health professional schools raises our attention to the importance of considering the priority health concerns of the communities in which we serve. Community engagement that considers equity and diversity has an impact on training health professions to be inclusive global citizens.

In order to understand the ways in which faculties of medicine can engage in social accountability to address global health issues, whether close to home or across the world, it is instructive to examine specific examples. In this paper the authors from three Canadian universities – Northern Ontario School of Medicine, Dalhousie University and the University of Saskatchewan – and Ghent University in Belgium, describe social accountability activities at their academic institutions as examples of different approaches to integrating global health into medical education.

Dalhousie University

The Dalhousie University Faculty of Medicine is committed to social accountability through equity, diversity and inclusion, community engagement and social justice.

Dalhousie's Global Health Office was established in 2001 to support the advancement of international activities, build service-learning programmes, strengthen diversity programmes, support international students, and ensure community engagement is pivotal to the advancement of curriculum and research. Operating through a social accountability framework, the Global Health Office is committed to train ethical leaders who strengthen health systems for marginalised populations in Canada and abroad.

Dalhousie identified significant gaps in enrolment of Indigenous and African Nova Scotian youth as well as those from rural and low income backgrounds within health and health professions and educational programmes. The Global Health Office worked with community partners to address such systemic deficiencies including role modelling and students' scarce interactions with people from the communities. This included the development of two pathway programmes for high school students that included mentorship, bursaries and support for Indigenous and African Nova Scotians upon entrance to study in a field of health at Dalhousie University.

Northern Ontario School of Medicine

The Northern Ontario School of Medicine (NOSM) in Canada opened in 2005 with a social accountability mandate focused on improving the health of the people and communities of Northern Ontario (Strasser *et al.* 2009).

Uniquely developed through a community consultative process, the holistic cohesive curriculum for the NOSM undergraduate programme is grounded in the Northern Ontario health context. In the classroom and in clinical settings, students are learning in context as if they are preparing to practise in Northern Ontario. Through community engagement, community members are active participants in various aspects of the school including: the admissions process; as standardised patients; ensuring that learners feel "at home" in their community; and in encouraging an understanding and knowledge of the social determinants of health at the local level. There is a strong emphasis on interprofessional education and integrated clinical learning distributed through over 90 communities, so that the students have personal experience of the diversity of the region's communities and cultures (Strasser *et al.* 2009, Strasser 2010, Strasser and Neusy 2010, Strasser *et al.* 2013, Strasser *et al.* 2015).

Ninety-two per cent of all NOSM students come from Northern Ontario with substantial inclusion of Indigenous (7 percent) and Francophone (22 percent) students. Sixty-two per cent of NOSM graduates have chosen family practice (predominantly rural) training (Strasser *et al.* 2013). Ninety-four per cent of the doctors who completed undergraduate and postgraduate education with NOSM are practising in Northern Ontario (Hogenbirk *et al.* 2016). The socioeconomic impact of NOSM included: new economic activity of more than double the school's budget; enhanced retention and recruitment for the universities and hospitals/health services; and a sense of empowerment among community participants attributable in large part to NOSM (Hogenbirk *et al.* 2015). There are signs that NOSM is successful in graduating doctors who have the skills and the commitment to practice in rural/remote communities and that NOSM is having a largely positive socioeconomic impact on Northern Ontario.

University of Saskatchewan

In 2010, the College of Medicine at the university established a Division of Social Accountability (DSA), building on a social accountability committee started in 2003. The DSA works to incorporate social accountability into all of the college's activities. Research by the DSA led to the description of social accountability through the "CARE model" (Meili *et al.* 2011b), with clinical activity, advocacy, research and education and training describing the key areas of activity of medical schools, and of the opportunity to incorporate social accountability (Meili *et al.* 2011a). This approach is used to work with individual departments and with committees addressing key issues such as global health, Indigenous health, and immigrant and refugee health.

The DSA offers the Making the Links Certificate in Global Health, described in detail in *Chapter 31*. This programme has been successful in teaching medical students the necessity of having a practical understanding of the social determinants of health in clinical practice (Meili *et al.* 2011a). As of 2013, the programme had trained 60 students. Of those, 34 had gone on to residency (the rest were still in training). Twenty-three of these students chose family medicine, with 18 selecting rural family medicine. Of the remaining students, ten chose general specialties (e.g., paediatrics, psychiatry) and one matched to dermatology. While social accountability is a part of all specialties, given the needs of Saskatchewan, the increased selection of rural family medicine (and enhanced preparation for that practice) is encouraging.

Ghent University

The undergraduate medical training programme at Ghent University (Belgium), has a strong focus on the social determinants of health that contribute to the increasing health gap (Marmot 2015) and on the important impact of income inequalities on the social health gap (Wilkinson and Pickett 2009).

The first year interdisciplinary module on "health and society" uses an interactive board game to explore how social determinants affect the life of individuals. In the third year, students put these insights into practice in a one-week "community oriented primary care" (COPC) experience (Rhyne *et al.* 1998). An interprofessional group of students (medicine, nursing, sociology, health promotion) participates in a COPC project in an underserved area of the city of Ghent, where groups of four students visit and interview a family living in poverty or in other difficult circumstances, attempting to understand the living conditions and their impact on health. Then they interview three healthcare providers working with this family (e.g., family physician, nurse, social worker and informal caregiver). The students bring together the information they collected in their interviews, and complement their findings with epidemiological and socioeconomic data about the community they are working in. This leads to the formulation of a "community diagnosis," looking at the upstream causes of ill health. Then the students contact non-governmental organisations and civil society organisations in the neighbourhood in order to formulate a proposal for an intervention. Finally, they present their findings to their peers and to stakeholders in the domain of health and welfare in the neighbourhood, including a proposal for a poster that could be used, and also write an advocacy letter to improve the living conditions of the family they interviewed (Art *et al.* 2008).

With augmented exposure to family medicine over the past decade, there has been a spectacular increase of graduates choosing family medicine, from 20 percent in 2006 to over 40 percent in 2016.

Moving forward

These examples of social accountability in action are part of a new approach to meet the changing health needs of societies with new orientations for the future workforce. In all countries, ageing populations, clearer recognition of the social determinants of health and the need for comprehensive primary healthcare delivered by skilled health workers require intersectoral action as indicated by the Sustainable Development Goals.

Moreover, apart from clerkships and training in hospitals, the community is now an important setting for undergraduate training of health professionals. This means that academic institutions will have to engage in local health policy and service delivery at the primary care level. Academic networks of community health centres may become as important as academic tertiary hospitals for the training of the physicians of the future. The WHO document "Improving Quality Primary Health Care" sets out the context of a health system focusing on primary healthcare (World Health Organization 2016). These new roles of institutions for health professional education will add a new dimension to their social accountability mandate, taking the lead in comprehensive care for specific groups in society, e.g., asylum seekers, refugees and ethnic/cultural minorities.

This kind of frontline experience will help academic institutions to participate in the debate on the need for change in the health systems, and to prepare undergraduate students to become change agents (Frenk *et al.* 2010). The Lancet Global Commission Report recommends "transformational education," which is based on health system and education system alignment through instructional and institutional reforms towards achieving health equity. An important opportunity in the process to train students to become change agents is the strengthening of student participation in the building and improvement of curricula (Dhaese *et al.* 2015).

Organisations like THEnet, the Network: TUFH, the AMEE ASPIRE group are challenged continuously to adapt the "multidimensional social accountability grid" in order to provide a framework that enables academic centres to assess their social accountability in relation to recruitment, training programmes, training context and their position in the global society.

The future of global health and social accountability is at a crossroads that will see integration of ethics, community engagement, health equity and determinants of health across all elements of our curriculum, research and service. The future of global health has moved beyond medical students doing clinical electives in low and middle income countries. Global health has incorporated social accountability with a focus on partnerships, shared learning and collaborations within our communities, locally and globally. This inclusive approach to global health and social accountability will frame the overarching competencies to guide our future healthcare professionals and strengthen health systems (Frenk *et al.* 2010).

In order to meet our Sustainable Development Goals, we need to train a health workforce that recognises its responsibility to serve the priority health needs of communities. The ongoing development of an international movement for social accountability in medical education bodes well for the education of all health professionals and the ability of these helping professions to contribute to achieving a healthier world.

References

Association of Faculties of Medicine of Canada (AFMC). 2010. The Future of Medical Education in Canada (FMEC): A Collective Vision for MD Education. Ottawa, Canada: The Association of Faculties of Medicine of Canada.

Association of Faculties of Medicine of Canada (AFMC). 2012. The Future of Medical Education in Canada (FMEC): A Collective Vision for Postgraduate Medical Education in Canada. Ottawa, Canada: The Association of Faculties of Medicine of Canada.

Art B, De Roo L, Willems S, De Maeseneer J. 2008. "An interdisciplinary community diagnosis experience in an undergraduate medical curriculum: development at Ghent University." *Academic Medicine* 83(7):675–683.

Boelen C, Heck JE. 1995. Defining and Measuring the Social Accountability of Medical Schools. Geneva, Switzerland: World Health Organization.

Buchman S, Woollard R, Meili R, Goel R. 2016. "Practising social accountability: from theory to action." *Canadian Family Physician* 62:15–18.

Dhaese SA, Van de Caveye I, Bussche PV, Bogaert S, De Maeseneer J. 2015. "Student participation: to the benefit of both the student and the faculty." *Education and Health* 28:79–82.

Drain PK, Primack A, Hunt DD, Fawzi WW, Holmes KK, Gardner P. 2007. "Global health in medical education: a call for more training and opportunities." *Academic Medicine: Journal of the Association of American Medical Colleges* 82: 226–230.

Frenk J, Chen L, Bhutta ZA, Cohen J, Crisp N, Evans T, *et al.* 2010. "Health professionals for a new century: transforming education to strengthen health systems in an interdependent world." *Lancet* 376(9756):1923–1958.

Global Consensus for Social Accountability of Medical Schools. Available at: www.healthsocialaccountability.org.

Hanson L, Harms S, Plamondon K. 2011. "Undergraduate international medical electives: some ethical and pedagogical considerations." *Journal of Studies in International Education* 15: 171–185.

Haq C, Rothenberg D, Gjerde C, Bobula J, Wilson C, Bickley L, *et al.* 2000. "New world views: preparing physicians in training for global health work." *Family Medicine* 32:566–572.

Health Canada. 2001. Social Accountability: A Vision for Canadian Medical Schools. Ottawa: Health Canada.

Hogenbirk Robinson JR, Hill ME, Minore B, Adams K, Strasser RP, Lipinski J. 2015. "The economic contribution of the Northern Ontario School of Medicine to communities participating in distributed medical education." *Canadian Journal of Rural Medicine* 20(1).

Hogenbirk JC, Timony P, French MG, Strasser R, Pong RW, Cervin C, Graves L. 2016. "Milestones on the social accountability journey: family medicine practice locations of Northern Ontario School of Medicine graduates." *Canadian Family Physician* 62: e138–e145.

Holland A, Holland T. 2011. First, Do No Harm: A Qualitative Research Documentary. https://vimeo.com/22008886.

Larkins SL, Preston R, Matte MC, *et al.* 2013. "Measuring social accountability in health professional education: development and international pilot testing of an evaluation framework." *Medical Teacher* 35:32–45.

Larkins S, Michielsen K, Iputo J, Elsanousi S. Mammen M, Graves L, Willems S, Cristobal FL, Samson R, Ellaway R, Ross S, Johnston K, Derese A, Neusy A-J. 2015. "Impact of selection strategies on representation of underserved populations and intention to practise: international findings." *Medical Education* 49:60–72.

Marmot MG. 2015. The health gap: the challenge of an unequal world. London and New York: Bloomsbury.

Meili R, Fuller D, Lydiate J. 2011a. "Teaching social accountability by making the links: qualitative evaluation of student experiences in a service-learning project." *Medical Teacher* 33(8).

Meili R, Ganem-Cuenca A, Leung J, Zaleschuk D. 2011b. "The CARE Model of Social Accountability: promoting cultural change." *Academic Medicine* 86:1114–1119.

Niemantsverdriet S, Majoor GD, Van Der Vleuten CPM, Scherpbier AJ. 2004. "I found myself to be a down to earth Dutch girl: a qualitative study into learning outcomes from international traineeships." *Medical Education* 38:749–757.

Palsdottir B, Neusy A-J, Reed G. 2008. Building the Evidence Base: Networking Innovative Socially Accountable Medical Education Programs. Education for Health. 21:2. Available from: www.educationforhealth.net.

Pinto AD, Upshur RE. 2009. "Global Health Ethics for Students." *Developing World Bioethics* 9:1–10.

Rhyne R, Bogue R, Kukulka G, Fulmer H, editors. 1998. Community-oriented primary care: health care for the 21st century. Washington, DC: American Public Health Association.

Ross S, Preston R, Lindemann I, Matte M, Samson R, Tandinco F, Larkins S, Palsdottir B, Neusy AJ. 2014. The training for health equity network evaluation framework: a pilot study at five health professional schools. *Education and Health* 27:116–126.

Schmidt HG, Neufeld VR, Nooman ZM, Ogunbode T. 1991. Network of community oriented educational institutions for the health sciences. *Academic Medicine* 66:259–263.

Strasser R, Lanphear J, McCready W, Topps M, Hunt D, Matte M. 2009. Canada's new medical school: the Northern Ontario School of Medicine – social accountability through distributed community engaged learning. *Academic Medicine* 84:1459–1456.

Strasser R. 2010. "Community engagement: a key to successful rural clinical education." *Rural and Remote Health* 10:1543. (Online). Available from: www.rrh.org.au.

Strasser R, Neusy A-J. 2010. Context counts: training health workers in and for rural areas. *Bulletin of the World Health Organization* 88:777–782.

Strasser R, Hogenbirk JC, Minore B, Marsh DC, Berry S, McCready WG, Graves L. 2013. Transforming health professional education through social accountability: Canada's Northern Ontario School of Medicine. *Medical Teacher* 35:490–496.

Strasser R, Worley P, Cristobal F, Marsh DC, Berry S, Strasser S, Ellaway R. 2015. "Putting communities in the driver's seat: the realities of community engaged medical education." *Academic Medicine* 90:1466–1470.

Stutz A, Green W, McAllister L, Eley D. 2015. "Preparing Medical Graduates for an Interconnected World: Current Practices and Future Possibilities for Internationalizing the Medical Curriculum in Different Contexts." *Journal of Studies of International Education* 19(1):28–45.

SARWGG – Strategic Advisory Board. 2015. Well-being, Health and Family for the Flemish Government. www.sarwgg.be/sites/default/files/documenten/SARWGG_20151217_New%20Professionalism_Vision%20statement_DEF.pdf.

The Training for Health Equity Network. 2011. THEnet's Social Accountability Evaluation Framework Version 1. Monograph I (1 ed.). The Training for Health Equity Network. Available at: www.thenetcommunity.org.

Wilkinson R, Pickett K. 2009. The Spirit Level: why greater equality makes societies stronger. London: Bloomsbury Press.

World Health Organization. 2016. Sustainable Goals. www.un.org/sustainabledevelopment/sustainable-development-goals/.

18 A new form of neocolonialism?

International health partnerships, missions, experiences, research and electives

Akshaya Neil Arya

Website: www.routledge.com/9781138236332

This online chapter begins with an exploration of neocolonialism as a child of colonialism, with biomedical components aswell as the economic. It examines the God, Gold and Glory elements of the colonial enterprise, to review whether this might also be part of the current global health one. Evidence for gold or profit with medical electives and missions as well as with research are presented, the glory in fulfilling personal and policy goals is highlighted. Although individuals may have mixed motivations, even those with good intentions can do harm; the chapter reviews reasons for change including damage done, but also distress among trainees. Throughout the book we provide suggestions and models for clinical experiences, medical missions and service projects, so this chapter concentrates on less addressed elements with suggestions as to ways to improve assessment of the quality of experiences and to move beyond neocolonialism in research.

Part III
Host perspectives

.

19 Host experience

A brief survey of the literature

Akshaya Neil Arya and Elysée Nouvet

The perspectives of hosts have been poorly represented in publications, conferences and forums in the Global North; recently a number of researchers have been seeking to understand host experiences and opinions (Lasker, 2016, Larsen, 2015). Depending on the context, "the hosts" may be patients, members of the community, students, research facilities, clinical programme, non-governmental organisation (NGO) leaders and "the setting" projects, short-term medical missions, research, or clinical electives. We describe the limited literature on host perceptions of learners involved in international health programmes which might broadly fall into five categories: (1) qualitative research aimed at understanding how clinical personnel perceive foreign learners doing medical electives with them; (2) research on community perceptions of learners working within the context of a large multinational NGO; and (3) research on "beneficiary" and host community perceptions of short-term medical missions (STMMs) that include learners; and (4) evaluations of Global South partner experiences in north–south research partnerships; and (5) opinions of partners but for specific purposes in the north (see Table 19.1). We then elaborate on three main challenges or limitations with such international health programmes, as highlighted in these explorations of host perceptions.

Local clinical personnel dealing with medical electives

This first category is reflected in *Chapter 20* and *Chapter 23* that follow. The sparse literature related to host perspectives includes a few "studies" by students of their host preceptors immediately as they were finishing their rotation and are of limited value. These will not be included here, save an exceptional McMaster University medical student-led multicountry anonymised questionnaire, distributed directly by individual McMaster students, but returned by mail or sealed envelope after an international preclinical elective. Conducted in 2011–12 they received 39 responses from 22 countries, 23 of which came from 12 low and middle income countries (LMICs). Themes included perception of mutual benefit (reciprocal educational benefit to Canadian students as well as host supervisors and institutions), consideration of negative impacts (drainage of resources in host countries and health risks for Canadian students) and *ideas to improve future collaboration* (minimising harm through increased preparation and communication). Many sought formal partnerships and bidirectionality (Bozinoff *et al.* 2014). None of hosts received compensation supervising, in contrast to Canadian supervisors. Although not discussed by the authors, the limited mention of harms may have been impacted by respondents' desire to maintain positive relations with McMaster and lack of trust in anonymity. While the mixture of LMIC and high income country (HIC) supervisors might have diluted findings somewhat, this was still a relatively large and varied sample of host supervisors.

Sometimes perceptions of what is proper behaviour may result from misunderstanding of the capability of foreigners or cultural differences. Radstone (2005) interviewing 39 hospital staff in the Solomon Islands in the early 2000s discovered that they generally believed that visiting medical students from England should be able to diagnose (94.9 percent), prescribe for (84.6 percent) and treat patients (89.7 percent) without supervision. While those other than qualified physicians such as nurses might commonly engage in such practices on the Islands, this would be considered beyond competence for the students coming from England, Whether this was a reflection of a lack of knowledge of what was allowed in England or the skillset of the student as opposed to a difference in values of patient consent and autonomy is unclear.

The study by Kraeker *et al.* (2014) study of 32 Ugandan medical trainees who had worked alongside students from the north using locally trained interviewers, found themes of benefit for north and south. While findings will be discussed in more detail later, they saw their compatriots treated as objects for hands-on training because of looser local standards, felt international trainees had less integration and interaction with themselves than desired, and there was no real balance or reciprocity of opportunity for learning.

Such responses seem more negative than those articulated by nine healthcare professionals interviewed in July 2011 at the University of Namibia School of Medicine (Kraeker and Chandler 2013). This convenience sample of those who had come into contact with foreign health professionals (trainees or teachers) included four physicians, two medical trainees, one pharmacist and two university lecturers. The study of benefits, harms and ethical implications identified "three main narratives that shaped participant perceptions of visits: (1) culture, context, and concern, (2) expectations, intentions, and miscommunications, and (3) partnership and the desire to share and gain knowledge" (p. 483). Although "(p)articipants did not vocalize any negatives associated with a medical trainee completing a short-term global health experience within their environment." (p. 485), at the same time they articulated concerns that those from outside with little understanding of cultural or local contexts attempted to impose their vision. They pushed back. "I tell him first to observe, learn, identify the needs of this community ... because you know the needs, behaviors, social needs, economic, even of the environment where you are working in." (p. 484). Recommendations included actively seeking out information regarding cultural and environmental context before visiting, completing a needs assessment to ensure that activities are needed and relevant, attempting to formulate long-term sustainable relationships and travelling with appropriate attitudes.

Kumwenda conducted 14 semistructured interviews with hosts at seven elective sites in Malawi, Zambia and Tanzania (Kumwenda *et al.* 2015). They used convenience sampling to get known hospital and clinic directors to give permission to contact one clinical and one administrative respondent at each sub-Saharan African site. Face-to-face interviews were conducted with 14 respondents, including ten responsible for providing direct clinical supervision to elective students (six "western trained" doctors and four locally trained) and four administrative staff, two from the Global North. The interviews were wide-ranging including sites' elective structure, student selection and assessment, pros and cons of hosting electives, capacity and drain on existing resources, communication challenges, reciprocity, sustainability, collaboration with western partners and recommendations for alternative elective models. Respondents were pleased to be involved "nurturing a group of professionals who will understand the provision of health care from a global perspective" and "generating potential future staff" (p. 623), but wished for greater student preparation. They also wanted more contribution from sending institutions to support teaching, supervision and patient care. In under-resourced settings they felt that training of local students needed to be prioritised and that the quality of supervision ought to be judged according to the local context. Variations between the urban or teaching hospitals and rural or mission hospitals were present but not detailed. Concerns cited in the literature with regard to safety and ethics of clinical activities did not emerge as issues for these hosts. The impact of most respondents being from the Global North was not discussed in any detail.

These themes found for medical student supervisors, administrators and trainees above were similar to those receiving researchers, students and short-term medical missions in each of the following sections.

Local community dealing with a large multinational NGO sending students

For her Stanford undergraduate thesis, Tiffany Kung conducted 45-minute, semistructured, qualitative face-to-face interviews with local doctors, social workers/NGO directors, homestay families and programme coordinators working with Health Education Abroad (HEA), a US-based global health education organisation in Bolivia and India, working with Child and Family Health International (CFHI) to gather their impressions of the benefits and challenges presented by visiting students. These were later put into a paper (Kung *et al.* 2016). Host community perceptions were largely positive, with benefits of hosting the foreign students cited by participants, including increased prestige for community hospitals and local NGOs, "This opportunity makes me feel important" (Kung *et al.* 2016, p. 4 of 9) but also serving a greater global purpose, broadening world views, resource enhancement with local economic development, and network building, but there were other less desirable effects which will be discussed later (Kung 2013). Although Kung was a student, supervised by CFHI people, she was granted more independence than most from sending organisations. Funding for independent evaluation should be considered by more larger sending organisations and their donors.

Local community dealing with STMMs

Short-term medical missions, as noted in the preceding *Chapter 18*, are big business. Maki *et al.* cited below, found 543 organisations from the USA spending at least $250 million on STMMs annually (Maki *et al.* 2008). However their hosts' opinions are rarely voiced in the literature.

Attempting to gauge community perspectives on short-term medical missions through a variety of relevant actors, Green *et al.* (2009) engaged in exploratory in-depth, semistructured interviews with 72 individuals affected by or participating in one such programme in Guatemala, including local healthcare providers and health authorities, foreign medical providers, nonmedical personnel working on health projects, and parents of children treated. The perceived impact was variable, including issues of power and colonial legacy, with implications for local and foreign medical team members, project planners and coordinators, and health authorities which are discussed in more detail later in this chapter.

McLennan (2014) conducted qualitative research master's and PhD in Honduras beginning in 2005, along with participant observation individual and group interviews conducted with medical voluntourists. For the master's ethnographic study she used interviews with ten Hondurans who were recipients of services and with eight host medical professionals, government representatives, NGOs, health and development workers, following this with a PhD including field work, online data collection, conference observation and over 50 interviews. McLennan's study found issues related to long-term relationship building, entrenching paternalism related in part to voluntourists' ignorance of underlying inequitable relationships, power and privilege. She reflected that short-term missions, worse than being a bandaid, could create dependency, compromise dignity and make inequities worse.

DeCamp and colleagues conducted 20 semistructured interviews in July 2012 with those receiving care from Medical Ministry International (MMI), an international faith-based Christian NGO operating short-term medical programmes in a Dominican Republic community for more than three decades (DeCamp *et al.* 2014). Many interviewees expressed appreciation of the medical aid provided in the absence of other options. One core challenge of perceptions studies with recipients of medical attention from missions identified by DeCamp and colleagues was trouble distinguishing the Global North researcher from the Global North volunteer. What might lie at the core of recipients being reluctant to discuss programme improvement directly, as DeCamp notes, was that they frequently misidentified the researcher as a caregiver, stating "I would say that an institution like yours [MMI] should build a hospital here." In half of the interviews, the participant did not know the name MMI, and many simply referred to the volunteers as "the Americans."

Chapter 22 on gratitude, highlights difficulties researchers have with getting host opinions. As DeCamp found, researchers may not be seen as independent and it seems that many fear criticism may result in a withdrawal of resources. Furthermore, it is more difficult to contact those who have disengaged and in some contexts language may be a barrier.

North–south research partnerships

Interestingly, the area of research partnerships is rarely researched. Thus a workshop report such as that by Kohrt *et al.* (2014) could be published in the literature. Conducted with HIC and LMIC investigators in cross-cultural psychiatric epidemiology, health services research, randomised controlled trials, and projects with war and disaster-affected populations in complex humanitarian emergencies including child soldiers and refugees with the Transcultural Psychosocial Organization (TPO) in Nepal (article also informed by similar workshop in Haiti), they reported on lessons learned as they attempted to produce mental health "research, interventions, and policies that are relevant, feasible, and ethical." Concern that global mental health and cultural psychiatry literature was dominated by HIC investigators, the authors discussed reasons stated for lack of participation of academics related to skills, language, or token representation exemplified by a workshop participant declaring "I've been on your papers, but some of them I've never actually read." In addition, field researchers and translators were excluded from authorship because "If they knew the hypotheses and research questions, it would bias the results. The researchers would only give you what you wanted to find" (Kohrt et al 2014).

Agnandji and colleagues conducted interviews (2009–10) with a core group of researchers at the long-standing Medical Research Unit of the Albert Schweitzer Hospital in Lamboréné, Gabon. They found several reflections that might be considered viewing research as neocolonial. While research was seen as of limited value to the research centre itself, technology and financial resources came from the Global North partner scientific institutions and scientists and the main contents and models of scientific activities are elaborated predominantly by them (Agnandji *et al.* 2012). "Research activities in sub-Saharan Africa may be limited to delegated tasks due to the strong control from Western collaborators, which could lead to scientific production …. In transnational collaborations, a sub-Saharan research institution may be limited to producing confirmatory and late-stage data with little impact on economic and social innovation."

These findings are similar to those discussed in Standish's *Chapter 14* and *Chapter 18* on neocolonialism. Local researchers wish to study issues of local concern and be true authors and partners even if capacity building is required.

"Host perspectives," but for non-host goals

Other papers, ostensibly studies of hosts, are for specific purposes not identified with finding their interests. These do not seek to find out what hosts feel about their guests or the impact of programmes but are designed for a particular purpose. A couple of these failed to live up to the great potential to help understand host perspectives by limiting their scope to Global North priorities.

Maki and colleagues surveyed five mission directors, 43 personnel, ten local hosts and 55 patients in Brazil, Honduras, Ecuador, Namibia and Zimbabwe, regarding an evaluation tool to determine measures of quality of STMMs such as cost, impact, education, efficiency, sustainability and preparedness (Maki *et al.* 2008). In order to "gain insight into student learning processes" (primarily experiential) during such electives, Niemantsverdriet *et al.* (2006) conducted semistructured interviews with five external supervisors of 6-week community oriented clinical and public health international electives undertaken by Dutch undergraduate students in Kenya, Mexico and the Philippines. This study was focused on pedagogy and did not explicitly examine the goals of the supervisors or the relationship. Interestingly, productive learning was often impeded by sociocultural differences, especially when the differences between the national cultures of the host country and the student home country were substantial, with students explaining differences as being due to unwilling and/or incompetent supervisors (Niemantsverdriet *et al.* 2006).

Three key challenges

Regardless of whether clinical, research or short-term medical missions, three key challenges of hosting foreign medical learners and volunteers emerged as most significant in these reports of host experiences. These included: (a) foreign learner/volunteers' pressure on limited resources; (b) cultural differences; and (c) paternalistic relations between hosts and learners/volunteers. Each of these challenges are unpacked in turn below and we will concentrate on Kraeker's Ugandan informants clinically, Kung's in terms of local NGO hosting students, Green's in terms of STMMs, which seem to have more direct quotes from interviewees.

Impact of foreigners in a resource constrained environment

Hosting students often involves a great deal of attention and uses precious resources such as time and translation services for hosts in the Global South, often with their most highly trained and educated personnel. Green *et al.*

Table 19.1 Host perceptions of international projects and trainees

Author	Location/Setting	Sample	Method	Themes/Findings
A. Medical Electives				
Bozinoff 2014	22 Countries (12 LMICs) taking McMaster preclerkship medical students	39 (23 LMICs) supervisors of students	Convenience sample Questionnaires given immediately post elective	Mutual benefits Consideration of negative impacts (resource use, patient care) Ideas to improve collaboration – formal partnership, bidirectional flow
Radstone 2005	Solomon Islands UK clinical students	39 Hospital healthcare staff	Interviews	Perceptions students could do more without supervision than allowed to do in England
Kraeker 2014	Uganda Makerere where Canadian clinical students came	32 Medical trainees	Locally trained interviewers	Looser standards – patients as objects, 'museum of disease' Little integration or reciprocity
Kraeker 2013	Namibia School Medicine clinical	9 Healthcare providers dealing with students and teachers	Semistructured interviews	Nil negative regarding trainees coming. "Participants' comments supported actively seeking out information regarding cultural and environmental context before visiting, completing a needs assessment to ensure that activities are needed and relevant, attempting to formulate long-term sustainable relationships, and traveling with the appropriate attitude."
Kumwenda 2015	Convenience sampling Malawi Uganda Tanzania	14 Elective hosts (10 clinical, 4 adminstrative at 7 sites more than half trained inor from Global North	Interviews (face to face)	Committed … but wanted greater student preparation and contribution from sending institutions

(continued)

Table 19.1 (cont.)

Author	Location/Setting	Sample	Method	Themes/Findings
B. Student Volunteers with Health NGO				
Kung 2013, 2016	Bolivia India NGO Health Education Abroad (HEA) with US volunteer students sent by Child and Family Health International	35 Local physician preceptor; social workers/NGO directors, home stay families and programme coordinators	Qualitative interviews	Largely positive – serving a greater purpose, improvements in job satisfaction, prestige, global connectedness, broadening world views, network building leadership skills, resource enhancement. BUT Processes driven from the north, lack of local participation, wished improvements in HIC trainee attitudes and behaviours
C. Short-Term Medical Missions				
Green 2009	Guatemala US NGO	72 Local healthcare providers and health authorities, foreign medical providers, non-medical personnel working on health projects, and parents of children treated	Exploratory in-depth, semistructured interviews	Burden on host Arrogance misunderstanding of visitors Preference of locals for foreigners creating resentment Lack of continuity
McLennan 2014	Honduras 2004–05, 2008–10 qualitative research for master's and PhD	Master's – 10 service recipients; 8 host-medical professionals, government, NGOs, health/development workers PhD 50+ interviews for projecthonduras. com online network bringing volunteers	Master's 8 hosts interviews- PhD interviews (individual or group) in field, at conference, online or participant observation	Difficulty with long-term relationship building Entrenching paternalism Ignorance of power, privilege and inequity STMM as bandaid could create dependency, compromise dignity and make inequities worse

Study	Country / Organization	Participants	Method	Findings
DeCamp 2014	Dominican Republic religious NGO MMI (Medical Ministry International) 2010	20 Recipients of care	Semistructured interviews	Researcher frequently misidentified as a care provider; Politeness, fears of loss of resources; Acceptance of neocolonial assumptions or genuine feelings of gratitude?
D. Research				
Kohrt 2014	Nepal Transcultural Psychosocial Organization (TPO) research	Participants in meeting conducted with HIC and LMIC investigators	Workshop	Lessons learned from collaborative writing; Often none or token representation; Exclusion or lack of participation of local academics in writing publishing with "fear of biasing results," "blinding," or related to skills, language
Agnandji 2012	Gabon Lamboréné research	Researchers Medical Research Unit hospital	Interviews	Research of limited value to the research centre itself, given complicated and demanding tasks "main contents and models of scientific activities are elaborated predominantly by those from the North"
E. Host but Specific Purpose				
Maki 2008	Brazil Honduras Ecuador Namibia Zimbabwe	Five mission directors, 43 personnel, ten local hosts, and 55 patients	Survey	Tool validation regarding STMM cost, Impact, education, efficiency, sustainability and preparedness
Niemantsverdriet 2006	Kenya, Mexico and Philippines	Five host supervisors of Dutch medical students	Semistructured interviews	Goal-learning processes and safety and cultural issues for students

(2009) noted burdens on host organisation/community with one Guatemalan project coordinator of short-term medical volunteers who lamented that he was "half project coordinator and half tour guide. I have to arrange transportation, accommodation, food, and translators for all of the volunteers." (Greene *et al.* 2009, p. 8/13).

Green also lamented that some would attribute differences in healthcare practices and decisions to different cultural beliefs, rather than to lack of resources and basic services quoting Paul Farmer, to "conflate poverty with culture." (Green *et al.* 2009, p. 11/13). There were concerns that dependence on foreign providers could affect the development of public health infrastructure and short-term medical missions failing to address root causes. One Guatemalan surgeon working at a large national hospital summed up the problem: "[Foreign] surgical teams only work on the tip of the iceberg when it comes to addressing the medical problems of this country. The problems of Guatemala – corruption, lack of resources, lack of education – all come from poverty. So poverty is the root of the problem, and surgery does not address poverty" (Green *et al.* 2009, p. 5/13). DeCamp's informants were similar with almost half (nine) of those interviewed taking the opportunity of the interviews to emphasise social determinants of their health and the consequent value of STMMs: "One of the things that most affects this country is poverty. The small amount of development. There are no jobs for the poor .... That is what most affects us" (DeCamp *et al.*, 2014).

Lack of recognition of causes of disparity, and the impact of trainees on such disparities would be problematic, if not incorporated into training and planning of exchange.

Culture and colonial legacies

Students might judge institutional or social practices in a host community as inferior, or report these upon their return as based in "culture," a common shorthand these days for "beyond logic." Such reductionist coding of "other" healthcare world's feeds into historical legacies of the north assuming superior practices and logics as compared to the south, and obscures the complex constellations of factors that underlie healthcare norms, including, for example, the availability of resources, information flows, local epidemiological patterns, caste and class systems, norms of gender and family relations, and/or distinct belief in para-medical treatments (whether spiritual, nutritional or massage-based). Cultural differences may be assumed, perceived or noted outside racist and colonial tropes.

Some schools in the Global North teach about mismatches in communication style between grad students and supervisors from other cultures, high power distance, low context and high context cultures, more and less direct and indirect communication styles and approaches to conflict, and mono and polychronic approaches to time (Dimitrov, 2009), but often with a tacit assumption that the northern perspective is more advanced or enlightened than merely different. Such differences in expectation could also result in conflict in exchanges with students and programmes from the north and south. The Dutch Maastricht study (Niemantsverdriet *et al.* 2006), while not focused on understanding hosts, found poorer outcomes with four dimensions of sociocultural mismatch in the student–supervisor dyad, national cultures: individualism versus collectivism (how to learn versus how to do), difference in power distance relationships (whether students could contradict or criticise teachers), comfort with or avoidance of uncertainty (less or more) and masculinity versus femininity.

DeCamp's Dominican Republic study produced some troubling responses, "Also, they are reading the word of God in order to cleanse our hearts, and they make us feel good;" whether this represented politeness, fears of loss of resources, acceptance of neocolonial assumptions or genuine feelings of gratitude. Student involvement was viewed as not just positive for their professional development, but also as beneficial to the communities because of the care delivered (e.g., "they take your blood pressure"), and as part of future non-specific benefits to the community: although this assumption is questionable in many contexts, the investigators chose to view this as possible in a setting with long-standing relationships with local community members and the government. Volunteers work closely with local pastors and community church members and where supervision is emphasised (DeCamp *et al.* 2014).

Studies such as Maki's and Niemantsverdriet's could be strengthened and opportunities to understand issues of importance and priority to hosts in the Global South by ethics boards mandating piggybacking of such questions.

In any case understanding more about the colonial legacy and training about the culture context is important for sending organisations and those participating in international experiences.

Power and paternalism or partnership

Participants often expressed concerns about processes being driven by the Global North without consulting partners. One physician interviewed by Kung stated "Who are the people on the board of HEA? Anybody from the grassroots? No. Are any local coordinators on the board? No. Are any local physicians on the board? No. You are managing the organization from a dry room. Unless you have people from the grassroots on the board, you will not know what the realities of life are in the communities HEA wants to help" (Kung 2013, p. 55).

She found concerns with finance. "[CFHI] is gathering the medical directors [and US staff] and flying them in for one night, during the peak holiday time. And paying for the hotel stays and food .... I don't think that, as a socially responsible organisation, we should do that." (Kung 2016, p. 6/9) but also attitudes, administrators not wanting to disrupt their own Christmas family time but expecting locals to disrupt theirs', using money as allowing disrespect of locals and lack of transparency with funds and participation in decision-making. On the other hand association with the Global North provided prestige, which a homeopathic physician termed "racial advertisement" (Kung 2016, p. 4 of 9). Said another "White skin is an advantage for us ... we should use it." (Kung 2016, p. 4 of 9).

Kumwenda and colleagues (2016) found issues with individuals "some students do come with an attitude that because they are Western medical students they will know much more than what our clinical officers know. They will find that they are not right and they have to learn to respect the Malawian clinical officers, respect their decision making." (p. 629) but also institutions with regard to power "students from [name of institution] are selected by their university; I don't have any choice of which students can come. And I have to say some of the students who come on this programme are quite a disappointment in their attitude. I am certainly going to terminate that programme." (p. 627).

Green and colleagues (2009) drew attention to the danger of a level of arrogance or elitism of visiting personnel, "Is it paternalism or cooperation? Is it charity or aid? Is it experimentation or quality care? Have all stakeholders been properly identified?" (Green *et al.* 2009, p. 10/13)? The feeling that foreigners might be better was sometimes shared by patients. A Guatemalan surgeon working in a private clinic and government hospital declared: "Guatemalan patients, especially those with less education, tend to put more faith in a blonde haired, blue eyed, white skinned foreign physician than their own Guatemalan physicians." (Green *et al.* 2009, p. 8/13). However, this might be mitigated as "when foreign providers work in coordination with the local healthcare providers, it reflects an acknowledgement that the local providers are competent" and can be visible to the local patient population (Green *et al.* 2009, p. 8/13).

Green also noted that assumptions of superiority might lead to a lack of consultation by foreign medical groups to assess needs and impacts appropriately or ensuring continuity of care. A Guatemalan physician interviewee working at a government health post in a community that was recently devastated by a natural disaster described practices s/he viewed as problematic: They "saw patients over a weekend and provided medications without any records or understandable explanations to the patients of why they needed the medication. He said those same patients came to his health post the following week, unable to explain what was done and why they were taking medication, forcing him to repeat their exams without any benefit to the patient or the system." (Green *et al.* 2009, p. 9/13). Other examples of "particularly misguided interventions which reflect the lack of coordination and consultation with the local healthcare community" included "de-worming campaigns" in areas without clean drinking water sources; groups that provided free eye glasses without an eye exam; or groups that indiscriminately handed out vitamins (Green *et al.*, 2009, p. 9/13).

Kraeker's Ugandan medical trainees were very blunt in discussing the power imbalance. "I think most people look at Africa as a museum of disease.

So whatever they write about, they see the stages of disease here. There are tropical diseases which I am assuming they do not have back home." (Kraeker *et al.*, 2014, p. 2). "I think here because of the lax in our laws, that's why they come here because they get the opportunity to touch the patient, to do the procedures and everything." (Kraeker *et al.*, 2014, p. 3). "Sometimes we work on projects with them while they are here but the tendency is when they go, they never really get back to us with what happened. It's quite a common thing." (Kraeker *et al.*, 2014, p. 3). "Yes, maybe the part I'd like to add, is the part where we see a lot of them, but very few of ours go there…" (Kraeker *et al.*, 2014, p. 4).

Agnandji described "… from the perspective of the core-periphery model, the scientists at the MRU may be considered as the "field workers" who collect data following the study protocol design and implementation by Western partners" (Agnandji *et al.*, 2012).

Sometimes even the right course of action may be viewed as objectionable, pointing to the importance of communication. Kung's Indian informants interpreted the desire to observe, "hesitancy" meant they didn't want to get their hands dirty "… they want to sit in a glass cubicle and look at people." (Kung *et al.* 2016, p. 5/9), which is due, at least in part, to ethical norms not to "practice on the poor" something that particularly disturbed Kraeker's medical trainees.

The issues of mutual benefit, but also involvement at all stages has been addressed in community development, community-based participatory (action) research and now service learning literatures over years (see *Chapter 10* and Chapter *11*). Social desirability bias, as well as the historically entrenched and neo-geopolitically reinforced power relations within which health electives are embedded, may bias host community feedback on international electives towards the positive. Chan and Nouvet point out in *Chapter 22* that reports of satisfaction gathered by northern students working with partners in the Global South may not do justice to experiences of host communities.

The articulation of negative perceptions in Kung's study may reflect a comfortable level of locals stating the negative without fear of retribution, with a sending organisation valuing their input, and putting resources into studying and reporting such findings. How much valuable feedback would be missed by organisations without the foresight to study and the bravery to publish, than CFHI?

Conclusions

Although it is difficult to summarise the complex feelings of various participants in the Global South with regard to trainees from the Global North, this literature review and the other chapters in this part give some direction. The sentiment regarding power, colonial legacies and resource constraints was common to all settings and the desire for true partnership. The difficulty separating the researchers from the sending institution, more marked with some study designs, might lead to an under-representation of negative feelings.

Creating more equitable international electives requires more than additional training. It requires shifting the discourse and measures of quality in international health electives and programmes, to foreground listening first to those on the receiving ends. This section was conceived in response to that gap we perceive in critical consideration of international electives for medical students. While reflection on international medical electives among students and faculty from the Global North may be growing, the literature on host perspectives of HIC international elective students is sparse but merits more space in considerations of what and how international medical electives work.

By clarifying on what bases individuals and institutions in the Global South have experienced these electives as beneficial or problematic, our aim is to move the assessment of these programmes beyond anecdotes towards more structured questions and debate. This volume's landmark 17 host, 14 country study, *Chapter 20*, with interviews in various contexts demonstrates similar unfulfilled desires for equity and reciprocity among hosts.

Acknowledgements

Thank you to Kelly Anderson, Jill Allison and Kate Standish for reviewing early drafts and suggesting references, and to Rebekah Baumann and Melissa Whaling for help with referencing.

References

Agnandji ST, Tsassa V, Conzelmann C, Köhler C, Ehni H. 2012. "Patterns of biomedical science production in a sub-Saharan research center." *BMC Medical Ethics* 13(1):3. doi: 10.1186/1472-6939-13-3.

Bozinoff N, Dorman KP, Kerr D, Roebbelen E, Rogers E, Hunter A, O'Shea, Kraeker C. 2014. "Toward reciprocity: host supervisor perspectives on international medical electives." *Medical Education* 48(4):397–404. doi: 10.1111/medu.12386.

DeCamp M, Enumah S, O'Neill D, Sugarman J. 2014. "Perceptions of a short-term medical programme in the Dominican Republic: voices of care recipients." *Global Public Health: An International Journal for Research, Policy and Practice* 9(4):411–425. doi: 10.1080/17441692.2014.893368.

Dimitrov N. 2009. *Western Guide to Mentoring Graduate Students Across Cultures.* London, ON: The University of Western Ontario Teaching Support Centre. Online edition. www.uwo.ca/tsc/resources/pdf/PG_3_MentoringAcrossCultures.pdf.

Green T, Green H, Scandlyn J, Kestler A. 2009. "Perceptions of short-term medical volunteer work: a qualitative study in Guatemala." *Globalization and Health* 5:4. doi: 10.1186/1744-8603-5-4. 13 pages on line.

Kohrt BA, Upadhaya N, Luitel NP, Maharjan SM, Kaiser BN, MacFarlane EK, Khan N. 2014. "Authorship in global mental health research: recommendations for collaborative approaches to writing and publishing." *Annals of Global Health* 80(2):134–142. doi: 10.1016/j.aogh.2014.04.007.

Kraeker C, Chandler C. 2013. "'We learn from them, they learn from us': Global health experiences and host perceptions of visiting health care professionals."

Academic Medicine 88(4):483–487. doi: 10.1097/ACM.0b013e3182857b8a. www.
africa.upenn.edu/asc/welearnfromthem.pdf.

Kraeker C, Khalifa A, Delahunty-Pike A, Waiswa M, O'Shea T, Damani A. 2014.
"Host perspectives of visiting medical trainees: a qualitative analysis of global
health electives." *Journal of Global Health Perspectives* Nov 16. http://jglobalhealth.
org/wp-content/uploads/2014/11/Kraeker_Christian.pdf.

Kumwenda B, Dowell J, Daniels K, Merrylees N. 2015. "Medical electives in sub-
Saharan Africa: a host perspective medical education." *Medical Education*
49(6): 623–633. www.researchgate.net/publication/277025324_Medical_electives_
in_sub-Saharan_Africa_A_host_perspective.

Kung T. 2013. "Voices of International Host Communities: The Impact of Global
Health Education Programs." Undergra. duate thesis, Stanford University.

Kung TH, Richardson ET, Mabud TS, Heaney CA, Jones E, Evert J. 2016. "Host
community perspectives on trainees participating in short-term experiences in
global health." *Medical Education* doi: 10.1111/medu.13106.

Larsen MA (Ed.). 2015. International Service Learning: Engaging Host Communities
(Routledge Research in International and Comparative Education). New York:
Routledge.

Lasker JN. 2016. *Hope to help: The Promises and pitfalls of global health volunteering (The Culture and politics of health care work)*. Ithaca, NY: Cornell
University Press.

Maki J, Qualls M, White B, Kleefield S, Crone R. 2008. "Health impact assessment
and short-term medical missions: a methods study to evaluate quality of care."
BMC Health Services Research 8:121. doi: 10.1186/1472-6963-8-121.

McLennan S. 2014. "Medical voluntourism in Honduras: 'helping' the poor?"
Progress in Development Studies 14(2):163–179. doi: 10.1177/1464993413517789.
www.academia.edu/5872943/Medical_voluntourism_in_Honduras_Helping_
the_poor.

Niemantsverdriet S, Cees P, van der Vleuten M, Majoor GD, Scherpbier AJAA. 2006.
"The learning processes of international students through the eyes of foreign supervisors." *Medical Teacher* 28(4):e104–111. doi: 10.1080/01421590600726904.

Radstone SJJ. 2005. "Practising on the poor? Healthcare workers' beliefs about the
role of medical students during their elective." *Journal of Medical Ethics* 31(2):109–
110. doi: 10.1136/jme.2004.007799.

20 Voices from the host

Findings from interviews at institutions hosting Canadian medical trainees in 14 countries from the Global South

Akshaya Neil Arya and Carolyn Beukeboom

Website: www.routledge.com/9781138236332

Host community perspectives remain poorly understood, and programme voices have rarely been heard by the global health community, let alone integrated into developing placements. To help address this issue, interviews were conducted with preceptors of Canadian medical trainees, administrators of programmes and coordinators of international activities in facilities hosting Canadian medical trainees from all Canadian medical schools. Although genuine pleasure in taking Canadian trainees was apparent, with benefits seen not just to the trainees themselves but local trainees, programmes and global health generally, several concerns, related to the training of students (particularly language and cultural), expectations of sending institutions, and issues of reciprocity, tempered such enthusiasm. A desire for formal memoranda of understanding was expressed, longer term relationships were seen as beneficial and there was a wish for collaborative research in areas of common interest such as health issues relevant to the local context. This pilot project gives a baseline in order to guide collaborative research on the impact of electives and planning incorporating Global South host preceptors, programmes and communities and to suggest practices that would be more ethical and beneficial to all.

21 Structures and functions of international volunteer programmes

My experience from the field

María del Carmen Valdivieso

Volunteer experiences including international health or development may involve investment of money and time, and for me they have resulted in wonderful and productive interactions and relationships. As a host organiser, I have also encountered many difficult moments in which basic principles do not seem to have been followed including equity in relationships, honesty and follow-through. This has even resulted in legal proceedings, raising basic questions as to whether such programmes are "good" or "bad" for our community partners and even for participants.

This chapter is a brief reflection of the product of 13 years of experience with two different volunteer and non-governmental organisations (NGOs) in the Sacred Valley of the Incas – Urubamba, Cusco, Peru.

In one district in 2014, there were 34 NGOs, many of them offering international "volunteer" programmes (IVPs) to support their projects, recruiting "volunteers to change lives." To examine such programmes critically, we must look at perspectives of, and relationships among, the various stakeholders: NGOs, universities, volunteer agencies, participants in IVPs and, of course, host communities. Unfortunately, the literature is dominated by professionals who are neither part of the receiving organisation, nor born or live in the host community (or the country).

As a Peruvian, I share some history with the communities in which we work, yet I, too, have not lived in the most isolated ones, and have never lived more than 10 months in a row in any single one; and with my background and privilege cannot completely put myself in their shoes. Therefore, I sometimes fail to understand certain community decisions.

Once a colleague relayed the following: "there was a Master's student in Agriculture, who wanted to do crop research in a community. His plan was to stay there for 6 months and then use the information to develop different options to benefit the community, such as seed protection and better prices for the crops. After presenting his ideas to the Community Assembly, his project was approved, but on one simple condition: he needed to buy a tractor for the community." Sensing my rising frustration as he relayed this story, my colleague went on, "We need to remember that Andean people living in precarious circumstances must remain practical. They truly do believe 'He might help us,' but the reality is that, in all likelihood we will remain in the same situation, when he returns to his old life in his own country, enriched by knowledge which will increase employment and other opportunities for him. You know in your heart that this is true."

Genuinely "helping," supporting community needs, requires profound changes in the relationships among stakeholders, in terms of the level of participation and responsibility. Moreover, I believe impacts of these programmes have their roots in the relationships established among sending institutions (including universities), "volunteer" agencies and the local NGO.

In order to generate better programmes, we might begin with a few questions:

1. Why are there so many IVP opportunities and so many who choose to participate? Do "volunteers" seek to help the people with greatest needs, or is this merely "voluntourism" seeking adventure and experience?
2. As most IVP participants are university students or graduates, although universities might not fund or promote a specific programme, do "higher education" institutions bear certain responsibilities? Are they taking into account the scholarship of engagement (Boyer, 1990), described later in this chapter.
3. How does increased emphasis on learning components of IVPs, often customising programmes in order to recruit more participants, affect communities? To whom and how are organising NGOs accountable?
4. And finally, is the term "volunteer" accurate to describe participants in IVPs? Do they possess the qualities of an ideal "volunteer"?

In essence, to limit damage to the lives of community members and to contribute to the education of the participants' IVP, such basic considerations in programmes must be addressed. If not, harms of such programmes will not be only for host communities, but equally to global society, as their structures reflect relationships of developing countries with developed ones.

Relationships among IVP stakeholders

Relationships vary in type, scale, strength and number. The needs of the various stakeholders are different and each of them has different capacity to fulfil them, as well as power. IVPs are an example of how unequal relationships, having been established, may be maintained by one who holds more power. What instruments give them that power? Is it only money?

Money may be a tool for an IVP participant to be part of a programme and decide on goals; money may be the motive for a programme provider to organise the programmes; money could also be the tool for the university to decide, if and when they wish to have a programme and what its components are; and last, but not least, money (or the consequences of it) may be the motive for the communities to accept IVP participants. It is naive to expect that in the near future money will cease to be a crucial instrument for any stakeholder in IVPs, or that it will no longer give disproportionate power to one of the parties; hence, what we can actually do is improve and reinforce relationships in order to establish them in fairer ways for all.

Reflecting on relationships leads us to consider responsibilities: some responsibilities in the IVP world are readily identified, others require deeper discussion. Can we mitigate the risks generated by these activities? To what extent is the university responsible for the impact of its students? Can we determine host community responsibilities based on equity? Are stakeholders are being supervised? If so, to whom and how?

Realising the importance of defining relationships and responsibilities can lead to a more open dialogue, not purely for legal or liability concerns, but to develop a different type of commitment among stakeholders, thus, better programmes.

Let us focus on the following relationships within the IVP world:

1. Sending institution (i.e., university) and programme provider (i.e., NGO);
2. Sending institution and host community;
3. IVP participants and host community;
4. Programme provider and host community.

Sending institution and programme provider

Currently, people interested in doing volunteer work may apply through several channels. Some platforms offer potential participants countless opportunities in various fields in almost every part of the world. University programmes may involve their students with individual programmes (often called "internships") or groups (alternative spring breaks, for example). Typically, each offers their participants opportunities to go abroad, learn and support communities. Lasker's *Hoping to Help* (2016) describes the current situation of "volunteerism" and its possible consequences and provides in depth description of different IVPs, especially those related to global health.

Group programmes tend to be short term and an opportunity to work in hands-on projects. Whereas some universities have been working on improving preparation of their students, their impact has been criticised as lacking in sustainability and benefits to communities. A thoughtful, well organised group programme has the potential to support host communities achieve tangible results and to strengthen the ties between the programme provider and the host community.

In contrast, individual programmes seek learning opportunities to complement book knowledge. Often universities include different IVP opportunities for their students, but do not know about the development of their programmes or the impact of their participation. Posting and funding of programmes does not guarantee the university awareness of their students work plan in the field, impact of their participation or knowledge about the community.

Whether a programme is for one person or for a group, this relationship impacts the host community and the IVP participants. Establishing a relationship with an NGO unlike with a business, and those with organisations whose main goal is to provide programmes and create opportunities for IVP participants are different from those which provide IVPs primarily to receive support for their projects. Nor are relationships with organisations favouring engaging foreigners over local people the same as those that do the opposite.

"Building Ethical Global Engagement with Host Communities: North–South Collaborations for Mutual Learning and Benefit" (Karim-Haji *et al.* 2016) produced by Western and Aga Khan Universities with Pamela Roy Consultancy for Global Higher Education is a very good starting point to improve North–South work. It opens up the discussion about the internationalisation of education emphasising, for instance, the importance of interculturality, stresses the importance of acknowledging and addressing mental health of IVP participants (something that has led to issues in our programme), highlights the asymmetrical nature of partnerships between universities and host communities and provides useful pre-departure information.

Sending institution and host community

Although the main purpose of IVPs should be the support of communities with the greatest needs, sending organisations often do not have the time to develop ties with host communities and merely trust programme providers to have strong relationships. A deep, solid relationship can help achieve sustainability.

The best way to inform one's self about the impact of projects on a community is to visit it. Yet, it is unusual for sending institutions to visit communities; thus they have limited specific information about the project, such as the number of inhabitants, the weather, etc. Such information seems insufficient genuinely to understand the reality and challenges of host communities.

Sending institutions do not have to be constantly present in the communities – that is the work of the NGO, but visiting does represent commitment and sends a message that the NGO is being supported by an "external" actor, with prestige, money and academic connections.

Generally, a stronger relationship between a sending institution and host community could allow better understanding and selection of appropriate participants for programmes, leading to fewer unilateral changes, and accountability among all partners, programme providers, sending institutions and the community.

IVP participants and host community

In terms of the impact of participants, the quality of personal bonds between participants and community members is important. I have seen strong, positive relationships with adult community members when there are: 1. Strong values of respect, interculturality and compassion; 2. Free (but supervised) space to develop responsible relationships. Consequently, the results of such relationships can enhance or damage initiatives, although sometimes caution must be exercised, depending on the context.

Under these circumstances, I have been pleased to observe how this relationship between the community and IVP participants can improve the trust between the community and programme provider.

IVPs also provide an opportunity for host community members to get a glimpse of how the "others" live. While they, too, wish to preserve their culture, at least in the area I work, host community members appreciate when others share with them other cultures and traditions.

The relationship between IVP participants and community children is a delicate one, due to the vulnerability of children. Close personal ties between IVP participants and children can cause long-term damage to children (when participants leave) and should be avoided, or at least closely monitored by programmes. Ironically, many of the most "attractive" IVP programmes promote the opportunity to work on a daily basis with children.

All things considered, host participant interactions are a central focus of IVPs. Properly managed, an IVP can enhance the experience for those most marginalised, and for eager, young participants.

Between programme provider and host community

Programme providers, be they NGOs or volunteer agencies, link host communities to sending organisations and their participants, and need to be in constant communication and work with each.

In essence, regardless of relationships, the fundamental value, sometimes difficult to achieve fully, is equity. Without equity, relationships and responsibilities will not be fairly established, nor will it lead to great outcomes that are beneficial for all stakeholders.

When we establish relationships with host communities, our actions are premised on the assumption that we can do more and provide more than they can alone. While we may have had more opportunities and privileges than our community partners, often we do not appreciate their capacities and their own potential. Unlearning this assumption can lead to genuine respect, which is fundamental to just relationships.

We called them "volunteers"

What is a volunteer? As a Peruvian, the first image that comes to mind, is a volunteer firefighter. In Peru, an ideal volunteer characteristically is thought of as a committed and responsible individual who does an unpaid job to help with the fulfilment of the needs of a society, is member of an organisation (or "brotherhood" as Peruvian firemen called the bond among them) and has a reputation for honour in recognition for their contribution to our society. To sum up, a volunteer works to support the others; the organisation relies on his work to achieve its goals; this gives the volunteer pride, meaning and joy. About this last characteristic, Bernardo Kliksberg described the last characteristic beautifully: "There must be a reason why oriental wisdom – coinciding with Biblical views – says: 'The fragrance always remains in the hand that gives the rose'." (Sen and Kliksberg 2007)

Volunteers for Amnesty International, OXFAM, TECHO (A Roof for My Country, an organisation created in Chile that works in Latin America and the Caribbean aims to combat poverty) seem to fit this definition. But how do IVP participants measure up? I will share some questions, comments and anecdotes to help answer this.

Thanks to a former colleague, our team always remembers what Margaret Mead once said, "Never doubt that a small group of thoughtful and committed citizens can change the world. Indeed, it's the only thing that ever has." The commitment to a cause and organisation is premised on the volunteers' identification of membership within an organisation, contributes to the effectiveness of volunteers, and probability of success is lower without this. How many former participants in IVPs still identify as members of their organisation and are they more committed to their cause/organisation than to building a resumé or obtaining university credits?

Many so-called "volunteers" from NGOs or volunteer agencies pay a fee, generally, to cover personal and organisational expenses. Not all "donations" are used in the same way. Henceforth, how can we be sure the programme provider offers these opportunities to support communities rather than to generate income?

Typical IVPs are not structured with "the fulfillment of specific needs of a society" as a unique goal, making this more difficult to ensure the outcomes of their programmes. However, with IVPs which charge a fee, participants may understand payment as a way to legitimise decisions which are based on more personal goals. While I have experienced, first hand, the positive impact of "volunteers," the outcomes of their participation depend on many different factors: the support of the NGO, the relationship with the host community, and the support of their universities.

IVP participants are often poorly regarded in Peru. One participant once said: "I came to Peru so I wouldn't have to follow rules that I need to at home." What gives them the "right" to expect this? Such attitudes make it highly unlikely that they care about their organisation's reputation. Another time, I had to fire two "volunteers" from our programme, for conduct contrary to our principles, not to mention Peruvian and North America laws. Despite the fact that our terms and conditions clearly stated that participants asked to leave would forfeit their fee, and regardless of the fact that the university was aware of their students' behaviour, a university representative asked us to reimburse them the money. What lesson did this teach the students?

IVP participants often assert their rights to a good experience while seeking minimal responsibility to, and maximum flexibility from, the organisers.

A year later, another "volunteer" suddenly decided to terminate her programme in midstream, for no particular reason. As she had returned for a second time, she knew our rules, but having studied law, rather than recognising the extraordinary lengths we had gone to to help her obtain funding, she decided to sue our organisation claiming we had promised to finance language training, despite the fact that she never paid for that service and that we actually facilitated the classes for her. Whereas the prosecutor found no proof for her allegations and said she was acting in "poor faith," dealing with this lawsuit cost our organisation heavily financially and emotionally. The next year she was awarded a US government fellowship. Neither the government, nor the funding institution for the 10-month programme, sought our opinion about her participation in Peru. What is the underlying message? That students can do what they wish abroad in a developing country, as it is very unlikely their future employees or university staff will know what happened.

To what extent should an organisation depend on IVP participants? And does the university bear some responsibility? On one occasion a university department and our organisation decided to collaborate on a specific project, with the university sending a group of students each year. After a successful first year, despite confirming participation for another year, the university, cancelled before their expected arrival. Apparently, the students preferred Tanzania over Peru. Such lack of reliability is not restricted to foreigners. After fieldwork with a group of students from a Peruvian university, our organisation was to meet with the students to finish the work. As the meetings were about to begin a professor declared that the students could not meet us without her supervision, as she was beginning a month-long vacation. At a later feedback session, a university staff member said that we needed to understand that our organisation was merely a "logistics provider."

Perhaps organisations should limit reliance on IVP participants, inserting them in specific, sustainable projects and activities. Maybe we need to accept the fact that IVPs are very useful for learning and growing, but not always to support the host communities, and that the projects could be realised at a fraction of the cost of the resources devoted to giving "volunteers" that experience.

The task to define and differentiate who and what is a volunteer is, or is not, may seem tedious, but is necessary if we wish to improve what are called "international volunteer programmes" or to find a new term based on their characteristics.

Currently many participants are more learners than volunteers. So why don't we call them by that name? One of the reasons may be that the perception that sending "volunteers" from developed countries to developing ones is to "help" but not to learn? A few years ago, I was awarded a UnitedStates State Department fellowship, which allowed me to learn more about economic empowerment. Although all of us were professionals and could have shared our knowledge with our American peers (and some of us did), the programme was for us to learn rather than to "volunteer" in their organisations (some with similar goals to ours). Similarly, programmes run by NGOs may offer similar opportunities for students to learn about the field, but the majority of them are still being called "volunteer" programmes. Is it safe to say that the difference in definition is the direction of migration – that when one goes from a developing country to participate in such programming we are fellows with the main goal of learning, but whenever participants from a developed country come to ours they are "volunteers"?

Improving IVPs

How can we address these flaws?

First we need to understand the nature of IVPs and how they started. Possibly an NGO/programme provider perceived a need: the interests of young people to go out to volunteer and took the opportunity; some of those programme providers wanted to do good, some to make money. These young people's interest may be rooted in religious background, altruistic values, a better resumé, university credit or notions of social justice. But I cannot help but wonder if the support of host communities is so important for them and for sending institutions, why is it that only a fraction of the millions of dollars generated seems to support those communities. Since interest from young people is unlikely to disappear (and is admirable), we need to begin with this reality and develop the best outcomes, not just for learning/religious/academic purposes for IVP participants or universities but for host communities as well.

In my experience, the best "sending institution" partners are those who are eager for their students to learn and reflect during the programme. Those with the greatest interest tend to be administrative staff as opposed to academics. Professors of international development or Latin American studies while kind were rarely involved in any of the programmes or promoted the link between the campus-based learning with what was happening outside and had limited interest unless the research component was a programme priority. Boyer (1990) declared that "Research and publication have become the primary means by which most professors achieve academic status, and yet many academics are, in fact, drawn to the profession precisely because of their love for teaching or for service – even for making the world a better place." Although research is of course very important, service/civic engagement is undervalued, unrecognised and there is little time devoted. If this imbalance were addressed, imagine how positive the impact might be. Is research the only or best way for universities to support communities, at home and abroad, especially those with the greatest need? What about if they go beyond what is found in campuses? The reality Boyer was describing in 1990 remains elusive two decades later and applies to those academics who are not developing the scholarship of engagement: "connecting the rich resources of the university to our most pressing social, civic and ethical problems, to our children, to our schools, to our teachers, and to our cities (...) the scholarship of engagement also means creating a special climate in which the academic and civic cultures communicate more continuously and more creatively with each other."

Learning components of programmes need to include more about context and well-structured reflection sessions. This will allow participants to ask more critical questions about the system under which we live, the causes of the problems based on the reality they have experienced, and the opportunity to which they will be exposed.

Pre-departure and orientation sessions, delivered by sending institutions or the NGO/programme provider, must go deeper than training on how to be polite (or politically correct) in interactions with communities with a different culture, background, history. We must motivate trainees, first to be compassionate – not just to show empathy – to unlearn understanding of what appears to be the only possible reality or solution to a problem, to develop interest in the context and to be critical about factors that perpetuate injustice for communities, and last but not least, genuinely to include the support of those communities as their main goal. This last one is difficult to achieve if the IVP structure is too weak to bear the load of personal interests or motivations underlying the programmes.

We need more discussion and reflection about privilege. I have met young people not only courageous enough to discuss uncomfortable situations, but often more willing to accept their privilege than their university professors and administrators.

Interculturality must be a part of the core values for every IVP, but it is barely understood, and often neglected. For instance, once during the halloween party (not an Andean tradition), a group of directors of an American non-profit organisation which offers internship programmes to do research and different impact evaluation work chose as halloween costumes the dress of typical Andean "mamitas." Their social media posts generated much mirth among their friends and colleagues. Although comments might not have been against "mamitas," using these costumes demonstrates a lack of awareness of Peru's colonial history and the impact of their behaviour. Additionally, participants and organisers of IVPs often seem to confuse respect with pity and regret regarding colonial wrongdoing, which unconsciously may be the opposite of respect, a sense of superiority.

While sending organisations are careful in choosing participants and signing legal documents describing terms, conditions and insurance, they are less interested in those with programme providers. As indicated above, the reason might be the lack of trust in the future partner, but lack of trust in this relationship will damage the dynamics within the programme, and as a result the outcome of it. If parties agree on the terms, with legalprotections, this can reinforce the relationship, and hopefully improve mutual trust. Moreover, these contracts may start the discussion of accountability in the IVP world, who is responsible to and for what.

Nonetheless, IVPs may not be genuinely volunteer programmes as I explained above, they have the potential to do much good with examples of great impact of volunteer forces around the world including Latin America (Sen and Kliksberg, 2007). Further research on this topic is necessary, preferably joint, between at least a sending organisation and a programme provider. We must have genuine understanding of the perceptions of each stakeholder, including those with different backgrounds and cultural values. To prove IVPs can have an impact on participants, in particular emotionally, we must follow their careers longitudinally after their participation. We can then correct aspects to allow optimal outcomes to "use" these experiences to do better work, become real change-makers and committed global citizens. Following the career paths of former participants, I can see how knowledge accumulated in the field has had a major impact on their careers. Out of the approximately 600 participants I have met, and in spite of the fact that I maintain contact with less than 10 percent of them, there are currently 15 people continuing education in the world's best universities, or developing careers that make a difference. I wish I could have followed more.

While I appreciate the effort of researchers and academics who have interests in and are critical of IVPs, I believe it is crucial to listen to and know all parties involved. IVPs have been criticised for being an end in themselves, as a solution. They may contribute, but are mainly a source to train future development practitioners, policy makers, social scientists and a tool to generate awareness of communities which they may only visit once in their lives.

These brief reflections from the field hopefully can contribute to the improvement of IVPs, which is a duty for all stakeholders involved. Some have more power to do so, but if all parties recognise their limitations and responsibilities and want to work together to achieve the goals, the outcomes will be beneficial for all. Furthermore, we also need to do so to avoid becoming another industry, damaging to the spirit of idealistic young people. We must seek the right partners and reinforce and improve our relationships. I and hopefully many other NGO/programme providers are determined to do so. I encourage you to work with us, so we can move down the path together.

References

Boyer, Ernest L. 1990. *Scholarship reconsidered: Priorities of the Professoriate.* Princeton, NJ: Carnegie Foundation for the Advancement of Teaching.

Karim-Haji, Farzana, Roy, Pamela and Gough, Robert. 2016. *Building Ethical Global Engagement with Host Communities: North-South Collaborations for Mutual Learning and Benefit.* Resource Guide presented at the 10th Annual Global Internship Conference, June 15–17. Boston, MA, USA. http://international.uwo.ca/pdf/Ethical%20Engagement%20Guide_2016.pdf.

Lasker, Judith. 2016. *Hoping to Help: the promises and pitfalls of Global Health Volunteering.* The Culture and Politics of Health Care Work. ILR Press.

Sen, Amartya and Kliksberg, Bernardo. 2007. *Primero la Gente. Una mirada desde la ética del desarrollo a los principales problemas del mundo desarrollado.* España. Deusto: Grupo Planeta (GBS).

22 Critically engaging host communities' praise for foreign healthcare volunteers

Lessons from Nicaragua

Elizabeth Chan and Elysée Nouvet

Setting the scene

In 2013, we conducted a study of beneficiary perspectives on the performance of humanitarian healthcare missions in Nicaragua. The aim of the study was to provide organisations and volunteers supporting foreign medical missions in Nicaragua with feedback on the performance of their organisations from the perspective of local "beneficiary" community members, as a means of contributing to reflection and quality improvement in Nicaraguan-directed but also other transnational medical care.

Fifty-two Nicaraguans, including physicians, nurses, patients, community leaders, family members of patients, as well as three individuals who did not access the short-term medical mission, were asked about their expectations and experiences of short-term surgical and/or primary care missions that had recently visited their area. Participants were sought based on their ability and willingness to discuss three missions in particular, all led by US founded and funded non-governmental organisations (NGOs) and serving largely peri-urban and rural populations in a non-emergency setting.

Overall findings from this study have been published elsewhere (Nouvet *et al.* 2015, Nouvet *et al.* 2016). Here, we unpack one key finding from this perceptions study: Nicaraguans' overwhelmingly positive accounts of short-term medical missions (STMMs). We summarise key elements within these positive accounts, and elaborate the connection of Nicaraguan expressions of gratitude towards STMMs and foreign volunteers to local and transnational norms of unequal access to healthcare resources. This unpacking aims to act as a sort of interruption within the concerted effort in this section attending to host experiences. By drawing attention to the political and social complexities that may underlie host accounts of what foreign medical volunteers are doing right or wrong, our hope is to contribute to a broader discussion about how we measure the benefit of short-term medical missions. Is this in the individual experience of those on the receiving end? Or must this always be evaluated in terms of the broader impacts of short-term medical missions; for example, the potential impact of these on local healthcare systems and local trust in those systems?

Expressions of gratitude

Any critical analysis exploring the impact of STMMs necessitates highlighting the limitations of generalising from a single qualitative study. Each "global health" volunteer project differs from the next in an infinite number of ways, which results in the difficulty of drawing comparisons of perceptions across different missions. The context in which volunteer missions are delivered or implemented will greatly impact the way the mission is perceived – both by the volunteers and the beneficiaries. Volunteer missions have highly varied objectives, places of operation, target populations, funding, capacities, duration, and scope of services provided. Missions are led by different institutions and volunteers can differ in training. The organisation through which the volunteer mission is delivered may be a more established and trusted presence in the communities in which they operate, or they may be new and/or suspect.

Core to the accounts of expectations and experiences of foreign medical missions gathered in the course of this study were expressions of gratitude and appreciation. Nicaraguan physicians, nurses, patients and community members emphasised the many ways the foreign healthcare missions were "doing good." They shortened long waiting lists for surgeries in under-funded public hospitals, and filled hundreds of otherwise unaffordable prescriptions. They provided free specialist consultations to the rural poor who otherwise face serious challenges accessing specialists in the Nicaraguan public health system, as these are based in urban centres and require the patient travelling first to seek an appointment, then returning at least one more time and often more for their consult, as the timing of these can be changed without notice.

Many patients and relatives of patients praised the foreign clinicians' smiles and gentle touch: humanising treatment they claimed they were routinely denied in the public healthcare system because of their poverty. These foreign humanitarian medical missions provided a different standard of care to the norm. From the perspective of these patients and their family members, short-term medical missions are most certainly "doing good."

The pleasure afforded to some patients within the context of "kind" and "caring" foreign STMMs regardless of clinical outcomes is not insignificant (Nouvet *et al.* 2016). Analysis of STMMs often assumes benefit can be measured in the number of patients served or operations completed. In contrast, many healthcare ethicists argue that benefit should be measured with attention to what care is provided, as well as how care is provided (Slim 2002).

Still, in the Nicaraguan context of this study, expressions of gratitude towards STMMs and their volunteers merit closer attention. Troubling power dynamics were often apparent within Nicaraguan patients' of medical missions accounts of these. Thus, for example, one study participant, "Ronald" (not his real name), stated, "Beggars can't be choosers!," in reference to not receiving the walker he had hoped for during the recent visit of an STMM in the community. This particular mission provided primary care and lasted a total of 6.5 hours. This appears to illustrate the lack of decision-making power on the part of beneficiaries in the healthcare they are able to access, both regarding local healthcare services and those provided by foreign humanitarian missions. These expressions of gratitude make visible a relationship of deep inequality between foreign STMMs and the Nicaraguans these sought out. Despite not receiving the care he hoped for, Ronald, like many others interviewed, greatly appreciated the friendliness and respect afforded him by the foreign medical volunteers.

While many Nicaraguans situated their praise within the context of a strained local healthcare system, not one participant signalled an expectation that things would change within this system any time in the near future. In addition to feelings of gratitude, positive perceptions often extended to the hope that missions would continue coming to their communities with more frequency and an expanded range of services. This hope for more is in conflict with the reality that short-term humanitarian missions are by nature not able to provide follow-up care or address long-term chronic health needs. Combined with positive experiences of foreign medical volunteers and their healthcare clinics – however temporary – such hopes for more foreground the risk of such fly-in programmes engendering long-term harm alongside any short-term benefits.

Dependency, discontent, and the politics of transnational caring

A consistent criticism of short-term medical missions that appears in the literature is the issue of dependency (McLennan 2014). Harvey and Lind (2005) in their report defined dependency on humanitarian aid as when a person "cannot meet immediate basic needs in the absence of relief assistance." This is indeed the case in many contexts (Barret 2006), often in emergency settings. The potential harms of dependency is a major concern prevalent in all humanitarian aid discourse. There are many potential long-term implications of fostering dependency on aid, such as undermining the local government and infrastructure, acting as a disincentive for the local government to meet the needs of their own populations, and disrupting development. Dependency is not limited to that of the individual beneficiary on aid in this perspective: it also references structural or systemic dependencies of governments and/or their health systems on foreign monies, staff and programmes. This concern about propagating dependency on aid and the inherent unsustainability of such aid impacts programming and policy regarding how aid is provided, especially in situations in which aid is provided on a prolonged basis.

Positive experiences of STMMs and their volunteers may aggravate points of discontent between users of a publicly funded healthcare system and those in charge of those systems at the national level. Such discontent has the potential to feed into demands or moves for national healthcare reform that may be needed and important to global health equity. There is no guarantee that experiences of "different and better" healthcare from foreigners will translate into calls for a stronger local health system.

In terms of the main subject of this chapter, short-term medical missions, the issue of dependency can be explored in terms of its impact on the local health system. Montgomery's seminal paper (1993) criticises the delivery model of a short-term medical mission, and whether it is appropriate for healthcare delivery in low income settings. It highlights the inability of short-term medical missions to provide preventive care, and thus its inability to improve or make an impact on health outcomes such as the prevalence and incidence of disease. Montgomery goes on to state that there is a potential danger if recipients of short-term medical missions wait to seek care from these missions, rather than seeking care locally, thereby delaying needed treatment. In this way, short-term medical missions may divert patients from accessing the local health system. These missions may also disrupt the daily work of local healthcare workers, relating to the concern that short-term medical missions may undermine the existing services that the local health system provides (Montgomery 1993, McLennan 2014).

Relating to dependency is the inequitable power relationship between volunteers and beneficiaries. A qualitative analysis of short-term medical missions in Honduras identifies a lack of decision-making power of the beneficiaries, in which the beneficiaries do not have a say in when, where, and how long the medical mission occurs. The lack of decision-making power contributes to an inequitable power relationship (McLennan 2014). The idea that volunteers are "helping" erases the global economic inequalities that render such travel by volunteers from richer countries to countries such as Nicaragua. In casting such efforts as "helping," thus locating the core of such missions in the individual good will of the volunteer, the volunteer is cast as simultaneously morally exceptional (Nouvet *et al.* 2016). Such casting of the good of "helping" also reaffirms a neoliberal logic in which each individual and each country is privately responsible for their own wellbeing. The foreign volunteers in Nicaragua are "helping" because they are moral, not because of any moral obligation or responsibility to redress transnational health and resource inequity.

Much of the literature calls for the need to integrate long-term aims and foster long-term relationships with beneficiary communities (Montgomery 1993, McLennan 2014, Green *et al.* 2009) in short-term medical missions. There is some evidence that this view is penetrating into the larger humanitarian relief community (ALNAP 2015); however, the three missions whose work in Nicaragua we studied still function within the traditional short-term medical mission framework, in which there is little to no consideration of addressing long-term needs.

The inability to address long-term care needs, the potential for undermining the existing health system, and the often unequal power relationship between the beneficiary and the short-term medical mission providers fosters dependency in the Nicaraguan case as in other contexts. While undoubtedly being lived as doing good in Nicaragua, short-term missions may be doing as much or even more harm than good in the long run. This is just one case that highlights the complexities of assessing the ethics of transnational medical initiatives.

Conclusion

There is currently no single established method of evaluating STMMs. Objectively measuring the impact of STMMs is complex especially when considering all the varying meanings that "benefit" and "impact" can encompass. In 2014, Sykes published a systematic review of the evidence on the impact of short-term medical missions, which included 67 qualitative and quantitative studies. Most studies identified in the review (80 percent) assessed surgical missions specifically. The review concluded that there was both a lack of empirical evidence and low quality of available evidence on the work of STMMs. As Sykes notes, there is a lack of a standard in measuring impact and effectiveness, in which the methods and outcomes used to evaluate these are highly varied and inconsistent. This is due in part because organisations responsible for these missions do not place rigorous evaluation as a top priority (Sykes 2014). Nonetheless, short-term medical missions do provide another avenue for beneficiaries to access needed healthcare services and do fill a gap that local health services may not provide (Montgomery 1993). Many Nicaraguans sincerely experience themselves as lucky to have received anything over nothing through the "good will" of foreign medical volunteers. People like Ronald do not always get what they hope for or need in this system, but they have no buying power to go elsewhere. Herein lies the key, in our view, to critically engaging host perceptions of foreign medical volunteers. The effect of foreign volunteers stepping into gaps in national or regional healthcare systems needs to be considered alongside any discrete evaluations of what particular programmes accomplish for particular members of the population.

Addressing the gap

This raises the question of what can be done to address this gap between the beneficiary and those involved in foreign medical missions. The following are suggestions based on findings from Nicaragua, in addition to existing literature:

1. *Improved collaboration and communication across all stakeholders*
    The medical missions included in this Nicaraguan study functioned outside the local health system. There was a general lack of information given to local healthcare providers; nurses in particular stressed that they had no control or say in primary care missions. Community members also lacked information on details of a mission and had little notification

in advance of a mission coming. This impacts the number of people that could be served by the mission, and may also affect the beneficiaries' expectations of what could be done for them. It is also unclear how much collaboration and communication occurs between organisations working within the same region or set of communities offering these missions, as to avoid redundancy or overlap in the provision of healthcare services. Thus, improved communication between all involved stakeholders could be a way better to inform beneficiaries, potentially allowing for input by the communities on their needs and involving them in their own healthcare.

2. *Opportunity for teaching*

For healthcare workers in particular, there is the opportunity for collaboration and teaching. Many healthcare workers expressed their desire to learn from their foreign counterparts, and saw this collaboration as a partnership. The capacity of a foreign mission to accommodate increased teaching will depend on its time and resources, which will vary mission to mission and across different organisations leading the missions.

3. *Establishing rigorous methods of evaluation*

There is a definite need for rigorous data collection and establishing methods of evaluating impact (Sykes 2014). These can help to promote greater accountability and transparency to the beneficiaries as well as to the public at large. Academic research studies are presented here as a contrast to how volunteer missions currently function. Scientific research abides by a set of rules, in which rigorous monitoring and evaluation as well as ethical review are the norm. In particular, the field of global health research emphasises the need to establish a relationship and rapport with the beneficiary, and to work with the local health system and stakeholders as partners. There are also other commonalities between volunteer missions and global health research work, including that the majority of funding often comes from international donors and grants. There is a standard to be upheld in scientific research; the same standards should be considered for volunteer missions. Ways for missions to collaborate better with the local health system and complement it rather than being at a disconnect needs to be explored, in particular for those organisations that operate regularly in the same regions and locations.

4. *Improved training and debriefing for students and volunteers involved in global health initiatives*

For students at all levels, forms of pre-departure training are highly important in integrating learning about cultural competency, ethical issues, and other travel considerations. For example, the Canadian Federation of Medical Students (CFMS) Global Health Program since 2013/14 requires medical students to take pre-departure training and "debriefing" for their electives when they travel outside Canada/USA. This kind of formal training and debriefing programme is likely to be more prevalent and required for postgraduate trainees (AFMC Global Health Resource Group and CFMS Global Health Program 2008, Wallace and Webb 2014). However, an assessment of pre-departure training found that the training tends to focus on clinical aspects and there is much less time spent on discussing health inequities. There is room for improvement and increased monitoring to ensure that pre-departure training adequately addresses these contextual issues discussed in this chapter (Wallace and Webb 2014). As volunteers participating in humanitarian aid missions, there is an obligation to reflect on what "helping" and "doing good" means.

Considering host/recipients' positive perceptions of foreign humanitarian work and the context in which these perceptions arise are important in being able to think critically about one's own contributions to a volunteer mission. Pre-departure training provides a platform for integrating this kind of critical thinking and reflection on expectations and the implications of such work in both an academic and volunteer setting. It should not be assumed, however, that gathering and taking local perceptions into account provides a solution to intrinsic inequalities within most global health electives. The overwhelming positive characterisation of short-term medical missions and their volunteers among Nicaraguans interviewed in our study may or may not be echoed in future "local perceptions" of medical electives. Regardless of this, the findings in our study have clarified for us the possibilities and limitations of such perceptions-based evaluations of transnational medical initiatives. We remain convinced that engaging communities throughout the programming cycle is also an ethical project. When humanitarian organisations carve out time and space to ensure those on the receiving end of aid can be heard, these individuals are recognised as valuable knowledge holders and potential partners, rather than as passive victims. Recognition is not the same as power however. Global health programmes, including short-term medical missions but also global health electives, are overwhelmingly funded and thus controlled by the pockets, desires, and intentions of those in the Global North. Asking those on the "host" side of these relationships to provide input and even critiques on programming does not shrink the gap between those positions.

References

ALNAP. 2015. "The State of the Humanitarian System 2015 Summary." Accessed July 15, 2016. www.alnap.org/resource/21236.aspx.

AFMC Global Health Resource Group and CFMS Global Health Program. 2008. "Preparing Medical Students for Electives in Low-resource Settings: A Template for National Guidelines for Pre-departure Training." www.old.cfms.org/downloads/Pre-Departure%20Guidelines%20Final.pdf.

Barret, Christopher. 2006. "Food Aid's Intended and Unintended Consequences." Background Paper for FAO State of Food and Agriculture. http://barrett.dyson.cornell.edu/files/papers/MixedEffectsv2Mar2006.pdf.

Green, Tyler *et al.* 2009. "Perceptions of short-term medical volunteer work: a qualitative study in Guatemala." *Globalization and Health* 5:4. doi: 10.1186/1744-8603-5-4.

Harvey, Paul and Jeremy Lind. 2005. "Dependency and Humanitarian Relief: A Critical Analysis." Humanitarian Policy Group (HPG). www.odi.org/sites/odi.org.uk/files/odi-assets/publications-opinion-files/277.pdf.

McLennan, S. 2014. "Medical voluntourism in Honduras: 'helping' the poor?" *Progress in Development Studies* 14(2):163–179. doi: 10.1177/1464993413517789.

Montgomery, L. 1993. "Short-Term Medical Missions: Enhancing or Eroding Health?" *Missiology: An International Review* 21(3):333–341. doi: 10.1177/009182969302100305.

Nouvet, Elysée, Chan, Elizabeth and Lisa Schwartz. 2015. "Beneficiary Perspectives Regarding the Ethical Performance of Humanitarian Healthcare Missions (BPREP)." Hamilton, ON: Humanitarian Healthcare Ethics Research Group (HHERG). https://humanitarianhealthethics.net/home/research/hhe-research-studies/bprep/.

Nouvet, Elysée, Chan, Elizabeth and Lisa Schwartz. 2016. "Looking good but doing harm? Perceptions of short-term medical missions in Nicaragua." *Global Public Health* doi:10.1080/17441692.2016.12206.

Slim, Hugo. 2002. "By What Authority? The Legitimacy and Accountability of Non-governmental Organisations." International Council on Human Rights Policy. Accessed June 5, 2016. www.gdrc.org/ngo/accountability/by-what-authority.html.

Sykes, K. 2014. "Short-term medical service trips: a systematic review of the evidence." *Am J Public Health* 104:e38–e48. doi: 10.2105/AJPH.2014. 301983.

Wallace, Lauren J. and Allison Webb. 2014. "Pre-departure training and the social accountability of international medical electives." *Education and Health* 27(2):143–147. doi: 10.4103/1357-6283.143745.

23 Reflections on a decade of hosting international medical trainees in Uganda

Samuel Luboga

Health training institutions in the "Global North" increasingly are seeking opportunities for their students to spend some of their training time experiencing healthcare in low resource settings. While benefits to the students and the sending institution are easy to define, benefits and costs to the hosting institutions, students and communities are often less clear (Crump *et al.* 2010). All stakeholders in global health must critically reflect on and take steps to quantify the costs and benefits to the host institutions, as a relationship designed to benefit one partner but exploit the other, however inadvertently, is unacceptable.

Context

The experiences being shared were acquired during the author's tenure as Deputy Dean of Education in the College of Health Sciences at Makerere University from 2000 to 2007. The college has "internationalisation" as one of its core values, and as such has entered into several international collaborations with universities around the world. Although these collaborations are governed by memoranda of understanding (MOU), they are often primarily based on the desire of the sending institutions to give their students an international experience. The students typically spend 4–6 weeks in Uganda experiencing first-hand health systems and disease conditions of the type and/or scale that they would probably not see back home. However, little consideration is given, by everyone involved (sending institutions, visiting students and even the host institution), to the impact this may have on the lives of the patients, students and staff of the host institution. Typically, the host institution is very generous and so eager to be of help that they do not stop to think the potential price this will cost them. The sending institutions often show no indication that there will be any impact on the host community. In fact they may feel their presence will be very beneficial.

The process

Because of the increasing demand for international electives within Makerere College of Health Sciences, in 2007 an International Students Coordination Office was established to coordinate and oversee these visitors.

On average it handles 320 students per year. Prospective elective students typically send application letters endorsed by their elective coordinators at their home institutions. In their applications they indicate the disciplines or services, e.g., endocrinology or obstetrics/gynaecology, to which they prefer to be attached during their stay. To offset some of the costs of their placement, since 2007 the International Students Coordination Office has required elective students to pay a fee, which varies between US $250 and $500 depending on the length of placement. Upon arrival the students are collected from the airport and taken to their pre-arranged accommodation. During their first week, the International Students Coordination Office provides elective students with an orientation to life in Makerere, Mulago National Referral and Teaching Hospital, Kampala and Uganda. They then give elective students identity cards and letters of introduction to ward mentors/supervisors. During their stay students are given prearranged language, technical and sociopolitical lectures. The technical (health-related lectures) are given by faculty at the host institution. The sociopolitical lectures are outsourced from faculty from the Department of Social Sciences in the College of Humanities. On the wards, alongside their Ugandan counterparts and under the strict supervision and guidance of the elective supervisor, they clerk patients (take history, examine and suggest laboratory investigations and treatment plans). They receive teaching at the bedside and in the various outpatient clinics. Many also get a chance to attend and even assist in deliveries and theatre sessions. By the time they leave Uganda their scope of knowledge and skills has been greatly widened. And for many, this is a life-changing experience.

Elective students from resource endowed countries are often shocked by everything they see, from the overcrowded wards to the advanced presentation of many patients, to the comparative lack of resources. They may have never seen patients who are so sick or dying at such young ages. Many will not have seen such vast poverty and a hospital short of almost everything. Many students need debriefing and counselling to help them recover and come to terms with their cultural shock.

Elective student behaviour

Elective students are very enthusiastic and keen to learn. They ask very useful questions whose answers are beneficial to everyone. They also provide a different perspective and question the status quo. They are pro-patient advocates. The patients greatly appreciate the interest elective students show in them and their conditions.

Sometimes elective students feel tempted to offer clinical care well beyond their level of competence. Reasons cited for doing so include the fact that for the first time in their lives they are confronted with extreme need and they feel uncomfortable doing nothing to help. To prevent this occurring during the elective, students are given strict instructions not to intervene except under supervision by an appropriate supervisor. There is a danger that patients will think that these students are qualified expatriate doctors and will be only too willing to be treated by them.

Some students misinterpret and criticise situations of omission resulting from lack of resources to be negligence. For example, elective students often complain that doctors in Uganda do not spend enough time listening to and educating their patients. They do not realise that the doctor has upwards of 100 patients waiting to see him in the few hours he has at his disposal. They also may not understand that while a patient may need an X-ray examination or medication, that rather than it being the doctor's fault, they may not get them because they cannot afford them.

The elective students are helped to understand some of the local cultural sensitivities. When, for example, students are invited over to colleague or patients' homes we guide them to dress appropriately, perhaps more formally than in their countries. Use of some words such as "stupid" may be misconstrued to be abusive. In the community a visiting student's refusal of an offer of a gift may be regarded by the giver as rude and a sign of ingratitude.

Once a week visiting students participate in a feedback session with the local elective coordinator and faculty, at which they share their experiences and impressions. Many a time visiting students have expressed horror at what they thought to be insensitivity or lack of empathy on the part of the host health workers. An example is when they feel that a patient was not given adequate attention or explanation. Another is that very sick patients are expected to buy their own medication or pay for a laboratory test or X-ray. Explanation of such unfortunate realities helps students appreciate the enormous efforts of health workers in low resourced settings despite the many challenges they face.

Elective students often want to communicate their experiences and feelings to friends and family back home. In doing so some may be tempted to disregard patient privacy and the professional code of conduct. Pictures and stories posted on Facebook and other social media have in the past offended rather than strengthened collaboration. Elective students are cautioned to exercise judgement and consult their supervisors before communicating sensitive information.

Resource challenges

Hosting exchange students imposes additional demands on the host institution, for example:

- The physical number of people on the wards, which is already high (consisting of patients, patients' relatives, staff and local health professional students) is significantly increased by the addition of exchange students.
- Theoretically the use of sundries, such as drip sets, gloves, catheters, etc. will go up, increasing cost and environmental impact.

- The presence of elective students greatly increases the demand on the supervisor's time as he/she juggles patient care and managing local trainees with overseeing exchange student-related activities and answering their questions.
- Increased student–patient contact may further strain efforts to ensure confidentiality.

Some of these challenges can be mitigated by increasing funding support to the wards and providing an allowance for the key personnel on the ward. In the name of equity, this cost should be borne by the benefitting student or sending institution.

Reciprocity

For a long time elective student traffic has been mostly unidirectional: students, both graduate and undergraduate, from resource rich countries were coming to Uganda while very few were going from Uganda to these countries. Even when return visits are made to resource rich countries, students from Uganda are often generally not given the same opportunities for experiential (hands-on) training and learning as elective students from resource rich countries are given here in Uganda. The same discrimination is extended to specialists from Uganda. Many times when they visit all they can do is watch their colleagues work and under no circumstances are they allowed to participate. This has reduced interest among senior clinicians in going on such trips for any length of time beyond one or 2 weeks.

Were it to be possible for this situation to change, many mutual benefits would likely accrue from global health exchanges. It is important to realise that health professions continue to be greatly enriched by student exchange programmes. Such exchanges should be continued while we work on strategies for improvement of the experiences by both sending and host institutions.

Conclusion

While elective students are warmly welcomed and their presence among us is often extremely beneficial in providing different perspectives, hosting elective students represents a considerable investment of time and effort for the host supervisor, institution and community. Caution needs to be exercised to ensure that local culture and sensibilities are respected at all times, and ways should be found to reimburse costs borne by the hosts and ensure reciprocity.

Reference

Crump JA, Sugarman J; Working Group on Ethics Guidelines for Global Health Training (WEIGHT). 2010. Global health training: ethics and best practice guidelines for training experiences in global health. *American Journal of Medicine and Hygiene* 83(6):1178–1182.

Part IV
Contemporary conversations

24 Global health job opportunities in international settings

*Adam Hoverman, Quentin Eichbaum,
Caity Jackson, William Cherniak,
Yassen Tcholakov, Thomas Hall, Ginny DeFrank
and Elahe Nezami*

Introduction

Students pursue global health educational and service opportunities for a variety of reasons. This chapter will focus on the job market for students and professionals seeking to work in the field of global health, defined broadly and encompassing both international and domestic local-global activities. We describe the types of global health jobs available, ways to enter the job market, and types of global health-relevant training offered by academic institutions and sought by employers. We also describe what is known about the balance of supply and demand for personnel, as well as the match between qualifications employers seek and those job seekers possess. It should be noted that this discussion focuses mainly on job opportunities and the overall landscape for individuals from high income countries (HICs) who seek work abroad that is largely either located in lower and middle income countries (LMICs) or pertaining to development efforts in LMICs. There is another large cadre of workers who focus on global health across multiple sectors, including government, health services, education, law, business and beyond. These are individuals who are from LMICs and either train locally or go abroad to train and return to employment in their home country or region.

Background

Baker's landmark and original work describes jobs and explores the many perspectives and extent of career opportunities within international and global health work (Baker *et al.* 1984). Over time, the field has shifted from "international health" predominantly referring to a rich-to-poor exchange of health resources to "global health," indicating an approach to the questions and challenges surrounding health and healthcare for all (Peluso *et al.* 2012). Primary responsibilities of the global health workforce include identification of the global burden of disease, research on the origins and effects of existing and emerging conditions, and implementation of sustainable solutions to the causes of ill health and challenges to wellness.

206 Hoverman et al.

Consistent with an evolution from international health to global health is the shift from individual health services to comprehensive community-based programmes involving inter-agency collaborations that transcend barriers and silos. Two distinct workforces have emerged: one involved in clinical care (e.g., "health workers") and the second specifically trained to plan, develop, manage, monitor, research, or evaluate initiatives (both clinical and non-clinical) intended to address health challenges. The latter is the subject of this chapter that we will refer to as the global health workforce.

Job search entry points

Many entry points exist to the discipline of global health. Required skills can vary from engineering, law, anthropology, sociology, public health and clinical medicine. Entry positions are often auxiliary, supportive, and programme management fields in the global development sector. Many students access global health careers following a stint of volunteerism or work in evaluation, outreach, or education. Further professional development is often via unpaid and formative training experiences (Umoren *et al.* 2015).

Humanitarian aid has classically prompted the increased need for relief workers. Traditional development cycles, from crisis relief to stable social development, reflect the jobs at each specific phase. Emergency relief efforts frequently demand specific and time-limited skills in the acute crisis. The period immediately following emergency relief requires clinical disciplines to rely on public health expertise and address infrastructure needs (e.g., water and sanitation, nutrition, and human displacement over a prolonged timeframe) (Petak 1985).

When crises move past the acute phase, engineering specialties become critical, in particular mechanical, civil, and water and sanitation, while environmental health and agricultural skills restore infrastructure. Finally, sustainable development and societal function relies on jobs in the social sciences, law (e.g., human rights, social justice, human trafficking), business and administrative disciplines.

Although global health internships do not always affect a health professional's career or clinical skills, field experience can contribute to increased dedication to primary care and resource-conscious care in the home setting of the healthcare worker (Umoren *et al.* 2015, Ramsey *et al.* 2004, Palazuelos and Dhillon 2016). A wide range of relevant disciplines offers a common starting point for global health work via internship or work–study experiences. Internships frequently influence job placement and research directions (Gupta *et al.* 2015). Longitudinal, one to 2-year commitments modelled after the Peace Corps approach, such as the Fogarty International Clinical Research Scholars Program, the Global Health Service Partnership, Global Health Corps, HEAL Initiatives and a diverse array of WHO internships, provide intensive entry into academic and research positions (Gupta *et al.* 2015, Benzian 2002, Richards-Kortum *et al.* 2012). Additionally, non-governmental organisations (NGOs) rely on a volunteer workforce, especially those that originate in high income settings and address service provision, education, technical assistance, and community development in low income settings (Richards-Kortum *et al.* 2012). Reliance on volunteer labour is difficult to sustain and a long-term career in global health calls for a balance of motivations, lifestyle demands, reflection on one's relevance and expanding skill sets (Loh *et al.* 2015, Crisp and Chen 2014).

The evolution of needed competencies in global health reflects the epidemiological transition. Responsive global health work necessitates coordination among many stakeholders. Clinical expertise is frequently less sought after than community work experience and managerial skills (Crisp 2011, Eichbaum *et al.* 2015, Gupta *et al.* 2015). Social entrepreneurship and design thinking, computer science, engineering, urban planning, social sciences, business, architecture, and improvement science skills, all offer a diverse range of career options for developing and disseminating novel and cost-effective interventions within global health. Responsive organisations have concurrently shown an increase in jobs focusing on novel solutions to complex global health challenges (Bussiéres *et al.* 2000, Crisp 2011).

Methods and means for finding jobs

Networking and relationship building is essential for surveying available job opportunities at all stages of one's career in global health. Fellowships and conference participation emerge as key methods for developing the kind of peer and mentor relationships essential for "best fit" positions available. The Fogarty International Center maintains a directory of fellowships for pre-doctoral/graduate students, post-doctoral students, faculty and health professionals. Award programmes, open funding, grants, travel awards and fellowships are listed for review and discovery. Many offer longitudinal, one and 2-year fellowship and traineeship programmes that connect the global health learner with formative experiences and mentor networks that often lead to long-term employment opportunities. Early career support is vital for formalising skills. Many of these opportunities allow participants to work in settings not commonly accessible to trainees and often reflect the mission of the sponsoring organisation. Pre and post-doctoral level support as well as mid-career funding is often available through governmental and private funding.

Networks and organisations

Several annual conferences attract both global health employers and job seekers. These include Global Health Council, Consortium of Universities for Global Health (CUGH), Canadian Society for International Health (CSIH) and the Canadian Coalition for Global Health Research (CCGHR). As the collective voice of the global health community these organisations provide a freely accessible job board and sometimes permit job postings and the viewing of resumés. Membership organisations often post jobs, internships, fellowships and funding opportunities. Websites of such membership organisations, including the Consortium of Universities for Global Health are a significant source of job postings, along with the recommendations of friends and colleagues. Similar to job fairs, conferences offer the participants opportunity to vet employers and hires, and share insights and connections.

Journals

The journal *Global Health: Science and Practice* provides limited job listings. The recent jobs page offers a free site for searching and posting related jobs. For uploading a resumé, bookmarking a specific posting, or saving a job search, the site allows a free registration. Whereas the major medical journals (e.g., *NEJM, JAMA, Lancet*) frequently offer pages for making customised searches for global health jobs, the primary global health journal websites currently have no equivalent feature. We hope this option may be explored by more journals in the future.

Achievements, degrees, certificates and accomplishments desired

Despite the recognition of degrees provided from accredited institutions, international standardisation has been shown to be problematic (Saltman *et al.* 2012). From a cursory review of 178 job postings, 50 percent requested applicants have the knowledge and skills normally acquired in schools of public health, with 51 percent requiring at least a master's level qualification or doctoral degree (Eichbaum *et al.* 2015).

Types of jobs and organisations

Professional activities in global health positions include: monitoring and building programmes in LMICs, on-the-ground service delivery, epidemiological surveillance in epidemics, disaster response in humanitarian emergencies, systems financing, policy-making, governance, health workforce development, health information systems, and supply management systems. Many intergovernmental agencies within the World Health Organization and United Nations specifically address responsive policy for health-related issues. Most provide lists of vacancies, customisable by topic area and location, and some offer online application portals. However, securing a position online may be difficult, as there are thousands of international applicants per post; with many selected applicants having acted in the role prior to the selection process. Bilateral agencies, NGOs and faith-based organisations provide thousands of additional positions across a similar range of disciplines, each with specific and distinct human resource profiles and procedures (Table 24.1).

Challenges in training and qualifications

The global health workforce need–placement juncture becomes a sensitive metric for current training programmes to meet existing job market demands via competencies and assessment. It is hoped that these can better reflect community and population demand. Similarly, this juncture provides an opportunity to investigate the match in numbers of graduates with the numbers of existing jobs, as well as the match of skill sets and capacity needed. Much has been done to describe how global health competencies can meet local health system needs and the global burden of disease (Kerry *et al.* 2013). An equivalent inquiry into the responsiveness of the global health marketplace to the global burden of disease following the work of Baker *et al.* (1984), however, is long overdue. Funding has increased alongside advances in technology, therapeutics and awareness of the role of income inequality and human health. Furthermore, student interest continues to increase in response to the questions that define the discipline of global health. Almost two-thirds of matriculating US and Canadian medical students expect global health opportunities during medical school, residency and their early careers. Interest in global health careers among medical students, residents and fellows has never been higher (Nelson *et al.* 2012, Palazuelos and Dhillon 2016). Greater governance and alignment of licensure and professional recognition across jurisdictions and health systems is required. Health professional migration also demands a transnational governance response as the global supply of health professionals reflects an underlying interdependence between global and local health systems (Crisp and Chen 2014).

Global health work in the local context

Koplan defines global health as the "area of of study, research and practice that places a priority on improving the health and achieving equity in health for all people worldwide." However, it is clear that significant health gradients exist between and within countries (Koplan *et al.* 2009, Marmot *et al.* 2008). These health gaps compel many to commit their careers, or a portion thereof, to the service of local refugee, immigrant, homeless, and uninsured communities as a mechanism for overcoming the cultural/linguistic differences, power imbalances, and unique challenges that travel and international health settings frequently entail. It is clear that international service environments raise ethical dilemmas in the health professional's home community, especially when the international context can also draw their time, attention and skill set elsewhere (e.g., "the brain drain"). Resource limitations and standard of care disparities emerge as relevant dilemmas for the global health professional. Advocacy and policy in support of strengthening local health systems that best serve these communities can be viable avenues for choosing local service needs over international service (Loh *et al.* 2015).

Roland Robertson's introduction and amplification of the term "glocalisa-tion" in the early 1990s and his examples of how global processes are also local processes have prompted awareness of the global employment poten-tial within the provider's home community. Combining the terms global and local, the resulting term glocalisation reflects the Japanese concept of *dochakuka* (from the term *dochaku* "living on one's own land"). Within this space, a tension can arise when globalised trends are pitted against local pri-orities (Featherstone *et al.* 1995). In particular, the workforce deficit known as the "brain drain" adds undue pressure when local and critical health needs remain unmet (Crisp and Chen 2014).

The set of neighbourhood clinics and service populations where the local services might offer global health opportunities to address health equity chal-lenges vary immensely between and within healthcare systems. Often such clinics are nationally funded and managed via ministries of health. In other settings, funding arises via non-profit structures or an equivalent manner of community participation. In the United States, neighbourhood health centres were established under the Economic Opportunity Act of 1964 at the height of the War on Poverty (California Department of Community Services and Development 2015). More recently, section 330 of the Public Health Service Act in 1975 authorised community health centres to establish public–private partnerships to provide comprehensive primary care. In 1991, the addition of federally qualified health centres to Medicare and Medicaid benefits, established "safety net" clinics with the intent of "enhancing the provision of primary care services in underserved urban and rural communities." The safety net arena extends to prison health, migrant health, homeless health, the Indian health services and the many tribal health networks, consortia, agencies, and initiatives for addressing Indigenous health priorities (HRSA 2016). In Canada, provincial community health centres meet the needs of high-risk communities and Indigenous health is championed by the National Aboriginal Health Organisation, an Indigenously designed and controlled body supported by Health Canada (Health Canada 2016). Australia estab-lished the Indigenous Australians' Health Programme on 1 July 2014, which expanded community controlled health organisations to better meet the needs of child and maternal health and chronic disease prevention and manage-ment across the country (Australian Government Department of Health 2016). In Europe, the European Network of Homeless Health Workers pro-vides a forum for exchange and mutual learning among healthcare profes-sionals working with people who are homeless in Europe, along with the free clinics established within the existing health systems to serve the needs of recently expanded migrant populations (FEANTSA 2016). These are several examples, of many, in which global health work can be found in high income settings.

Table 24.1 An abbreviated list of global health employers and their related websites for job postings and career centres

Organisation	Description	Job postings info/career centre	Website
American Society of Tropical Medicine and Hygiene (ASTMH)	… dedicated to reducing the worldwide burden of tropical infectious diseases and improving global health.	http://jobbank.astmh.org	www.astmh.org/about-astmh
Bill and Melinda Gates Foundation	… we are impatient optimists working to reduce inequality.	www.gatesfoundation.org/Jobs	www.gatesfoundation.org
Centers for Disease Control and Prevention (CDC)	CDC works 24/7 to protect America from health, safety and security threats, both foreign and in the USA.	http://jobs.cdc.gov	www.cdc.gov
Doctors without Borders (Médicins sans Frontiéres)	Médecins Sans Frontiéres (MSF) is an international, independent, medical humanitarian organisation that delivers emergency aid to people affected by armed conflict, epidemics, natural disasters and exclusion from healthcare.	www.msf.org/en/work-msf/how-apply	www.msf.org
Global Health Hub	The Global Health Hub is a website that connects global health implementers to the information they need to do good work.	www.globalhealthhub.org/jobs-grants-listings/	www.globalhealthhub.org/
Global Health Service Partnership (GHSP)	We strive to strengthen health education and delivery in places facing a dire shortage of health professionals by working with partner countries to meet their long-term healthcare human resource needs.	http://seedglobalhealth.org/apply-2/	http://seedglobalhealth.org

(continued)

Table 24.1 (cont.)

Organisation	Description	Job postings info/career centre	Website
Johns Hopkins Bloomberg School of Public Health	Every day, the Bloomberg School works to keep millions around the world safe from illness and injury by pioneering new research, deploying knowledge in the field and educating tomorrow's public health leaders.	www.jhsph.edu/offices-and-services/career-services/	www.jhsph.edu/about/
Liverpool School of Tropical Medicine	… we work across the world, often in very difficult circumstances, to fulfil our mission of reducing the burden of sickness and mortality in disease-endemic countries.	www.lstmed.ac.uk/vacancies	www.lstmed.ac.uk
London School of Hygiene and Tropical Medicine	Our mission is to improve health and health equity in the UK and worldwide; working in partnership to achieve excellence in public and global health research, education and translation of knowledge into policy and practice.	https://jobs.lshtm.ac.uk	www.lshtm.ac.uk/index.html
Oxfam International	We use a combination of rights-based sustainable development programmes, public education, campaigns, advocacy, and humanitarian assistance in disasters and conflicts.	www.oxfam.org/en/work	www.oxfam.org/
Population Council	Our work allows couples to plan their families and chart their futures. We help people avoid HIV infection and access life-saving HIV services. And we empower girls to protect themselves and have a say in their own lives.	www.popcouncil.org/careers	www.popcouncil.org/

Organisation	Description	Jobs/Recruitment URL	About URL
Royal Society of Tropical Medicine and Hygiene	We organise academic conferences and other events for people committed to changing the face of global health.	https://rstmh.org/jobs	https://rstmh.org/
Saving Lives at Birth	We invite bold ideas for science and technology advances that prevent, detect or treat maternal and newborn problems at the time of birth.	https://savinglivesatbirth.net/apply	https://savinglivesatbirth.net/
SEED Global Health	We strive to strengthen health education and delivery in places facing a dire shortage of health professionals by working with partner countries to meet their long-term healthcare human resource needs.	http://seedglobalhealth.org/about/jobs/	http://seedglobalhealth.org/about
Tulane School of Public Health and Tropical Medicine	The academic programme … is designed to provide a comprehensive, practice-based, global health-focused education at both the undergraduate and graduate level.	www2.tulane.edu/jobs/	www2.tulane.edu/publichealth/academics/index.cfm
UK Agency for International Development (DFID)	DFID leads the UK's work to end extreme poverty, building a safer, healthier, more prosperous world … we're ending the need for aid by creating jobs, unlocking the potential of girls and women and helping to save lives when humanitarian emergencies hit.	www.gov.uk/government/organisations/department-for-international-development/about/recruitment#jobs	www.gov.uk/government/organisations/department-for-international-development/about
United Nations Childrens' Fund (UNICEF)	Working to improve the lives of children and their families. UNICEF also lobbies and partners with leaders, thinkers and policy makers to help all children realise their rights –especially the most disadvantaged.	www.unicef.org/about/employ/index_vacancies.html	www.unicef.org/about/

(continued)

Table 24.1 (cont.)

Organisation	Description	Job postings info/career centre	Website
United Nations Framework Convention on Climate Change (UNFCCC)	The ultimate objective of the convention is to stabilise greenhouse gas concentrations "at a level that would prevent dangerous anthropogenic (human induced) interference with the climate system."	https://unfccc.int/secretariat/ employment/recruitment	http://unfccc.int/2860.php
United States Agency for International Development (USAID)	USAID is the lead US government agency that works to end extreme global poverty and enable resilient, democratic societies to realise their potential.	www.usaid.gov/work-with-us/careers/ vacancy-announcements	www.usaid.gov/who-we-are
University of Washington Department of Global Health	The US Department of Global Health was established in 2007, bridging the schools of medicine and public health, with a mandate to harness the expertise and interdisciplinary power of all 16 UW schools and colleges.	http://globalhealth.washington. edu/about-us/jobs	http://globalhealth.washington. edu/about-us/who-we-are
Wellcome Trust	We support scientists and researchers, take on big problems, fuel imaginations, and spark debate.	https://wellcome.ac.uk/jobs	https://wellcome.ac.uk/about-us
World Medical Association (WMA)	The WMA's function has always been to constitute a free, open forum for the frank discussion, not of clinical problems, but of matters related to medical ethics, medical education, sociomedical affairs and medical topics generally.	www.wma.net/en/contact/ index.html	www.wma.net/

References

Australian Government Department of Health. 2016. Indigenous Australians' Health Programme. Accessed October 30, 2016. www.health.gov.au/internet/main/publishing.nsf/Content/indigenous-programme-lp.

Baker T, Weisman C and Piwoz e.1984. "us physicians in international health: Report of a Current Survey." *JAMA* 251(4):502–504.

Benzian H. 2002. Dental aid organisations: baseline data about their reality today. *International Dental Journal* 52(5):309–314.

Bussières JF, St-Arnaud C, Schunck C, Lamarre D and Jouberton F. 2000. The role of the pharmacist in humanitarian aid in Bosnia-Herzegovina: the experience of Pharmaciens Sans Frontieres. *Annals of Pharmacotherapy* 34(1):112–118.

California Department of Community Services and Development. 2016. "History." Accessed August 1, 2016. www.csd.ca.gov/AboutUs/History.

Crisp N. 2011. "Global health capacity and workforce development: turning the world upside down." *Infectious Disease Clinics of North America* 25(2):359–367.

Crisp N and Chen L. 2014. "Global supply of health professionals." *New England Journal of Medicine* 370(10):950–957.

Eichbaum Q, Hoverman A, Cherniak W, Evert J, Nezami E and Hall T. 2015. "Career opportunities in global health: a snapshot of the current employment landscape." *Journal of Global Health* 5(1).

Featherstone M, Lash S and Roland R. 1995. Global Modernities, Ch 2, Sage Publications Ltd.

Gupta R, Bush BP, Dorsey J, Moore E, van der Hoof Holstein C and Farmer PE. 2015. "Improving the global health workforce crisis: an evaluation of global health corps." *Lancet Global Health* 3(11):e679.

Koplan J, Bond CT, Merson MH, Srinath RK, Rodriguez MH, Sewankambo NK and Wasserheit JN. 2009. "Towards a common definition of global health." *Lancet* 373(9679):1993–1995.

HRSA. 2016. Dual Status-Health Centers that are both FQHC Look Alikes & Section 330 Grantees. Issued and last modified April 24, 2006. Accessed October 30, 2016. http://bphc.hrsa.gov/programrequirements/policies/pal200601.html.

Health Canada. 2016. Advancing the Health of First Nations. Accessed October, 30 2016. www.naho.ca/.

Kerry VB, Walensky RP, Tsai AC, Bergmark RW, Rouse C and Bangsberg DR. 2013. "US medical specialty global health training and the global burden of disease." *Journal of Global Health* 3(2):1–9.

Loh LC, Chae SR, Heckman JE and Rhee DS. 2015. "Ethical considerations of physician career involvement in global health work: a framework." *Journal of Bioethical Inquiry* 12(1):129–136.

Marmot M, Friel S, Bell R, Houweling T and Taylor S. 2008. "Closing the gap in a generation: health equity through action on the social determinants of health." *Lancet* 372(9650):1661–1669.

Nelson BD, Kasper J, Hibberd PL, Thea DM and Herlihy JM. 2012. "Developing a career in global health: considerations for physicians-in-training and academic mentors." *Journal of Graduate Medical Education* 4(3):301–306.

Palazuelos D and Dhillon R. 2016. "Addressing the 'global health tax' and 'wild cards': practical challenges to building academic careers in global health." *Academic Medicine* 91(1):30–35.

Peluso MJ1, Encandela J, Hafler JP and Margolis CZ. 2012. "Guiding principles for the development of global health education curricula in undergraduate medical education." *Medical Teacher* 34(8):653–658.

Petak W. 1985. "Four phases of emergency management: a challenge for public administration." *Public Administration Review* 45:3–7.

Ramsey A, Haq C, Gjerde C and Rothenberg D. 2004. "Career influence of an international health experience during medical school." *Family Medicine* 3(6):412–416.

Richards-Kortum R, Gray LV and Oden M. 2012. "Engaging undergraduates in global health technology innovation." *Science* 336(6080):430–431.

Saltman DC, Kidd MR, Jackson D and Cleary M. 2012. "Transportability of tertiary qualifications and CPD: a continuing challenge for the global health workforce." *BMC Medical Education* 12(51).

Umoren RA, Gardner A, Stone G, Helphinstine J, Machogu EP, Huskins JC, Johnson C, Ayuo P, Mining S and Litzelman D. 2015. "Career choices and global health engagement: 24-year follow-up of U.S. participants in the Indiana University-Moi University elective." *Healthcare* 3(4):185–189.

25 Standardising medical education's approach to global health

Are we moving forward?

Akshaya Neil Arya and Jill Allison

The changing landscape of global health in medical education

In 1995, the World Health Organization (WHO) defined the social accountability of medical schools as "the obligation to direct their education, research, and service activities towards addressing the priority health concerns of the community, region and the nation that they have a mandate to serve" (Boelen and Heck 1995). Socially accountable education prepares future health professionals to address the priority health concerns of society, often with a focus on vulnerable and marginalised populations. The commitment to strengthen global health capacity through community engagement, diversity and health equity has guided the development of new standards and practices. In Canada, new accreditation standards mandating service-learning for undergraduate medical education programmes increase the need to work with local partners to create opportunities based on community identified needs. This has lead to an increase in the development of programmes which require objectives and assessment as well as opportunities for reflection (CACMS 2015, p. 13).

International volunteer work has grown in popularity among students seeking admission to competitive programmes in the health field and medical students wanting to gain exposure to clinical experiences and find a competitive advantage to getting into a residency programme. Simultaneously, many have questioned the ethics, standards and frameworks that guide international and local experiences leading to the WEIGHT standards (see *Chapter 13*, Crump *et al.* 2010) and wide-reaching recommendations related to ethical reciprocal relations with hosts. Subsequently students have led the call to create guidelines around pre-departure training, recognising competencies, developing standards around local programming and developing global health offices, seeing this as the only way that clinical placements can advance the mission cited by Koplan *et al.* (2010) in defining global health as placing "a priority on improving health and achieving health equity for all people worldwide."

While interest in global health and international experiences has surged among undergraduates in recent years, structural factors contribute to patterns of uptake of global health electives within medical education. Despite this and literature describing positive effects of international experience on knowledge, skills and attitudes (Godkin and Savageau 2003, Thompson *et al.* 2003) at several schools in Canada, there has been a dramatic reduction in the number of medical students doing international electives during their training. Among the multiple factors contributing to this change are costs associated with international travel, safety concerns, students' recognition that international work can be challenging without proper supervision and/or training, and the commitment to learn about health equity in their own country and community. In addition, changing academic criteria and curricula can sometimes foreclose opportunities for "fitting in" a global health experience.

What standards for global health experiences miss

Internationalisation and accreditation standards can present challenges for students and faculty in medical education as well as the programming within the offices (i.e., international electives, service learning, diversity). Curricular and philosophical challenges are created when trying to locate appropriate opportunities for global health experiential (and sometimes even interprofessional) learning. The process is often shaped by neo-colonial assumptions that the community will benefit from the privilege, rather than acknowledging that the students are the beneficiaries.

While energy is spent conducting pre-departure training, less is spent looking at pedagogical value of experiences. For students issues such as reverse culture shock are widespread, yet post-return debriefing or support while intrinsically mandated is often neglected – seemingly overwhelmed by the logistics of bringing students together for group sessions or individual interviews. Even mandating reflection papers falls lower on the priority totem pole than clinical and class obligations, the need to prepare for residency match and to manage rotations away from the home school.

As universities explore, however haphazardly, the ethics of training relationships with the community in which they practise in Canada, there is little formal recognition of this overseas. There appears to be little real movement towards equity or discussion of true partnerships. The zeal to track and standardise, often inadequately resourced by the Canadian medical school, places a greater burden on the host. Asking host institutions to carry insurance for one or two preclinical students a year is prohibitive for some partners already bearing the costs of translation. Safety issues appropriately addressed for Canadian students can lead to discomfort with those working alongside partners without protective equipment such as gloves and masks. Long-standing relationships with non-academic partners may be negated or compromised.

In an effort to ensure standardised academic expectations, limitations are sometimes created around who is qualified to supervise. Many experiential opportunities might involve local healthcare experts such as nurses, or midwives, or clinical officers rather than physicians. Restricting supervisors of medical students to physicians, for example, forecloses opportunities to gain supervised experience within the scope of practice with other upskilled allied professionals, particularly in the preclinical years. This tacitly discounts inter-professional values and respect and undermines the learning opportunities around task shifting or sharing as a widely recognised strategy for cost saving, meeting human resources needs and addressing specific health needs in a community.

Ways forward

Aligning local and global

One of the challenges in developing and maintaining global health programming in educational institutions is trying to articulate experiences within a broader set of institutional values and philosophies. While global health programmes and opportunities are important elements in ensuring that diversity and global engagement are naturalised as part of the curriculum and within the pedagogical culture, there is still a gap in bringing global awareness locally. The impact of learning from local cultures and the values with which medical schools build their programmes must institutionalise the importance of such concepts as social accountability. Aligning the learning opportunities in a global health international elective, research or experiential opportunity with local activities reflecting the overarching values and mission of the medical school serve two important roles. First, it ensures that the institutional, community and political goals of medical service are aligned. Second, it ensures continuity across the learning continuum from global to local and back, rather than global health electives and teaching becoming a stand-alone interest in medical education. Drain *et al.* (2009) argue that global health training is most effective during residency where clinical skills and levels of practice afford a deeper engagement with patient populations. However, if perspective and a broader understanding of health systems, global health governance and the social inequities behind much of the burden of disease are the goals of global health programming it would seem that global health learning opportunities are important throughout medical training. In reality, global health is less about service delivery and more about understanding and addressing the deeper structural issues – economic, political, climatic, and conflict-related – that shape inequities on a regional and global level than obtaining particular knowledge and skills.

Partnerships

Together with national standards and policies related to competencies, ethics, codes of conduct and training, most institutions have developed their own set of standards around learning objectives, behavioural expectations and preparation and debriefing. Although much has been done to incorporate global health learning into the pedagogical framework of North American medical schools, there remains a dearth of research and literature on the interests and expectations of host communities, particularly in low and middle income countries (LMICs).

Global health standards should include a measure of engagement with receiving institutions ensuring that partnership and mutual benefit is built into any training opportunities for students. Rather than providing opportunities for students from the Global North to gain experience in a system built around presumed inequalities (*Chapter 18*), global health programmes should ensure that their students are embedded in a systemic partnership with mutual goals and expectations, objectives that meet the needs of all parties and include an assets-based approach to any international learning experience. Finding out what hosts want is one step along this process (*Chapter 20*). Co-development of a common agenda with communities to determine how such relationships might be mutually beneficial is predicated on strong relationships with the communities whom schools hope to engage.

Offering creative alternatives to standard clinical electives in undergraduate medical education can provide enrichment opportunities that establish transformative learning early in student careers. Collaborative approaches that allow students from one university to participate in programmes developed for and by other schools enriches the range of possibilities and fosters a deeper collaborative network among partners in LMICs and also locally.

Educational integration

The need for consistency and continuity in standards of global health education has become increasingly important as more and more students undertake training opportunities abroad as part of their medical education. Global travel is more accessible and students often feel they must incorporate an international experience within their programmes but often do not see it as a vital part of their career development. This is evidenced in the timing of many electives when students seek an international experience either before their clinical training begins or after they have been matched to a residency programme. This may suggest that they do not see the international elective as contributing to the strength of their residency application, but rather as a benefit to personal growth. While this, in itself, is an important objective, it is also imperative that global health experiences not be constituted as separate but rather embedded in the principles of health equity and health advocacy in the broader medical education framework.

Certificates

A number of medical schools in Canada and the USA have developed specific concentrations or certificate programmes that allow students to engage more deeply in the issues related to global health.

While concentrations offer students a deeper engagement and an opportunity for enriched and committed learning in global health, the objectives are generally focused on the students. Partner communities are engaged but sometimes expected to provide the experiences on a continuous basis even if their own circumstances change. Concentrations are attractive to students and provide opportunities for those who are committed to increasing their experience and knowledge. However, there must also be solid grounding on key issues in global health throughout the curriculum in order for all students to make concepts relevant to their practice in the future. Rowson *et al.* (2012) suggest that the "globalised doctor," "humanitarian doctor" and "policy doctor" each have different educational requirements. How can important skills attained in a global health programme such as engagement, awareness and global citizenship be measured? (Mill *et al.* 2010). There is a need for an evaluation framework to assess the long-term impact of undergraduate certificate programmes beyond the satisfaction and pedagogical competencies among students who participate.

Administrative structures

The administration of international global health electives may occur through a global health office, a clinical department or general undergrad office. As opposed to the USA, where global health offices may be university-wide or in schools of public health, across Canada, global health offices tend to be in medical schools or health sciences, where they have had a variety of configurations and staff. Many are organised around full-time faculty, often clinical faculty with experience in international health delivery and/or research. Some offices are stand-alone programmes with managers who may or may not have health backgrounds. The lessons from our experience may be equally appropriate to university-wide global health offices, to those in public health schools and other professional faculties, whichever entity is in a position to champion programming.

Global health offices provide consistency across the learning continuum, from undergraduate programmes to graduate or residency programmes, ensuring that learner and faculty experiences are consistent with the values and commitment that institutions want to convey in their global health engagement. Global health offices are also well placed to support local service learning programmes and opportunities, helping to frame these as part of the continuum towards health equity. This approach helps to reduce the image of the exotic in international experiences and bridge the gap between local and global.

Regardless of the structure, formal empowerment and a well-resourced programme are important. A global health office provides a number of advantages to faculties of health sciences, whether the offices are housed within a particular faculty or shared across an interdisciplinary set of programmes. The office facilitates the transmission of values related to equity and fairness, global citizenship across the range of global health programming whether it is pedagogical, research, or advocacy. It is a key function of global health structures to ensure that global health experiences are not separate adventures that risk being voluntourism experiences rather than ethically sound pedagogical opportunities rooted in partnerships, continuity and respect.

References

Boelen C and Heck JE. 1995. "Defining and Measuring the Social Accountability of Medical Schools. Geneva: World Health Organization." WHO document WHO/ HRH/95.7. http://apps.who.int/iris/bitstream/10665/59441/1/WHO_HRH_95.7.pdf.

CACMS. 2015. Committee on Accreditation of Canadian Medical Schools. Standards and Elements. www.afmc.ca/pdf/CACMS_Standards_and_Elements_June_2014_ Effective_July12015.pdf.

Crump JA, Sugarman J and the Working Group on Ethics Guidelines for Global Health. 2010. Training Ethics and Best Practice Guidelines for Training Experiences in Global Health. *American Journal of Tropical Medicine and Hygiene* 83(6):1178–1182.

Drain PK, Holmes KK, Skeff KM, Hall TL and Gardner P. 2009. "Global Health Training and International Clinical Rotations during Residency: Current Status, Needs, and Opportunities." *Academic Medicine* 84(3):320–325.

Godkin M and Savageau J. 2003. "The effect of medical students' international experiences on attitudes towards serving underserved multicultural populations." *Family Medicine* 35(3):273–278.

Koplan JP, Bond TC, Merson MH, Reddy KS, Rodriguez MH, Sewankambo NK and Wasserheit JN, for the Consortium of Universities for Global Health Executive Board. 2009. "Towards a common definition of global health." *Lancet* 373:1993–1995.

Mill J, Astle B, Ogilvie L and Gastaldo D. 2010. "Linking global citizenship, undergraduate nursing education, and professional nursing: curricular innovation in the 21st century." *Advanced Nursing Science* 33(3):E1–E11. doi: 10.1097/ ANS.0b013e3181eb416f.

Rowson M, Smith A, Hughes R, Johnson O, Maini A, Martin S, Martineau F, Miranda JJ, Pollit V, Wake R, Willott C and Yudkin JS. 2012. "The evolution of global health teaching in undergraduate medical curricula." *Globalization and Health* 8:35. www. globalizationandhealth.com/content/8/1/35.

Thompson M, Huntington M, Hunt D, Pinsky L and Brodie J. 2003. "Educational effects of international health electives on US and Canadian medical students and residents: a literature review." *Academic Medicine* 78(3):342–347.

26 Graduate global health practicums

Understanding the implications and opportunities

Shweta Dhawan, Emily Kocsis, Michelle Amri and Simone Mohrs

Introduction

As globalisation improves access to regions of the world, interest in global training opportunities has increased exponentially in a variety of disciplines (Kerry *et al.* 2011, Macfarlane *et al.* 2008). In the field of global health, the surge in interest for training opportunities that extend beyond the typical classroom setting is particularly acute. Many education institutions in high-income countries have responded by investing in academic global health pro-grammes that provide clinical and non-clinical placements in low resource settings as a complement to traditional curricula (Crump *et al.* 2010). This heightened enthusiasm for global health practicum opportunities – among students and university leaders alike – presents a myriad of complicated ethical implications.

Practicums are a standard component of many global health graduate training curriculums. Given the interdisciplinarity and breadth of the global health field, course-based graduate global health programmes, or public health programmes with a global health specialisation typically offer students the opportunity to pursue a "practice-based practicum," that is, neither clinical nor research oriented. Practice-based practicums typically range from 6 weeks to 6 months, and offer students the opportunity to pursue a variety of positions related to health, including working as epidemiologists, food tech-nologists, programme assistants, research assistants, health promoters, and numerous others. As more and more graduate programmes "internationalise" traditional curricula to include experiential learning opportunities abroad, it is both surprising and worrisome to note that in comparison to clinical place-ments, ethical considerations associated with practice-based practicums have received much less consideration.

We recognise that there is significant heterogeneity in the nature of practi-cums depending on local settings, and that students enrolled in non-health programmes also may conduct international practica on topics related to health. However, the focus of this chapter is to critically review the unique considerations of practice-based practicums pursued by global and public health graduate students in an international setting. The chapter is informed by the existing literature on this subject, but to a larger extent draws on the experiences and tacit knowledge of the authors, their colleagues, and their peers, through reflective practice, as both students and practitioners in global health. By drawing attention to the experiences of graduate students pursuing international practicums – a group that is woefully underrepresented in the literature – this chapter encourages efforts to reflect on global health practicums and develop and implement practices to mitigate their adverse consequences.

Key considerations

Broader implications may pose greater concerns and risk

I also had to interact with many cultures and backgrounds on a daily basis (although I had prior experience living abroad, it was generally an interchange between two cultures rather than a large melting pot (that) is the Asia Pacific Region).

(Personal communication 2016)

Global health by its very nature is an interdisciplinary field that views the health of communities through a myriad of lenses. Graduate studies in global health reflect this interdisciplinary nature, providing students with the opportunity to explore a number of disciplines related to global health, including: health policy, epidemiology, health promotion, and health systems management. Effectively this generalist approach gives student a "taste" of many different skill sets relevant to global health, providing the rudimentary foundation for multidisciplinary, multi-stakeholder interactions during practicum placements.

This broadened scope of interactions is unlike other fields where the nature of work and engagements is somewhat more niche specific. For example, medical students pursuing international clinical placements are confined to a particular healthcare setting, with the student engaged in one-on-one work with patients and local healthcare staff. Conversely, due to the interdisciplinary skills acquired during global health training and the nature of global health work, a much larger segment of society will likely interact with the student. In any given practicum, the student may interact in complex and unpredictable ways with patients, local community members, host organisation representatives, government employees, research teams, and various other stakeholders. While this affords students exciting opportunities to expand the scope of their learning, a poorly conceived practicum runs the risk of causing more generalised, community-wide impacts.

Overestimation or misunderstanding skills

When I explained to local community members that my degree was in global health, more times than not the next question was: "So you're a doctor of some kind?"

(Personal communication 2016)

In the case of international clinical electives, a familiar narrative involves host healthcare facilities overestimating or misunderstanding the students' skills. Students are given responsibilities beyond their capabilities, which may result in a variety of adverse consequences for both the student and medical facility. Although the circumstances are different, graduate students undertaking practice-based practicums abroad are by no means immune to this phenomenon.

The nascent nature of global health as an area of study lends itself to misinterpretation of what the students' actual skills and capabilities are. Given the history of medical service trips, communities in low resource settings have had considerable exposure to students with skills in clinical health. However, only relatively recently has this new type of health trainee, with expertise in a variety of non-clinical disciplines, existed in low resource settings. This may create a climate of misunderstanding, with students potentially placed in settings for which they are not yet prepared. In such cases, unwarranted or unethical actions may lead to stress, guilt, or dangerous situations on the part of the student, while the host organisation may compromise the standard of service it provides by hosting an unqualified student.

Risk of workforce displacement and dependency

> All work I did could have been completed by a local student as well[,] hence I have denied someone else a great opportunity.
>
> (Personal communication 2016)

Global health practicums offer graduate students a fascinating opportunity to broaden their learning and engage in a rewarding exchange of knowledge (Cole *et al.* 2012). In return, host organisations benefit from the unique perspective and skill set the graduate trainee has to offer. However, often disregarded during this seemingly beneficial exchange are the impacts associated with providing a "job" to an international student on the local workforce.

As temporary members of a local workforce, practicum students can significantly impact the ebb and flow of the local labour pool depending on the role and nature of their work. Graduate students who provide a specialised service may make significant contributions during their practicum, but it may be difficult to replace their service when the student departs, leaving a gap in service delivery (Crump and Sugarman 2008). Conversely, graduate students may take on logistical and supporting roles within organisations that could have been fulfilled by trained local personnel. As a result, local professionals are not only deprived of opportunities to learn, but also of future employment that may result from this engagement. The nature of these interactions has far reaching consequences on both the local personnel and the health system in offering sustainable health services to the community.

Lack of regulatory mandate

> I was ultimately responsible for my own growth and even created my own role in my placement.
>
> (Personal communication 2016)

"Internationalising" traditional curricula to include experiential learning opportunities abroad is a common structure across several clinical disciplines, including medicine, occupational therapy, physiotherapy, nursing, and various others (McInally *et al.* 2015). International clinical practicums conducted as part of these programmes are subject to multiple levels of oversight and review through professional colleges that protect and serve the public interest by maintaining the standards of practice of the profession. As such, when students in a regulated clinical profession go abroad to conduct an international practicum, their actions are not only the responsibility of their university, but also of an overarching regulatory body. Similarly, for students conducting research as part of their practicum, research ethics boards regulate the professional conduct during international research activities and are mandated to protect the rights of the participants in the study, ensuring that the highest ethical standards are met.

In the case of graduate global health practicums, however, formalised safeguards to protect the student and host organisation are largely absent. In most cases, a practicum coordinator oversees the selection of the practicum, and supports the student to create a learning plan and objectives for the placement. However, the degree of support offered is highly variable between institutions, and more importantly, institutions are not mandated to provide this type of regulation. As such, practice-based global health placements pursued by graduate students are situated in a precarious grey area, with little institutionalised regulation to prevent unethical consequences.

Rethinking global health practicums: reflective practice, mentorship and programme structures

The complicated nature of global health training opportunities presents an array of challenges and benefits to both students and host communities. While ethical challenges may sometimes be inevitable, there are also opportunities to implement practices that mitigate these risks. We highlight opportunities at individual, dyadic, and institutional levels to mitigate the potential ethical issues associated with international graduate practicums in global health.

Individual: the role of reflective practice

> Mandatory reflection pieces had to be submitted but there was no active dialogue or mentorship to support reflection.
>
> (Personal communication 2016)

Course-based global health programmes typically follow the structure of classroom-based learning supplemented by a practicum, with performance on both components evaluated based on assessments by course instructors or supervisors. While many students subconsciously reflect on their learning experiences, there is very little focus on using reflective practice as a tool for learning from one's own experiences.

As a tool, reflective practice can instruct graduate students pursuing global health practicums in two ways: reflecting-in-action during the practicum experience and reflection-on-action after completion of the practicum (Jenkins 2007). Both experiences start with describing the events that set the scene and answering questions such as: "How do you feel about the situation? How do your feelings relate to any action? If you 'step back' from this, does it look different? Are there ethical, moral, or social issues that might be explored?" (Morgan 2009). These questions provide the framework for interrogating the values, norms, and practices that inform the practicum, urging the student to view their experience through a more critical lens.

While there are certainly aspects of this narrative present within the global health arena, as a learning tool, reflective practice requires greater emphasis within the context of graduate global health practicums (Osterman and Kottkamp 1993). Graduate programmes that employ reflective learning can also support students to become critically engaged with ethical global health practice and respond to unfamiliar settings typically encountered in a global health practicum. Academic institutions can help promote this skill set by offering mandatory courses on reflective practice prior to practicums, providing tools to support reflections, and creating systems to actively review reflections in the presence of a mentor.

Between individuals: institutional structures to encourage mentorship

> I was provided with zero mentorship or pre training prior to my practicum. We were essentially instructed to find our own placements which could be anywhere in the world.
>
> (Personal communication 2016)

Through academic supervisors, on-site supervisors and staff, the supports required for institutional mentorship are already built into the academic learning environment. In preparation for the practicum, a mentor – often a supervisor engaged with the academic institution and knowledgeable about the student's academic activities – can play a pivotal role in information exchange and knowledge acquisition (Mullen 1994). Furthermore, mentors can offer safe spaces where students are exposed to diverse ideas and opinions, and are willing to open themselves up and admit their shortcomings (Cole *et al.* 2015). This open environment allows the mentor to help students identify their learning goals, exchange knowledge on host partners' objectives, and consequently act as a liaison in designing a practicum that would meet both of their expectations. During the placement itself, mentoring from a host institution may support the student in understanding the host's expectations, acquiring cross-cultural communication skills, and advancing their own learning goals.

Upon completion of the placement, timely follow-up and reflection under the supervision of both the academic and placement mentors may prompt active reflection on the sustainability and long-term implications of practicum activities. In addition to supporting activities within the practicum, the benefits of investing in mentorship structures may also extend to the institutional level, providing a solid foundation to build authentic, productive partnerships to build strong graduate global health programmes.

Beyond individuals: effective programme structures

In comparison to other disciplines, global health education is a relatively new field with constantly evolving learning processes and approaches. Higher education institutions around the world have approached this field from a variety of perspectives, resulting in diverse learning models and outcomes. While there is no infallible model for creating authentic, productive experiences for the student, institution, and host community, the unintended implications of graduate practicums may be prevented with programme structures designed to identify, mitigate and resolve problematic issues. Such programme structures may take on a variety of forms; however, we identify two key aspects for programme administrators to consider within the context of graduate practicums: personnel training and developing authentic partnerships.

First, increased resources should be directed towards training personnel, such as practicum coordinators, faculty supervisors, and on-site mentors. The training provided may include both competencies in mentoring and immersive learning opportunities that orient staff to practicum projects and their scope of engagement. Additionally, resources must also be diverted to providing students with financial support to afford them with the opportunity to engage in fair and equitable global health practicums. This is particularly important given the growing number of unpaid practicum opportunities overseas and financial barriers students face in pursuing longer-term practicums that may allow for delivering of greater quality or quantity of work.

Second, processes to create authentic partnerships with host organisations and communities should be further established and maintained. A 2015 study found that nine out of the 19 (47 percent) global health programmes reviewed did not conduct a formalised needs assessment of partner organisations during the process of finding practicum sites (Zaidi *et al.* 2015). Active discourse during the process of developing practicum terms, conditions, and learning objectives may mitigate some of the unintended consequences of global health practicums. Further, comprehensive guidelines should be developed around the roles and responsibilities of actors involved in the practicum, protocols for communication, timelines, monitoring, and the evaluation of outputs and outcomes.

Concluding thoughts

This review seeks to highlight some of the key ethical implications associated with graduate students engaged in practice-based global health placements. While there are similarities between graduate global health students engaged in international practicums and their counterparts in clinical or research-based programmes, the unique ethical dilemmas facing this group of students are often overlooked. As graduate global health programmes multiply, considerations around the scope of interactions during practicums, workforce displacement concerns, risk of overestimating or misunderstanding student skills, and the absence of regulatory fixtures require further critical discourse.

There is a pressing need to focus greater scholarly attention on this unique group of students by encouraging reflective practice, improving mentorship support, and improving programme structures. Like any emerging discipline, rethinking and refining the training standards that build the global health workforce will be a slow, iterative, and potentially difficult process. With concerted, authentic reflection and dialogue, we hope this will provide a more equitable, mutually beneficial practicum experience for institutions, students, and host communities alike.

Acknowledgements

Donald Cole, Stephanie Nixon, and the many peers and colleagues who honestly and openly shared their experiences.

References

Cole, D.C., Plugge, E.H., & Jackson, S.F. 2012. "Placements in global health masters' programmes: what is the student experience?" *Journal of Public Health* fds086. http://doi.org/10.1093/pubmed/fds086.
Cole, D.C., Johnson, N., Mejia, R., McCullough, H., Turcotte-Tremblay, A.M., Barnoya, J., & Falabella Luco, S. 2015. "Mentoring health researchers globally: Diverse experiences, programmes, challenges and responses." *Global Public Health* 1–16.
Crump, J.A., & Sugarman, J. 2008. "Ethical considerations for short-term experiences by trainees in global health." *JAMA 300*(12):1456–1458.
Crump JA, Sugarman J & the Working Group on Ethics Guidelines for Global Health. 2010. Ethics and Best Practice Guidelines for Training Experiences in Global Health. *American Journal of Tropical Medicine and Hygiene* 83(6):1178–1182.
Jenkins, K. 2007. "Thinking differently about reflective practice." *Public Health Research Education & Development (PHRED) Focus* 16(2): 1.

Kerry, V.B., Ndung'u, T., Walensky, R.P., Lee, P.T., Kayanja, V.F.I.B., & Bangsberg, D.R. 2011. "Managing the Demand for Global Health Education." *PLOS Med* 8(11): e1001118. http://doi.org/10.1371/journal.pmed.1001118.

Macfarlane, S.B., Jacobs, M., & Kaaya, E.E. 2008. "In the Name of Global Health: Trends in Academic Institutions." *Journal of Public Health Policy* 29(4):383–401. http://doi.org/10.1057/jphp.2008.25.

McInally, W., Metcalfe, S., & Garner, B. 2015. Enriching the Student Experience Through a Collaborative Cultural Learning Model. Retrieved from www.ncbi.nlm.nih.gov/pubmed/26376575.

Morgan, G. 2009. "Reflective practice and self-awareness." *Perspectives in Public Health* 129(4):161.

Mullen, E.J. 1994. "Framing the Mentoring Relationship as an Information Exchange." *Human Resource Management Review* 4(3):257. Retrieved from http://ezproxy.library.dal.ca/login?url=http://search.ebscohost.com/login.aspx?direct=true&db=bth&AN=5787353&site=ehost-live.

Osterman, K.F., & Kottkamp, R.B. 1993. Reflective Practice for Educators: Improving Schooling through Professional Development. Newbury Park, CA: Corwin Press.

Zaidi, M., Haddad, L., & Lathrop, E. 2015. Global Health Opportunities in Obstetrics and Gynecology Training: Examining Engagement Through an Ethical Lens. Retrieved from www.ncbi.nlm.nih.gov/pubmed/26324736.

27 Short-term experiences in global health in the digital world

Blogs, social media and more

Heather Lukolyo, Elizabeth M. Keating and Sabrina Butteris

Social media platforms (SMPs) are internet-based tools which support and promote the exchange of user-developed content, allowing individuals and communities to communicate electronically. They are becoming more a part of modern life and participation in SMPs by the general public has increased from 8 percent in 2005 to 72 percent in 2012 (Von Muhlen and Ohno-Machado 2012, Bernhardt *et al.* 2014). Even in 2010, social media use among US young adults was found to be as high as 86 percent (Madden 2010). A 2012 review of social media adoption by health professionals found rates of 64–96 percent among medical students and 13–47 percent among clinicians (Von Muhlen and Ohno-Machado 2012).

SMPs, include: Facebook (a social networking site), YouTube (a video sharing site), Instagram (a photo sharing application), Twitter (a microblogging application), Whatsapp (an instant messaging service), Linked-In (a professional networking site), and blogs (online journaling). New tools (e.g. Snapchat, an instant photo sharing application) are frequently emerging, making some older tools outdated (e.g., MySpace, a social networking site). While these tools can be used for personal communication and to enhance professional networking and education, they may present potential risks to patients and providers regarding the distribution of inaccurate or poor-quality information, damage to professional image, breaches of confidentiality, and violation of personal–professional boundaries (Ventola 2014, Lagu and Greyson 2010).

The proliferation of SMP use over the past decade has coincided with a continued surge of interest in global health by medical trainees (medical students, residents and fellows). While guidelines exist for SMP use in many US medical schools and residency programmes (Wells 2011, Kind *et al.* 2010), social media savvy medical trainees are pursuing short-term experiences in global health (STEGH) without specific guidance on how to conduct themselves in the digital world during their time abroad. Trainees are likely to experience a range of emotions during STEGHs such as social isolation, homesickness, culture shock, and frustration (Butteris *et al.* 2014, Dell *et al.* 2014). Some may wish to process these emotions with the digital community, which offers opportunities for experiential sharing and communication with others independent of location.

Challenges of social media in the global health setting

Even the most experienced travellers are likely to pass through stages of culture shock when they are immersed in a culture different from their own (Pedersen 1994, Butteris and Conway 2009). It is during the second and third phases identified by Pederson (the rejection where the new culture feels difficult and one can only see the differences between the two cultures, and regression where one glorifies one's home country and is critical of the new with a superior attitude) that one is at high risk for interpersonal conflict, cultural misunderstandings, culturally insensitive behaviours, and inappropriate judgements. When trainees turn to SMPs to help them process or cope, they may be unaware of their reactions to the new culture or environment. SMPs allow for real-time complete transparency of thoughts, which can be damaging in the context of reactions to culture shock. Even a well-intentioned post that lacks understanding of cultural nuances may come across as culturally insensitive and undermine professional relationships.

Trainees may also utilise SMPs to project a certain image of oneself to friends, family, and colleagues back home. For example, a trainee on a 2-week STEGH to sub-Saharan Africa may post about how grateful they are to "serve the children of Africa," even if the primary outcome of the experience was their own growth and education. Others may use SMPs to satisfy an eager audience back home who is awaiting updates. This audience, which may include parents who are nervous about sending their children abroad, may be eager to brag about the work their children are doing. Other trainees may feel so struck by what they see and experience that they turn to SMPs to try to share this with others back home.

At times trainees may violate boundaries via SMPs that one would not dream of in one's own country. This could be due to a lapse in judgement in which the trainee forgets that the same principles of privacy, confidentiality, and protection of vulnerable populations in their home institution should also apply abroad. They may erroneously presume that images or posts would never make it back to the communities in which they were taken. Whatever the motivation, SMP use by learners in the global health setting has unique challenges. See *Table 27.1* for examples of these challenges. Below, we discuss challenges posed by various types of SMPs.

Blogging

Increasingly, global health trainees and workers are creating blogs as a way to keep a network of friends and families updated on their experiences abroad. While blogging may be a way to process intense emotions, one may question whether this type of processing should be done on a public forum. It may unfairly colour the opinions of people at home of the trainee, that country, or the institution. A private, appropriate alternative to expressing oneself via blog would be personal journaling.

Some US training programmes use blogs written by global health trainees as a way to show both programme leaders and funders what their trainees are doing in-country (University of Minnesota 2016). While some of these are reviewed by US preceptors prior to posting, the preceptor still may not be able to view these entries through the lens of the global health setting they reference. This induces some bias that cannot be resolved without involving local staff. Alternatively, other US programmes specifically restrict or prohibit their trainees from maintaining blogs during their time abroad.

Social network posts

Social network platforms such as Facebook and Twitter, much like public blogs, offer the opportunity to share updates with friends via posts composed of text and audiovisual material. Posting on these pages is instant and can be impulsive. Often people will have a reaction to something and post it on their page before processing. For the current generation of trainees who have grown up expressing themselves on SMPs, it may be even more challenging to see how posting during STEGHs may be wrong. If posts are later realised to be inappropriate, they can be difficult to remove. If one is able to take down a post, in the interim others may have seen it and reflected negatively on the trainee or institution.

Instant photo sharing

Photography in low resource settings is rife with ethical conundrums; when photos can be shared instantly on photo or video sharing applications such as Instagram and YouTube, the risks are even greater. Even if a photographer thinks an image shared on social media will be viewed only by a network of friends, depending on privacy settings the photo may be viewable by the general public. A friend may share or take a screenshot image of the photo and share it with a much wider than intended audience, possibly allowing it to make its way back to the host community.

The safety and privacy of these vulnerable populations such as patients or children in orphanages are compromised by photographs that identify them and their locations (Devakumar *et al.* 2013). Current international guidelines for clinical photography are inconsistently applied or enforced, particularly for patients in the Global South (Macintosh 2006). Even if such guidelines exist locally, visiting trainees may not be aware of them and violate them unknowingly.

Even when verbal consent is obtained, there is an unequal balance of power between the photographer and those being photographed, which could result in subjects being taken advantage of. This power disparity is even more pronounced in low resource settings (Devakumar *et al.* 2013). Photography subjects are likely unaware how their photos will be used. Photography of children adds another layer of complexity, as they are unable to consent.

In addition, photographs of patients or suffering individuals such as in international disasters warrant special consideration. Often these photos would not meet ethical standards commonly applied in medical practice in developed countries (Calain 2013). Some have called these images of suffering "starvation pornography" or "pornography of poverty" (Nathanson 2013). These photos imply that the host community is a land of misery and suffering. They also imply that communities have failed in caring for their own people and that something must be done from outside the local setting. While drastic images of the "suffering other" may raise awareness of an issue, they also risk undermining both the human dignity of photo subjects and the host community.

Visitors who insert themselves into these types of photos during their STEGHs may reflect an interest in appearing to have had a positive impact abroad (Kascaksamp and Dasgupta 2016). Kascaksamp and Dasgupta (2016) explain, "They use their privilege to take a photograph that makes them feel as though they are engaging with the community, but instead they are making themselves the hero in a story about 'suffering Africa.'"

Instant messaging

The smartphone application called Whatsapp is an instant messaging service popularly used abroad as a cheaper, although less secure, mode of communication than text messaging due to lack of SMS fees. When a message is sent from a phone via Whatsapp, the data are first sent to commercial servers via the internet, where the recipient devices retrieve messages (Drake *et al.* 2016). In 2014, 4.6 million accounts on a similar instant messaging service were breached and relevant data posted online (BBC News 2016). Thus, when used by medical trainees to discuss clinical cases, the security of patient data is jeopardised. Care must be taken to ensure anonymity when using this service to discuss patient data.

Positive aspects of social media

While there are many potential drawbacks of social media use during global health experiences, there are also some possible benefits. The use of SMPs are not well studied in the context of culture shock and adjustment to a new environment. It is unclear to what extent being a member of an online social network may mitigate or propagate some of the emotions that individuals experience during their time abroad. While social media use when far from home may reduce feelings of homesickness, spending one's evenings looking at what friends back home are posting on social media may preclude trainees from actually interacting with locals in their host communities, something that international host preceptors have reported is important to them (Lukolyo *et al.* 2016).

Several SMPs, including Twitter and Whatsapp, have been documented as means for medical education and case discussion (Hossain *et al.* 2015, Johnston *et al.* 2015). Applications such as Whatsapp could be used as a tool to keep trainees on STEGHs connected with colleagues at other sites and/ or mentors back home, thereby potentially lessening social isolation. Some residents use Twitter and other forms of social media for medical education, as they can be accessed at times convenient for the trainee and are easily stored, searchable, and accessible (Cheston *et al.* 2013, Galiatsatos *et al.* 2016). Because social media can be accessed from anywhere in the world with an internet connection, this would enable trainees, even in remote settings, to access learning materials housed on social media.

Social media use has surged in both developed and developing countries making it a potential platform for raising awareness and advocacy to target audiences back home or in the global health setting (Pew Research Center 2016). There are increasing reports in the medical literature of successful social media-driven campaigns, from medical students using SMPs for health promotion as part of the Ebola response in Sierra Leone and Guinea (Chapman *et al.* 2016, Fung *et al.* 2016) to public health researchers exploring the use of social media to deliver HIV information to patients and combat stigma (Garett *et al.* 2016).

Guidelines for digital professionalism while abroad

To our knowledge, there are no existing guidelines in the medical literature for digital media use for trainees completing STEGHs. We draw upon several domestically focused guidelines to propose guidelines for responsible digital media use in an international setting (Icahn School of Medicine at Mount Sinai 2016, Baylor College of Medicine 2016, Regions Hospital 2010).
     Institutional policies and practices:

Social Media/Photography Contract

Consider having trainees sign a social media and photography contract prior to their STEGH (UW Health 2016) and require reading related to responsible photography (Unite for Sight 2016). This encourages critical thinking about the ramifications of social media use while abroad.

Speak for Yourself

Tell trainees to be clear that they are speaking for themselves and not on behalf of their institution on SMPs. Adding a disclaimer such as "the views expressed on this page are my own and do not reflect the views of my employer" is often appropriate. Ensure that trainees know that even if they utilise a disclaimer, especially when engaged in STEGHs, they will be perceived as an ambassador of their training programme and even their country.

Individual practices:

Use Good Judgement and Confirm Accuracy

Remind trainees that they are responsible for what they post on SMPs. Encourage them to be respectful and think about how others might perceive their postings. Tell them to check the accuracy of what they are posting. Ensure they know that inappropriate postings can damage relationships, undermine professional reputations for both them and their organisation, and discourage teamwork. If they are in doubt, tell them not to post it.

Appreciate Permanency

Remind trainees that once something is posted online it is difficult to remove it completely. Even if deleted later, it may be stored somewhere the trainee had not anticipated. Future employers can often access this information and may use it to evaluate the trainee.

Seek Guidance

Many hospitals and institutions have social media policies, communications departments, or global health programmes that may be well versed in digital media (see for example: Regions Hospital 2010, University of Michigan 2011, Baylor College of Medicine 2016). Consider contacting them for guidance.

Privacy considerations:

Protect Patient Privacy

Ensure trainees know that disclosing patient information, including photographs, without permission is unadvisable and may go against local policies as well as policies of the trainee's home institution.

Safeguard Trainee Privacy

Make sure trainees know the privacy policies of the sites where they are posting information. Even if they think they are posting to a few trusted people, depending on privacy settings the general public may still be able to access these photos. Further, content posted on SMPs or even private emails may be forwarded to a wider than intended audience. Privacy settings may not be easily accessible or changed, so be sure that trainees do their research prior to posting on a site.

Philosophical considerations:

The "Would-I-post-this-back-home?" Litmus Test

With all posts that involve host individuals, ask the trainee if he/she would feel comfortable posting the same photos of such people from their home institution. If the trainee would not post a photo containing patients' faces at his/her home institution, he/she has no business doing so in the host community.

Utilise Other Fora for Reflection and Emotional Processing

Although they may lack the immediate gratification and interactivity of SMPs, other avenues may be more appropriate for reflection and emotional processing during a STEGH. These include personal communication (e.g. a phone call) or a personal journal, as indicated above. Reflective practice has been shown to be beneficial for trainees in medical education and is acknowledged by the Accreditation Council for Graduate Medical Education as an important component of professional development (Wald and Reis 2010, Wald *et al.* 2009).

Conclusions

The world is more connected than ever before due in part to technological advances including SMPs. Although there may be some benefits to using SMPs while engaging in STEGHs, their use is fraught with challenges, especially in the context of culture shock and power imbalances. Users must critically analyse their participation in social media during their time abroad and consider its implications. Institutions that send trainees abroad may wish to develop guidelines to guide their trainees and ensure digital professionalism.

References

Baylor College of Medicine. 2016. "Baylor College of Medicine Social Media Policies." Accessed February 8, 2016. http://intranet.bcm.edu/?tmp=/pa/socialmedia.

BBC News. 2016. "Snapchat Hack Affects 4.6 Million Users – BBC News." Accessed August 22, 2016. www.bbc.co.uk/news/technology-25572661.

Bernhardt, Jay M., Julia Alber, and Robert S. Gold. 2014. "A Social Media Primer for Professionals Digital Dos and Don'ts." *Health Promotion Practice* 15(2):168–172.

Butteris, Sabrina, and James Conway. 2009. "Towards Best Practices in the Global Health Institute: Culture Shock and Communication –Avoiding Misadventures

Table 27.1 Global health digital professionalism case studies

Case	Unintended negative consequences
While working in Lesotho, a resident is asked to "friend" a patient on Facebook.	This is almost always inappropriate, unless the doctor–patient relationship has ended. If that is the case, it would be inappropriate to discuss health information.
A medical student on a STEGH in India blogs about the frustrations of working in a low resource hospital (delayed lab results, medicine shortages, power outages). Another blog post expresses frustrations that a local colleague always smells poorly, takes overly long lunch breaks, and is incompetent in the clinic.	If local staff were to see the post, it could be interpreted as judgemental and could damage professional relationships. His post is also inevitably coloured by his newness to the setting as well as his own culture shock. Further, this is an inappropriate forum to raise concerns about a colleague. There are appropriate ways for addressing concerns in the workplace, such as talking to a supervisor.
A paediatric resident on a STEGH in Zambia posts on Instagram a picture of a baby who was just discharged from the national referral hospital, expressing joy and best wishes to the family.	Without written patient/representative consent, this is a violation of patient confidentiality. Further, this may be in violation of local hospital policy. Individuals completing STEGHs must be aware of local policies and laws related to safeguarding patient privacy and confidentiality.
A resident completing a STEGH with an HIV organisation in Uganda posts an album on Facebook to share photos with friends and family of the setting in which he is working. Included in the album is a photo of the HIV clinic's waiting room, which includes patients' faces, not only disclosing their identity but also their HIV status to the public.	The resident did not obtain consent from the individuals in the photograph or from the HIV organisation with which he is placed. This is a violation of patient confidentiality and protection of vulnerable populations.
A medical student doing a surgical rotation in Tanzania posts photos of herself with the surgical and anaesthesia team in the operating room, with the patient on the operating table.	The patient asleep on the surgical table is not able to give consent. This is a violation of patient confidentiality, privacy, and professionalism.
A resident completing a STEGH in Senegal changes her Facebook profile picture to a photo of herself auscultating a child's chest at the clinic where she worked for 2 weeks. The child's face is visible. Dozens of family and friends comment on the profile photo to commend her for her work.	Not only does this violate patient privacy and informed consent, the motivations of posting this photo must also be considered. The resident's motivations may be more about constructing an image of herself as a saviour helping poor children in Africa. The same resident would probably never fathom posting such a photo from her continuity clinic at her home institution.
A visiting medical student writes a Facebook status that puts down the health system she has been working in for the past month while on a STEGH in Guatemala. A local colleague sees this and shows it to colleagues at the Ministry of Health. This causes a rift between the student's home institution and in-country partners.	This is unprofessional and illustrates the consequences that a rash Facebook post can have and how it can damage relationships with local partners.

in Cross Cultural Relations." Accessed August 26, 2016. http://ghi.wisc.edu/wp-content/uploads/2012/03/owards-Best-Practices-in-the-Global-Health-Institute.pdf.

Butteris, Sabrina M., Sophia P. Gladding, Walter Eppich, Scott A. Hagen, Michael B. Pitt, and SUGAR Investigators. 2014. "Simulation Use for Global Away Rotations (SUGAR): preparing residents for emotional challenges abroad – a multicenter study." *Academic Pediatrics* 15(5):533–541.

Calain, Philippe. 2013. "Ethics and images of suffering bodies in humanitarian medicine." *Social Science & Medicine* 98:278–285.

Chapman, Helena J., Victor J. Animasahun, Adesoji E. Tade, and Asad Naveed. 2016. "Addressing the role of medical students using community mobilization and social media in the Ebola response." *Perspectives in Medical Education* 5(3):186–190.

Cheston, Christine C., Tabor E. Flickinger, and Margaret S. Chisolm. 2013. "Social media use in medical education: a systematic review." *Academic Medicine* 88(6):893–901.

Dell, Evelyn M., Lara Varpio, Andrew Petrosoniak, Amy Gajaria, and Anne E. McCarthy. 2014. "The ethics and safety of medical student global health electives." *International Journal of Medical Education* 5:63.

Devakumar, Delan, Helen Brotherton, Jay Halbert, Andrew Clarke, Audrey Prost, and Jennifer Hall. 2013. "Taking ethical photos of children for medical and research purposes in low-resource settings: an exploratory qualitative study." *BMC Medical Ethics* 14(1):27.

Drake, Thomas M., Henry A. Claireaux, Chetan Khatri, and Stephen J. Chapman. 2016. "WhatsApp with patient data transmitted via instant messaging?." *Americal Journal of Surgery* 211(1):300–301.

Fung, Isaac Chun-Hai, Carmen Hope Duke, Kathryn Cameron Finch, Kassandra Renee Snook, Pei-Ling Tseng, Ana Cristina Hernandez, Manoj Gambhir, King-Wa Fu, and Zion Tsz Ho Tse. 2016. "Ebola virus disease and social media: A systematic review." *American Journal of Infection Control* [Epub ahead of print]. doi: 10.1016/j.ajic.2016.05.011.

Galiatsatos, Panagis, Fernanda Porto-Carreiro, Jennifer Hayashi, Sammy Zakaria, and Colleen Christmas. 2016. "The use of social media to supplement resident medical education–the SMART-ME initiative." *Medical Education Online* 21:29332.

Garett, Renee, Justin Smith, and Sean D. Young. 2016. "A review of social media technologies across the global HIV care continuum." *Current Opinion in Psychology* 9:56–66.

Hossain, Ibtesham Tausif, Umair Mughal, Bashar Atalla, Mustafa Franka, Sarim Siddiqui, and Mohammed Muntasir. 2015. "Instant messaging – one solution to doctor–student communication?." *Medical Education Online* 20:30593.

Icahn School of Medicine at Mount Sinai. 2016. "Mount Sinai Health System Social Media Guideline." Accessed February 8, 2016. http://icahn.mssm.edu/about-us/services-and-resources/faculty-resources/handbooks-and-policies/faculty-handbook/institutional-policies/social-media-guidelines.

Johnston, Maximilian J., Dominic King, Sonal Arora, Nebil Behar, Thanos Athanasiou, Nick Sevdalis, and Ara Darzi. 2015. "Smartphones let surgeons know WhatsApp: an analysis of communication in emergency surgical teams." *American Journal of Surgery* 209(1):45–51.

Kascaksamp Lauren, and Sayantani Dasgupta. 2016. "#InstagrammingAfrica: The Narcissism of Global Voluntourism." Pacific Standard. Accessed February 8, 2016. www.psmag.com/business-economics/instagrammingafrica-narcissism-global-voluntourism-83838.

Kind, Terry, Gillian Genrich, Avneet Sodhi, and Katherine C. Chretien. 2010. "Social media policies at US medical schools." *Medical Education Online* 15.

Lagu, Tara and S. Ryan Greysen. 2010. "Physician, monitor thyself: professionalism and accountability in the use of social media." *Journal of Clinical Ethics* 22(2):187–190.

Lukolyo, Heather, Chris A. Rees, Elizabeth M. Keating, Padma Swamy, Gordon E. Schutze, Stephanie Marton, and Teri L. Turner. 2016. "Perceptions and expectations of host country preceptors of short-term learners at four clinical sites in sub-Saharan Africa." *Academic Pediatrics* 16(4):387–393.

Madden, Mary. 2010. "Older Adults and Social Media." Pew Internet & American Life Project. Accessed August 20, 2016. www.pewinternet.org/Reports/2010/Older-Adults-and-Social-Media.aspx.

Macintosh, Tracy. 2006. "Ethical considerations for clinical photography in the global south." *Developing World Bioethics* 6(2):81–88.

Nathanson, Janice. 2013. "The Pornography of Poverty: Reframing the Discourse of International Aid's Representations of Starving Children." *Canadian Journal of Communication* 38(1):103.

Pedersen, Paul. 1994. *Five Stages of Culture Shock, The: Critical Incidents Around the World: Critical Incidents Around the World*. ABC-CLIO.

Pew Research Center. 2016. "Online activities in emerging and developing nations." 2016. Pew Research Center Global Attitudes Project. Accessed August 22, 2016. www.pewglobal.org/2015/03/19/2-online-activities-in-emerging-and-developing-nations/.

Regions Hospital. 2010. "Regions Hospital Social Media Use and Behavior." Accessed February 8, 2016. www.regionshospital.com/ucm/groups/public/@hp/@public/documents/documents/dev_057502.pdf.

Unite for Sight. 2016. "Ethics and photography in developing countries." Accessed August 26, 2016. www.uniteforsight.org/global-health-university/photography-ethics.

University of Michigan. 2011. "UMHS Policy 01-01-040 Use of Social Media for Business Purposes." Accessed February 8, 2016. www.med.umich.edu/prmc/services/socialmedia/policy.htm.

University of Minnesota. 2016. "Pediatric Global Health Track University of Minnesota Blog." August Accessed 25, 2016. Pedsgh.blogspot.com.

UW Health. 2016. "University of Wisconsin Global Health Elective Professionalism Agreement." Accessed January 15, 2016. www2.aap.org/sections/ich/Documents/toolkit/International%20Electives/Professionalism%20Agreement/2-%20U%20Wisc%20Professionalism%20Agreement%20and%20Cultural%20Competence.pdf.

Ventola, C. Lee. 2014. "Social media and health care professionals: benefits, risks, and best practices." *Pharmacy and Therapeutics* 39(7):491–520.

Von Muhlen, Marcio, and Lucila Ohno-Machado. 2012. "Reviewing social media use by clinicians." *Journal of American Medical Informatics Association* 19(5):777–781.

Wald, Hedy S., and Shmuel P. Reis. 2010. "Beyond the margins: reflective writing and development of reflective capacity in medical education." *Journal of General Internal Medicine* 25(7):746–749.

Wald, Hedy S., Stephen W. Davis, Shmuel P. Reis, Alicia D. Monroe, and Jeffrey M. Borkan. 2009. "Reflecting on reflections: Enhancement of medical education curriculum with structured field notes and guided feedback." *Academic Medicine* 84(7):830–837.

Wells, Katie M. 2011. "Social media in medical school education." *Surgery* 150(1):2–4.

28 Women's representation and leadership in global health

Caity Jackson, Désirée Lichtenstein, Katy Davis, Kelly Thompson, Kris Ronsin and Roopa Dhatt

In recent years, a greater emphasis has been placed on achieving global gender parity in health. International organisations and governments have committed to gender equality and women's empowerment in the Millennium Development Goals (MDGs), and again in the Sustainable Development Goals (SDGs) in recognition that gender parity in education is only one part of a gender equal world. The SDGs seek to "achieve gender equality and empower all women and girls" (United Nations 2015). These commitments are a step in the right direction but in order to achieve gender equality, equal gender leadership needs to be implemented within all levels of the system, including the workforce; particularly as gender equal leadership and planning results in gender equal outcomes. To recognise completely the importance of gender within health delivery mechanisms, progress in equity should be reflected from the top down and be considered a primary element for continued success and progress within this discipline.

Women play a large, if not under-recognised role in healthcare globally. In many countries, women comprise over 75 percent of the health workforce (Gender and Health Workforce Statistics 2016). Similarly, women are overwhelmingly present in health academia; for example, Harvard's global health student body is composed of 71 percent of women. In spite of this, women remain disproportionately under-represented at the most visible and highest levels of policy, management, and leadership, including executive positions and boards of directors (Silverman and Fan 2013, Johns Hopkins Bloomberg School of Public Health 2013). Overall, women represent only 22.6 percent of national parliamentarians (Women in National Parliaments 2016). This limited representation translates to the political health space where approximately 25 percent of ministers of health are women, and similar numbers are seen in the chief delegates to the World Health Assembly.

This lack of representation is preventing development. Existing research on gender parity in leadership and empowerment of women in other sectors makes an economic case for women's participation. For example, achieving gender parity is valued at $28 trillion, an increase of 26 percent in the global economy compared to projections for current gender unequal levels (McKinsey 2016). The achievement of women's rights, increased economic empowerment and involvement in leadership is good for everyone. However, the global health research community must advance the evidence base for gender parity in the sector to support a more expedited transformation of the sector's policies. In particular, the global health community must evaluate leadership at all levels and how it impacts health outcomes.

This chapter will delve into gender equity on both sides of healthcare – from those receiving services to those developing and implementing programming. It will review gender-based disparity in health and discuss why gender is such an important consideration in healthcare access, delivery and policy, and introduce various tools and methods being used across different sectors to work towards gender equality. It will outline the current state of gender parity in global health leadership, including new movements and initiatives, as well as presenting case studies and organisational profiles to help illustrate the current situation within the health and development field. This content serves to emphasise the importance of completely integrated gender equality, from healthcare to the health of the world.

The status of women in global health

Disparities in health

Health equity and the incidence of illness and disease are inextricably linked to a number of social determinants – defined as "the conditions in which people are born, grow, live, work and age" (World Health Organization 2016a). Of these determinants, gender and sex remain the most pervasive as they have the capacity to influence all other determinants. Biological (sex) and gender[1]-based (including social and political causes) differences result in health risks, disease incidence, health service needs, and ability to access healthcare and maintain even basic health.

Gender-based differences exist in all societies, influencing health-seeking behaviours, health status, and access to health services. Globally, morbidity and mortality rates differ between the genders due to a range of both social and physiological causes. Because of social or cultural norms and being perceived as lower status compared to men, women are more likely to suffer domestic abuse and greater risk of acquiring HIV. Men on the other hand are more at risk for toxic occupational exposure and to be the immediate victims in armed conflict (United Nations 2015). During adolescence, women – especially those living in developing regions – suffer more from pregnancy and childbirth-related diseases and HIV causes of death and morbidity, whereas adolescent men suffer more from injuries, violence, and self-harm, in both high income and low/middle income regions (United Nations 2015).

Biologically, women and men are affected differently in health and experience notable discrepancies in their health needs and risks over the life course. When these biological aspects of sex coincide with the societal constructions of gender, it can lead to poor health outcomes for both men and women.

For example, pregnancy remains a biological reason women suffer early morbidity and mortality, but risks extend beyond intrinsic factors. Female reproductive health is very much affected by social and political conditions, while men do not experience similar problems linking reproductive health to sociopolitical factors at this time in their lives. Family planning and antenatal care are extremely important aspects of comprehensive reproductive care and lack of access can have an adverse effect on pregnancy outcomes and over-all health and wellbeing (The World's Women 2015). Many countries neglect to develop or emphasise comprehensive care as a necessary component of population health, putting fewer resources into female-specific programmes and negatively affecting the outcome of women's health in general (United Nations 2015).

Current research that has analysed gender inequity in health has shown that the presence of gender inequality damages the physical and mental health of millions of girls and women across the globe (World Health Organization 2016). This trend translates into the leadership sphere, where the imbalance between each gender's influences and a lack of women's presence has an impact on health systems strengthening, its programme development and the overall effectiveness of care, from the community level all the way up to top levels of the health system. A review by Downs (2014) showed that women in leadership positions in governmental organisations implement different poli-cies and make different decisions than men. This gender-influenced decision-making had a direct influence on the health and wellbeing of women. In the study, women tended to invest in public works more closely linked to wom-en's concerns, such as clean drinking water, whereas men invested in works more aligned with men's activities, such as irrigation systems for farming (Downs 2014).

The bias and inequality present within systems needs to be addressed and challenged in order to improve health disparities, with the identification of the differences and inequalities paramount to resolving them. Once the problem has been identified, indicators can be developed to track programming and progress towards this important goal (Government of Sweden 2007). Public policy, on both national and global scales, needs to take into account the resulting evidence on gender as an important social determinant of health and adapt interventions, existing and subsequent policies to address the ineq-uities. These efforts will be even further strengthened if these reforms are led by a collaborative of people that truly reflect the cause, with equal representa-tion of leaders of all genders across all levels.

Strategies to ensure that the global health community considers gender a priority

New approaches to integrating gender equality have been developed, recognis-ing that both women and men (and others) require access to and control over resources and decision-making processes in order to achieve gender equality.

It has also become apparent that efforts to achieve this are most effective when they recognise that gender roles are interlinked. Such newer and relatively successful strategies include gender mainstreaming and the application of a gender lens.

Gender mainstreaming

Gender mainstreaming was adopted as a major global strategy for gender equality at the Beijing Platform for Action in 1995, defining gender mainstreaming as "a gender perspective and the process of assessing the implications for women and men of any planned action, including legislation, policies or programmes, in all areas and at all levels. It is a strategy for making women's as well as men's concerns and experiences an integral dimension of the design, implementation, monitoring, and evaluation of policies and programmes in all political, economic, and societal spheres so that women and men benefit equally and inequality is not perpetuated" (United Nations 2002).

The gender mainstreaming method is achieved by promoting gender equality as central in projects rather than as an add-on or auxiliary to the cause. As such, gender concerns should be prioritised and incorporated into all aspects of policy development and programming. Agreed priority approaches include:

- Analysing legislation by whether or not it reduces or increases gender equality from a holistic point of view, not only on paper.
- Prioritising policies and implementing initiatives that address women's special needs due to biological or gender-based discrimination.
- Ensuring active participation and equal representation of women in politics and decision-making institutions.
- Initiating shifts in culture and the process of organisational change, and identifying concrete steps towards further change (United Nations 2002).

The gender lens

The gender lens is an approach and tool to focus the user's attention on gender differences and identify aspects of care and disease that require further management (Ontario Women's Health Centre's Gender and Health Collaborative Curriculum Project 2009). This approach provides a health-based framework to consider how the following spheres contribute to an individual's gender:

- biology,
- social structure,
- education, and
- economic factors.

This framework applies not just to healthcare itself (Rodin 2013), but to policy, legislation and programming within and outside of health. There are several methods used to obtain a gender lens – one simple method used is the 4R method (Government of Sweden 2007). It involves analysing activities by considering:

Representation: Who does what? Are the roles the same? What is the distribution of men and women at each level?

Resources: How are resources (such as time, money and space) distributed? Who controls what?

Reality: What is the background to why it looks like it does? What are the norms and values and rights that affect the work, activities, and organisation? What are the economic, institutional, and social factors that underlie, support, and influence this?

Realisation: What is our action plan and how do we formulate new objectives and measures?

Women in organisational leadership

Health sector progress towards gender equal leadership has many notable milestones. In 1995, the Beijing Platform for Action called upon institutions to create a 50:50 gender parity at all levels of leadership. The Secretary General's Report on the Improvement of the Status of Women in the United Nations System in 2014 failed, however, to offer optimism that this is being achieved. It demonstrated that the number of women working in leadership in the United Nations increased only marginally between 2011 and 2013, with a persistent inverse relationship between the level and women's representation. The percentage of women in top positions in WHO and UNAIDS in 2013 were 26.7 and 33.3 percent, respectively (UN Women 2014b).

International non-governmental organisations (NGOs) and public development agencies show similar trends with the International Committee of the Red Cross and the International Federation of Red Cross and Red Crescent Societies having 32 and 33 percent of their current leadership positions held by women, respectively, and the United Kingdom's Department for International Development's leadership positions are occupied by women in 33 percent of positions (IFRC 2016, the Department for International Development 2015). Despite an organisation commitment and a global champion for women and girls, the Bill and Melinda Gates Foundation have only 25 percent of women on their executive leadership team (Easton 2015, Gates Foundation 2015). Whether in UN agencies, NGOs, public agencies, or completely private development foundations, women rarely make up even one third of leadership teams.

The movement to address gender disparity in global health leadership has rapidly gained momentum, very aptly spearheaded by current women leaders. In 2014, a twitter campaign, the "#WGH100," was spearheaded by Ilona

Kickbusch of the Graduate Institute of International and Development Studies, Geneva, with the intention of identifying exceptional women in the field and bringing them to the world's attention. The #WGH100 list was published in the *Lancet*, leading to the #WGH200 and the #WGH300 (*The Lancet* 2015, p. 318, Graduate Institute Geneva 2015). Similar initiatives/ organisations have drawn focus to gender equality, including the work of UN Women's He For She campaign, and the All Male Panel (2016) tracker. Many of these groups advocate not only for the increased presence and activity of women in global health, but for increased visibility.

One supranational organisation that is making more visible steps on this front is the Pan American Health Organization (PAHO). In 2011, they achieved 50/50 gender parity in their 51st Directing Council, with women representing half of the ministers of health, chief medical officers, and other heads of national delegations as well as the senior leadership from PAHO and the WHO (PAHO WHO 2016b). This was a significant improvement since 1948, the first time when women appeared at all in an official PAHO photo of the Sixth Pan American Conference of National Health Authorities. From three women out of 25 attending members, it took 53 years to reach parity among women and men. Subsequent directing councils have not seen this trend of complete gender parity continue but the percentage of women leaders within the highest level of leadership is consistently higher than the norm we find in other organisations. PAHO's gender equality policy by the directing council for attaining gender equality and empowerment of women in "Health for All" approved in 2005 marked a crucial turning point and real commitment towards gender equality in healthcare leadership (Bacon 2015, PAHO WHO 2016a).

The next generation of women's leadership

Kelli Rogers reported in a blog for Devex in 2015 that women hold less than 25 percent of leadership positions in the global health field despite the majority of students working in and entering the field being women. In 2012–13, the Johns Hopkins MPH programme, saw a student intake that was 63 percent women. Rachel Silverman and Victoria Fan wrote that "it's hard not to notice the relative paucity of women at the top ranks of academia and global health institutions, despite obvious majorities of women in global health student bodies and among junior researchers." All of this conversation has spurred even more exploration of, activity and advocacy around, the issue (Silverman and Fan 2013, Johns Hopkins Bloomberg School of Public Health 2013).

In their article, "*Who Runs the (Global Health) World?*," Silverman and Fan refer to the "desired cohort effect," or the trickle-up of these predominantly women student bodies to the global health leadership level, a concept that many place passive hopes upon. The group Women in Global Health looked at this scenario and examined the leadership structures of the International Federation of Medical Students' Association (IFMSA) to prove or disprove this theory. The IFMSA connects and represents medical and other health-related students from national member organisations (NMOs) in 116 countries to educate, advocate, and campaign for global health issues. The IFMSA represents the current cadre of incoming medical professionals and should be representative of that group, yet has had an average of only 27 percent of women on its executive board for the past 4 years, despite over-representation of women in its general membership. Similarly, only 30 percent of the IFMSA's national member organisations are led by women (International Federation of Medical Students Association 2016). It may be that this imbalance needs time, however, only two out of the last ten presidents were women and historically only 15.6 percent of presidents were women. The data by period (from 1951 to 2016), for the last 10 years was 20 percent and the last 20 years was 30 percent women presidents. Women in Global Health were able to demonstrate that the current leadership gender composition will not in fact just naturally transition out and be replaced by that which we find in public health classrooms, where women dominate (Women in Global Health 2016). This analysis served to emphasise the need for more active participation and advocacy in this area of work.

Role models, leadership, and the way forward

When we look at leadership in a field, we look not only to those who are seen at the highest levels or associated with position, but to those that are catalysts to their organisation's accomplishments and general societal advancements. Those at the highest level of leadership are often the ones who become the face for the field, issue, or campaign and when there is such an imbalance of gender within this top leadership, the workforce and outside world receive a message about the field and who represents it. When speaking about leadership, many may not believe they are meant to be sitting at the decision-making table if they do not see someone that they can relate to, someone that represents them. If we do not see women in leadership positions, we assume that there is no place for them, for what other reason could there be? If you want more women to be in leadership positions you need to support their development and bring more visibility to those in the sector.

Women in global health

Women in Global Health (WGH) is a global movement that brings together all genders and backgrounds to achieve gender equality in global health leadership. We believe that everyone has the right to attain equal levels of participation in leadership and decision-making regardless of gender. WGH creates a platform for discussions and collaborative space for leadership, facilitates specific education and training, garners support and commitment from the global community, and demands change for gender transformative leadership.

Note

1 Gender vs. Sex? Sex refers to biological differences, such as chromosomes and reproductive systems, whereas gender refers to the social construction of sex, the characteristics formed by the norms, roles and relationships between men and women. Gender roles vary over time and between cultures but sex varies very little (Ontario Women's Health Centre). To be able to generalise we will discuss only men and women in this chapter; however, gender contains men, women and identities that do not fit into those labels such as non-binary, including a gender, intersex and gender fluid. However, it is good to know that people that do not fit into the typical cisgender and binary gender roles, such as non-binary and trans people, are a vulnerable population that usually have poorer health than the general population, are more likely to commit suicide, more likely to have HIV and have worse mental health.

References

All Male Panel. 2016. Tumblr. Accessed February 3, 2016. http://allmalepanels.tumblr.com/.

Bacon, Lauren. 2015. *"The Odds That a Panel Would 'Randomly' Be All Men Are Astronomical."* The Atlantic. October 20. Accessed March 4, 2016. www.theatlantic.com/business/archive/2015/10/the-odds-that-a-panel-would-randomly-be-all-men-are-astronomical/411505/.

Department for International Development. 2015. *"Department Organogram."* Taken March 7, 2016. https://data.gov.uk/organogram/department-for-international-development-0.

Downs, JA. 2014. "Increasing Women in Leadership in Global Health." Academic Medicine 89:8.

Easton, Nina. 2015. *"Melinda Gates on Bill, ending poverty, and her plans to invest in women and girls."* Fortune Magazine. May 21. Accessed February 5, 2016. http://fortune.com/2015/05/21/melinda-gates-plans-to-invest-in-women-and-girls/.

Gender and Health Workforce Statistics. 2016. *"Resource Spotlight: Gender and Health Workforce Statistics."* Accessed March 19, 2016. www.hrhresourcecenter.org/gender_stats.

Graduate Institute Geneva. 2015. Global Health Programme: *"300 Women Leaders in Global Health."* Accessed January 5, 2016. http://graduateinstitute.ch/files/live/sites/iheid/files/sites/globalhealth/ghp-new/publications/300%20Women%20Leaders%20in%20Global%20Health%20-%20final.pdf.

Government of Sweden. 2007. *"Gender Mainstreaming Manual – A book of practical methods from the Swedish Gender Mainstreaming Support Committee."* (JämStöd) (15). Accessed January 10, 2016. www.government.se/contentassets/3d89b0f447ec43a4b3179c4a22c370e8/gender-mainstreaming-manual-sou-200715.

International Federation of Medical Students Association. 2016. *"Past Officials."* Accessed March 4, 2016. http://ifmsa.org/past-officials/.

IFRC. 2016. *The governing board.* Accessed March 5, 2016. www.ifrc.org/en/who-we-are/governance/the-governing-board/.

Johns Hopkins Bloomberg School of Public Health. 2013. *"Student demographics of 2012–2013."* Accessed January 20, 2016. www.jhsph.edu/academics/degree-programs/master-of-public-health/prospective-students/student-demographics.html.

McKinsey. 2016. "*McKinsey Global Institute Report.*" Accessed April 24, 2016. www. mckinsey.com/global-themes/employment-and-growth/how-advancing-womens-equality-can-add-12-trillion-to-global-growth.

Ontario Women's Health Centre's Gender and Health Collaborative Curriculum Project. 2009. "*Looking Through a Gender Lens.*" Accessed February 7, 2016. www.genderand-health.ca/en/modules/introduction/introduction-genderasadeterminantofhealth-Shayna-06.jspand Health Collaborative Curriculum Project.

PAHO WHO. 2016a. "*The Changing Face of Leadership.*" Last updated 2011. Accessed March 4, 2016. www.paho.org/hq/index.php?option=com_content&view=article&id=6019%3A2011-the-changing-face-leadership&catid=1443%3Aweb-bulletins&Itemid=135&lang=en.

PAHO WHO. 2016b. "*Directing Council.*" Accessed March 2016. www.paho.org/hq/index.php?option=com_content&view=category&layout=blog&id=1259&Itemid=1159.

Rodin, Judith. 2013. "Accelerating action towards universal health coverage by applying a gender lens." *Bulletin of the World Health Organization* 91:710–711. Accessed March 6, 2016. doi: http://dx.doi.org/10.2471/BLT.13.127027.

Silverman, R. and Fan, V. 2013. "*Who Runs the (Global Health) World?*" Centre for Global Development Blog. Accessed January 5, 2016. www.cgdev.org/blog/who-runs-global-health-world.

The Lancet. 2015. "Twitter campaign highlights women in global health." *Lancet* 385:318. Accessed January 5, 2016. www.thelancet.com/pdfs/journals/lancet/PIIS0140-6736(15)60104-0.pdf.

The World's Women. 2015. United Nations statistics division. 2015. Accessed January 6, 2016. http://unstats.un.org/unsd/gender/worldswomen.html.

United Nations. 2002. "*Gender Mainstreaming: An Overview (Report).*" New York: United Nations. Accessed April 4, 2013.

United Nations. 2015. "*Sustainable Development Goals 2015.*" Accessed January 6, 2016. https://sustainabledevelopment.un.org/?menu=1300.

UN Women. 2014a. "*Beijing Declaration and Platform for Action.*" Accessed January 4, 2016. www.unwomen.org/~/media/headquarters/attachments/sections/csw/pfa_e_final_web.pdf.

UN Women. 2014b. "*Improvement in the status of women in the United Nations system: Report of the Secretary-General.*" Accessed January 7, 2016. www.unwomen.org/digital-library/publications/2014/8/improvement-of-the-status-of-women-in-the-un-system-2014.

Women in Global Health. 2016. Accessed February 2, 2016. www.womeningh.org.

Women in National Parliaments. 2016. Last updated November 1, 2016. Accessed December 13, 2016. www.ipu.org/wmn-e/world.htm.

World Health Organization. 2016a. *What are Social Determinants of Health?* Retrieved March 4, 2016. www.who.int/social_determinants/sdh_definition/en/.

World Health Organization. 2016b. "*Commission on Social Determinants of Health.*" Accessed October 30, 2016. www.who.int/social_determinants/thecommission/finalreport/en/.

29 Global LGBT health

Current challenges, opportunities and tools for global health practitioners and educators

Sahil Angelo

Introduction

In nearly every country around the world, lesbian, gay, bisexual and transgender (LGBT) populations face stigma and discrimination that often create and perpetuate disparities in health (World Health Organization 2013).[1] In recent years, the public health community has devoted more attention to improving global LGBT health, and has made considerable headway – particularly around HIV prevention and care as it relates to men who have sex with men (MSM) and transgender women. However, significant barriers remain.

Global health educators and practitioners must include LGBT health into their respective pedagogy and programming, in order to ensure the needs of these populations are properly met. To this end, this chapter provides an overview of global LGBT health, and includes a case study as well as tools that global health practitioners can leverage in the future. The information presented draws from an extensive literature review and interviews with experts in this field.

A brief overview of global LGBT health

LGBT populations share a history of stigma and discrimination, which often leads to a common set of health inequities. Research shows that LGBT persons, when compared to their heterosexual counterparts, have a higher risk of depression, suicide, substance abuse, and non-communicable diseases like cancer, obesity and hypertension. They are also at higher risk of contracting sexually transmitted infections (STIs) and relevant co-infections with diseases like tuberculosis (Institute of Medicine 2011).

These health risks are biological and behavioural, but are often exacerbated by social discrimination and structural violence specific to sexual and gender minorities. Sexual and gender minorities are subject to institutionalised prejudice, social exclusion, violence, rape and internalised shame about their sexuality (Daulaire 2014, Pan American Health Organization 2013,Kates 2014, Obama 2011, Hard and Mackadon 2012, Carroll and Itaborahy 2015, Tat *et al.* 2015). Numerous reports from around the world – including from the USA – reveal that fears of rejection, discrimination, or substandard care often cause LGBT individuals to conceal their sexual preferences or gender identity from healthcare providers (World Health Organization 2013, Smith 2015, United States Agency for International Development 2014).

Sexual and gender minority status creates health disparities that are further exacerbated by other social determinants of health, like race, socioeconomic status, homelessness, age, and religion (Institute of Medicine 2011). For example, LGBT individuals are more likely to be poor, particularly when violence, stigma, and criminalisation affect access to education, employment and other economic opportunities, and essential health services (Badgett *et al.* 2013, Swedish International Development Cooperation Agency 2012, United States Agency for International Development 2014, Stonewall International 2016). Age further impacts the ways in which LGBT individuals may encounter unparalleled difficulty: elder LGBT individuals are more likely to be isolated without social support as they age, which places them at a higher risk of poor health and financial insecurity (Fredrikson-Goldsen *et al.* 2015, Fredrikson-Goldsen *et al.* 2014, Hard and Makadon 2012). Overall, these broad health inequities among LGBT persons can lead to higher mortality when compared to heterosexual adults (Stall *et al.* 2016, Cochran *et al.* 2016).

There is still a dearth of data about the health of LGBT individuals, making it difficult for health practitioners to understand the burden of unequal health outcomes and tailor interventions accordingly. Further, each sexual and gender minority has unique health challenges, but there is very little disaggregated research. The majority of existing research focuses primarily on MSM – particularly in the context of HIV and other sexually transmitted infectious (Trapance *et al.* 2012, Killen *et al.* 2012, Coulter *et al.* 2014, Institute of Medicine 2011, Boehmer 2002).

Furthermore, most studies examine health in developed western nations such as the USA, partially because LGBT individuals have more freedom to disclose their status openly and participate safely in studies. There is often a paradox, particularly in repressive environments, where a lack of usable information on LGBT persons hampers data collection and the creation of health interventions for sexual and gender minorities (Stahlman *et al.* 2016). The unique health needs of each group are summarised below.

Disaggregating LGBT health

MSM around the world are extremely vulnerable to contracting STIs, due to biological, social and structural factors (Stahlman *et al.* 2016, Mayer *et al.* 2012).[2] Most research focuses on HIV among MSM: studies show that this group comprises more than 75 percent of the prevalent HIV infection in upper-income countries. In low and middle income countries (LMICs), MSM are 19 times more likely than others to contract HIV (Beyrer *et al.* 2012). They are also more susceptible to anal human papilloma virus (HPV), hepatitis and herpes. These viruses can progress into anal cancer, liver cancer, and

Kaposi sarcoma, respectively. The risk of disease progression is especially salient among men co-infected with HIV (Mayer *et al.* 2012, Blondeel *et al.* 2016). Despite engaging in same-sex relations, many MSM may have wives or intimate encounters with other women, which poses a risk to non-MSM populations.

The sparse research on lesbian individuals and women who have sex with women (WSW) reveals that this group is at higher risk for non-communicable diseases like asthma, obesity, arthritis, cervical and breast cancer when compared to their heterosexual counterparts (Simoni *et al.* 2016, Quinn *et al.* 2015, Brown and Tracy 2008). WSW populations are also at risk for sexually transmitted diseases like HIV, genital herpes, and HPV, particularly if they also have sex with men either on a recreational or transactional basis (Tat *et al.* 2015). In certain regions of the world, like in southern Africa, sexual violence against and/or "corrective rape" of lesbian women is pervasive, highlighting one example of how being both a woman and a sexual minority can exacerbate discrimination (Tat *et al.* 2015).

There is even less information on transgender health. Transgender persons experience many of the same risk factors as MSM and WSW, but these may be exacerbated by more extreme stigmatisation. The scant data that do exist primarily discusses transgender women in the context of HIV, who are 50 times more likely to be infected with the disease than any other adults spanning the same reproductive age (Baral *et al.* 2013), with their worldwide HIV prevalence rate estimated at a staggering 19 percent (Poteat *et al.* 2015, Stahlman *et al.* 2016, Reisner *et al.* 2016).[3] Even less is known about transgender men (Reisner *et al.* 2016). It is important to note that transgender individuals may also require hormone therapy or genital surgeries in order to express their identity adequately. These services are often costly in high income countries, and do not exist in many LMICs (Bredeson 2015).

A case study: LGBT health in Uganda

Uganda's recent wave of homophobic legislation illustrates the ways repressive laws and social environments can impact LGBT health. In early 2014, the President of Uganda, Yoweri Museveni, signed the Anti-Homosexuality Act 2014 (AHA), legislation that elevated the penalty for same-sex conduct to life in prison. The legislation also made aiding, abetting, sponsoring, and failing to report homosexuality a crime punishable with up to 7 years in prison (Downie 2014). The law was overturned 6 months later due to a procedural technicality.

Despite the law's short duration, the AHA undermined public health efforts to serve LGBT individuals. Prominent LGBT activists were threatened and attacked, and LGBT individuals avoided health facilities out of fear of being reported. Furthermore, service providers and other organisations that traditionally served LGBT populations were also targeted under the broadly defined "promotion of homosexuality" clause (Burki 2014). In April 2014, a US-funded HIV research facility that also provided HIV services to MSM was raided by police allegedly for "training youths in homosexuality." The project re-opened after the US intervention, but two other HIV testing facilities closed after the AHA was passed (Burki 2014).

It is important to note that Uganda's case is an extreme example of the ways stigma and discrimination can tangibly impact the health of LGBT populations. The health impact of other subtle, pernicious behaviour – like healthcare providers making LGBT patients feel uncomfortable – cannot be overemphasised.

Global LGBT health: the way forward

There is a widening schism in the way countries approach LGBT issues. On one hand there has been remarkable progress: 118 countries have decriminalised same-sex acts and 20 have legalised gay marriage. On the other hand, homosexual acts are still criminalised in 76 countries, and punishable by death in eight – in addition to the recent wave of anti-homosexual legislation in countries like Uganda (UN High Commissioner for Human Rights 2015). Furthermore, there are non-state actors, including terrorist groups like Daesh (ISIS), who execute sexual and gender minorities.

This global divergence is reminiscent of the early phases of the HIV epidemic. It took strong international leadership from UNAIDS, the US President's Emergency Plan for AIDS Relief (PEPFAR), and the Global Fund to Fight AIDS, Tuberculosis, and Malaria slowly to bridge the divide.

Similarly, strong leadership and a coordinated global strategy will be required to improve global LGBT health. The World Health Organization (WHO) is typically the institution to set global norms, vision, and strategic guidelines; however, a core group of African and Middle Eastern nations, in partnership with Russia, have hampered the WHO's efforts to substantively and technically address LGBT health (Daulaire 2014). Fortunately, entities like PEPFAR, The World Bank, United Nations High Commissioner for Refugees (UNHCR), and the Global Fund to Fight AIDS, Tuberculosis, and Malaria have stepped up and are working to provide this global leadership and unity.

Despite these institutions' best efforts, there remain many barriers that hamper the ability for health practitioners to serve the LGBT population effectively. In light of these vastly different political, legal, cultural, social, and economic environments, the health community must develop an expansive toolkit that can be applied to promote LGBT health in the local context. As a result, it must include a mix of public health, economic development, and human rights tools that are leveraged simultaneously. These include:

- Educating students and colleagues about the unique health needs of LGBT populations. Formally teaching and training students and colleagues about the health needs specific to LGBT populations is imperative. Creating classes that focus on LGBT health, and integrating these courses into broader global and public health curricula is a critical next step for educators. The next generation of practitioners needs to know how to serve this vulnerable population sensitively and skillfully both in terms of healthcare delivery and research. There are resources from institutions like the Williams Institute at UCLA and the Fenway Institute in Boston – as well as a growing number of academic journals – that can assist educators in the course development (Harrington Park Press).[4]

- Students and trainees conducting global health fieldwork must make themselves aware of the study countries' social, political, and cultural views on LGBT health. It is of utmost importance that all practitioners – both students and experts – listen to the concerns and advice of members of the LGBT community in each country prior to intervention. These individuals have the most insight into their local context and their vulnerability – their wishes and advice, as with all communities, must be respected.

- Delivering essential services. It is imperative that healthcare workers either begin or continue providing healthcare to LGBT persons. Withdrawal of these services, particularly as a form of political protest, could adversely impact LGBT individuals' health-seeking behaviour and are unlikely to change government policies (Downie 2014, Beyrer *et al.* 2012). A key component of service delivery is ensuring providers are trained on the unique facets of LGBT health, which will foster trust and improve the quality of care (Hard and Makadon 2016). For example, in Ethiopia, LGBT citizens distrusted public facilities, but spoke highly of private clinics that were "LGBT friendly," as they offered a safe space to learn effective public health interventions and receive tailored, respectful care (Personal communication 2015).

- Improving data collection and research on LGBT health. Health practitioners are uniquely positioned to build the evidence surrounding LGBT health. Including LGBT-specific questions in health surveys and analyses will be invaluable for generating disaggregated data and identifying new correlations between sexual/gender minorities and health. This information can then be used to grow the body of implementation science, which will help determine best practices.

- Data will be particularly important in building the case for LGBT health and human rights. As mentioned earlier, this will continue to be a challenge in environments where anti-homosexuality laws and practices risk the safety of staff and study participants. Countries that provide legal protections for sexual and gender minorities, particularly in the Global South, will become increasingly important locations for research. Partnering with local and regional scientific communities will help circumvent some of the challenges involved in LGBT research.

- Engaging in global health diplomacy. Global health practitioners should engage government officials on LGBT health. Many have used the HIV platform as an entry point to provide services to vulnerable populations such as MSM, arguing – with varying degrees of success – that providing prevention and care is essential to turning the tide of the epidemic. However, these arguments need to extend beyond HIV to make the case to health officials that all LGBT individuals deserve care, as a matter of social justice.
- Ideally, successful health diplomacy results in government health officials convincing other sectors like the judicial system and the ministries of finance to protect and invest in the wellbeing of LGBT persons. Global health practitioners with high-level access should lean on ministers of health to put LGBT health back on the table at international meetings and to agree on a coordinated, international strategy, which is desperately needed. Changing perspectives on LGBT individuals will require patience, persistence, and a truly inclusive dialogue.
- Identifying, supporting, and including LGBT civil society. Civil society plays an essential role in providing information and services, as well as establishing accountability. These groups need to be actively involved in shaping donor strategies, developing policy, fostering coordination, and identifying solutions as they usually have the best sense of the local environment. For example, after the AHA was passed, many activists in Uganda requested that the USA work behind the scenes for fear that strong and continual public statements would jeopardise these activists' physical safety. In addition to providing insight into the local context, civil society will play a major role in sustaining gains as donors eventually withdraw.
- It is important that donors create new partnerships with civil society organisations that are traditionally overlooked. Practitioners should ensure different organisations are represented to ensure inclusion and avoid in-fighting or competition among groups that are supporting LGBT rights.
- Expanding and strengthening efforts to ensure the safety of LGBT individuals. The Uganda case study briefly highlighted some of the security challenges facing the LGBT community, such as violence and sexual assault. During the AHA, there were reports of confusion about where to go for assistance and how quickly it could be provided (Kates 2014). Establishing and communicating safety contingencies in-country will help protect LGBT persons and ensure their health needs are met, particularly during times of crisis.
- Engaging faith leaders. The faith community can be both beneficial and detrimental to LGBT health. There are numerous instances in which faith-based organisations provide essential services to vulnerable LGBT populations and actively fight stigma (Fleischman 2015). At the same time, there are many religious based groups who promote discrimination

against LGBT persons. Engaging faith leaders is critical for combatting the stigma and discrimination that perpetuate inequities for LGBT populations and promoting inclusion.

• Tapping into the private sector. The private sector has played a significant role in global health, but remains an untapped resource for addressing global LGBT health and human rights. There is a growing body of economic research showing the financial gains of LGBT inclusion, and the private sector can play an important role in generating and disseminating that information (Badgett 2014, Badgett *et al.* 2014). Multinational corporations currently seem reluctant to leverage their business assets or take a stand on global LGBT rights, but doing so could be a powerful catalyst for a more inclusive environment.

• Documenting violence and discrimination against LGBT individuals. Maintaining a record of infringements provides justice for the families and friends of victims, and helps to ensure accountability and transparency. Healthcare workers are in a unique position to document these abuses when patients attend local clinics or hospitals.

• Creating new high-level international champions for LGBT health and human rights. Claims of western imperialism can undermine international efforts to push for LGBT rights. It is important that new champions tackle this issue, particularly from the Global South. In this regard, governments, multilateral organisations, global health practitioners, and activists should not solely focus on the bad eggs, like Uganda or Russia, but also countries like Nepal, Malta, or Malaysia, who are making progress (Reid 2016). Furthermore, appointing high-level LGBT special representatives or ambassadors can serve to elevate these issues politically.

Conclusion

We are presently faced with a unique set of challenges and opportunities for improving LGBT health worldwide. There has been remarkable progress in some parts of the world, but those gains – and subsequent optimism – have been tainted by rising violence and discrimination towards the LGBT community in other regions. Inaction and complacency perpetuate the biological, social, and structural inequities and the daily suffering afflicting LGBT individuals. The ability for sexual and gender minorities to access quality, safe, and friendly care is key measurement of our progress towards global health equity. In our continued fight for global health and human rights, it is imperative that the global health community continues to consider the unique challenges faced by LGBT individuals as we craft policies and programmes that ultimately seek to achieve health and justice for all.

Acknowledgements

The author would like to thank the following individuals for their time, generosity, and expertise: Dr Jennifer Kates, Director of Global Health and HIV Policy, The Kaiser Family Foundation; Maeve McKean, Senior Advisor to the Assistant Secretary, Office of Global Affairs, US Department of Health and Human Services; Dr Kenneth Meyer, Medical Research Director and Co-Chair, Fenway Institute; Mark Bromley, Council Chair, The Council for Global Equality; Dr Nicholas Thomson, IAS-NIDA Fellow, Johns Hopkins University; Dr Stefan Baral, Director, Key Populations Program, Johns Hopkins Bloomberg School of Public Health; Todd Summers, Senior Advisor, Global Health Policy Center, Center for Strategic and International Studies; Dr Phillip Nieburg, Senior Advisor, Global Health Policy Center, Center for Strategic and International Studies; and Amara Frumkin, Emory University School of Medicine.

Notes

1 There is controversy over the term "LGBT," and in light of this debate, the author has selected the "LGBT" classification to be consistent with the US government.
2 Not all men who have sex with men (MSM) identify as gay or bisexual.
3 Transgender women sex workers have a HIV prevalence as high as 27.3 percent.
4 The Harrington Park Press is a company that specialises in publishing scholarly journals, books and academic papers focused on LGBT issues. For more information, please visit: http://harringtonparkpress.com/lgbtg-core-research-journals/.

References

Badgett, Lee M.V., Durso, Laura E., Schneebaum, Alyssa. 2013. *"New Patterns of Poverty in the Lesbian, Gay, and Bisexual Community."* The Williams Institute UCLA. http://williamsinstitute.law.ucla.edu/wp-content/uploads/LGB-Poverty-Update-Jun-2013.pdf.

Badgett, Lee M.V., Nezhad, Sheila, Waaldijk, Kees, Rodgers, Yana V.D.M. 2014. *"The Relationship between LGBT Inclusion and Economic Development: An Analysis of Emerging Economies."* The Williams Institute, UCLA School of Law. http://williamsinstitute.law.ucla.edu/wp-content/uploads/lgbt-inclusion-and-development-november-2014.pdf.

Badgett, Lee M.V. 2014. *"The Economic Cost of Homophobia: How LGBT Exclusion Impacts Development."* World Bank, Washington D.C. Presentation delivered March 3, 2014. http://live.worldbank.org/economic-cost-of-homophobia.

Baral, Stefan D., Poteat, Tonia, Stomdahl, Susanne, Wirtz, Adrea L., Guadamuz, Thomas E., Beyrer, Chris. 2013. "Worldwide burden of HIV in transgender women: a systematic review and meta-analysis." *Lancet Infectious Diseases* 13:214–222.

Beyrer, Chris, Baral, Stefan D., van Griensven, Frits, Goodreau, Steven, Chariyalertsak, Suwat, Wirtz, Andrea L., Brookmeyer, Ron. 2012. "Global Epidemiology of HIV infection in men who have sex with men." *Lancet* 380:367–377. www.thelancet.com/journals/lancet/article/PIIS0140-6736(12)60821-6/abstract.

Blondeel, Karen, Say, Lale, Chou, Doris, Toskin, Igor, Khosla, Rajat, Scolaro, Elisa, Temmerman, Marleen. 2016. "Evidence and knowledge gaps on the disease burden in sexual and gender minorities: a review of systematic reviews." *International Journal for Equity in Health* 15(16). http://equityhealthj.biomedcentral.com/articles/10.1186/s12939-016-0304-1#CR24.

Boehmer, Ulrike. 2002. "Twenty Years of Public Health Research: Inclusion of Lesbian, Gay, Bisexual, and Transgender Populations." *American Journal of Public Health* 92(7):1125–1130.

Breedesen, B. 2015. "From brutes to butterflies: Inside Thailand's sex-change industry." *The Nation*.

Brown, Jessica, and Tracy, Kathleen. 2008. "Review Article – Lesbians and cancer: an overlooked health disparity." *Cancer Causes and Control* 19:1009. http://link.springer.com/article/10.1007/s10552-008-9176-z.

Burki, Talha. 2014. "The changing tide in Uganda's HIV control." *Lancet Infectious Diseases* 14(7). www.thelancet.com/journals/laninf/article/PIIS1473-3099(14) 70815-1/fulltext.

Carroll, Aengus, and Itaborahy, Lucas P. 2015. *State sponsored homophobia 2015: a world survey of laws: criminalisation, protection and recognition of same-sex love.* ILGA.

Cochran, Susan, Bjorkenstam, Charlotte, Mays, Vickie M. 2016. "Sexual orientation and all-cause mortality among US adults, age 18–59 years, 2001–2011." *American Journal of Public Health* 96(12):931–947. http://ajph.aphapublications.org/doi/pdf/10.2105/AJPH.2016.303052.

Coulter, Robert W.S., Kenst, Karey S., Bowen, Deborah J. 2014. "Research Funded by the National Institutes of Health on the Health of Lesbians, Gay, Bisexual, and Transgender Populations." *American Journal of Public Health* 104(2):e105–e112. www.ncbi.nlm.nih.gov/pmc/articles/PMC3935708/#__ffn_sectitle.

Daulaire, Nils. 2014. "The Importance of LGBT Health on a Global Scale." *LGBT Health* 1:8–9.

Downie, Richard. 2014. *Revitalizing the Fight against Homophobia in Africa.* Center for Strategic and International Studies.

Fleischman, Janet. "The Nexus of Faith and Health." *Smart Global Health* 2015. www.smartglobalhealth.org/blog/entry/the-nexus-of-faith-and-health/.

Fredriksen-Goldsen, Karen, Cook-Daniels., Loree, Hyun-Jun, Kim, Erosheva, Elena A., Emlet, Charles A., Hoy-Ellis, Charles P., Goldsen, Jayn, Muraco, Anna. 2014. "Physical and Mental Health of Transgender Older Adults: An At-Risk and Underserved Population." *The Gerontologist* 54(3):488–500. http://gerontologist.oxfordjournals.org/content/54/3/488.abstract?ijkey=fda5921331760cd45ac461527b7073300c56d7a7&keytype2=tf_ipsecsha.

Fredrikson-Goldsen, Karen, Hyun-Jun, Kim, Shiu, Chengshi, Goldsen, Jayne, Emlet, Charles A. 2015. "Successful Aging Among LGBT Older Adults: Physical and Mental Health-Related Quality of Life by Age Group." The Gerontologist 55(1):154–168. https://gerontologist.oxfordjournals.org/content/55/1/154.

Hard, Kevin L., and Makadon, Harvey. 2012. *Improving the Health Care of Lesbian, Gay, Bisexual, and Transgender People: Understanding and Eliminating Health Disparities.* The Fenway Institute. www.lgbthealtheducation.org/wp-content/uploads/12-054_LGBTHealtharticle_v3_07-09-12.pdf.

Institute of Medicine. 2011. *The health of lesbian, gay, bisexual, and transgender (LGBT) people: building a foundation for better understanding.* Washington: National Academies Press.

Kates, Jennifer. 2014. "The U.S. Government and Global LGBT Health: Opportunities and Challenges in the Current Era." *The Kaiser Family Foundation Issue Brief.*

Killen, Jack, Harrington, Mark, Fauci, Anthony S. 2012. "MSM AIDS Research Activism, and HAART." *Lancet* 380(9839):314–316. www.thelancet.com/journals/lancet/article/PIIS0140-6736(12)60635-7/fulltext.

Mayer, Kenneth H., Bekker, Linda-Gail, Stall, Ron, Grulich, Andrew E., Colfax, Grant, Lama, Javier R. 2012. "Comprehensive clinical care for men who have sex with men: and integrated approach." *Lancet* 380:378–387.

Obama, Barack. 2011. *Presidential Memorandum – International Initiatives to Advance the Human Rights of Lesbian, Gay, Bisexual, and Transgender Persons.* White House Office of the Press Secretary. www.whitehouse.gov/the-press-office/2011/12/06/presidential-memorandum-international-initiatives-advance-human-rights-l.

Pan American Health Organization. 2013. *Addressing the causes of disparities in health service access and utilization for lesbian, gay, bisexual, and trans (LGBT) persons.* CD52/18.

Poteat, Tonia, Wirtz, Andrea L., Radix, Anita, Borquez, Annick, Silva-Santisteban, Deutsch, Madeline B., Khan, Sharful Islam, Winder, Sam, Operario, Don. 2015. "HIV Risk and preventative interventions in transgender women sex workers." *Lancet* 385(9964):274–286. www.thelancet.com/journals/lancet/article/PIIS0140-6736(14)60833-3/fulltext.

Quinn, Gwendolyn P. Sanchez, Julian A., Sutton, Steven K., Vandaparampil, Susan T., Ngyuen, Giang T., Green, B. Lee., Kanetsky, Peter A., Schabath, Matther B. 2015. "Cancer and Lesbian, Gay, Bisexual, Transgender/Transsexual, and Queer/Questioning Populations." *CA Cancer Journal Clinicians* 65(5):384–400. www.ncbi.nlm.nih.gov/pmc/articles/PMC4609168/#R56.

Reid, Graeme. 2016. "Equality to Brutality: global trends in LGBT rights." *World Economic Forum.* www.weforum.org/agenda/2016/01/equality-to-brutality-global-trends-in-lgbt-rights/.

Reisner, Sari L., Poteat, Tonia, Keatley, JoAnne, Cabral, Mauro, Mothopen, Tampose, Dunham, Emilia, Holland, Claire E., Max, Ryan, Baral, Stefan. 2016. "The Global Health Needs of Transgender Populations: A Review." *Lancet* 388(10042):412–436. www.thelancet.com/journals/lancet/article/PIIS0140-6736(16)00684-X/abstract.

Simoni, Jane M., Smith, Laramie, Oost, Kathryn M., Fredriksen-Golden, Karen. 2016. "Disparities in Physical Health Conditions among Lesbian and Bisexual Women: A Systematic Review of Population-Based Studies." *Journal of Homosexuality* accepted author version posted April 2016. www.tandfonline.com/doi/abs/10.1080/00918369.2016.1174021?journalCode=wjhm20.

Smith, Riley. 2015. "Healthcare experiences of lesbian and bisexual women in Cape Town, South Africa." *Cultural Health Sex* 17(2):180–193.

Stahlman, Shauna, Beyrer, Chris, Sullivan, Patrick S., Mayer, Kenneth H., Baral, Stefan D. 2016."Engagement of Gay Men and Other Men Who Have Sex with Men in the Response to HIV: A Critical Step in Achieving an AIDS-Free Generation." *AIDS Behavior.*

Stall, Ron, Matthews, Derrick D., Friedman, M Reuel, Kinsky, Suzanne, Egan, James E., Coulter, Robert W.S., Blosnich, John R., Markovic, Nina. 2016. "The Continuing Development of Health Disparities Research on Lesbian, Gay, Bisexual, and Transgender Individuals." *American Journal of Public Health* 106(5):787–789.

Stonewall International. 2016. *The Sustainable Development Goals and LGBT Inclusion*. www.stonewall.org.uk/sites/default/files/sdg-guide_2.pdf.

Swedish International Development Cooperation Agency. 2012. *Human Rights of Gay, Bisexual, and Transgender persons – conducting a Dialogue*. www.globalequality.org/storage/documents/pdf/sida%20dialogue%20paper%20on%20development.pdf.

Tat, Susana, Marrazzo, Jeanne M., Graham, Susan M. 2015. "Women Who Have Sex with Women Living in Low-and-Middle-Income Countries: A Systematic Review of Sexual Health and Risk Behaviors." *LGBT Health* 2(2):91–104. www.ncbi.nlm.nih.gov/pubmed/26790114.

Trapance Gift, Collins, Chris, Avrett, Sam, Carr, Robert, Sanchez, Hugo, Ayala, George, Diouf, Daouda, Beyrer, Chris, Baral, Stefan D. 2012. "HIV in Men who have sex with Men 4: From Personal Survival to public health: community leadership by men who have sex with men in the response to HIV." *Lancet* 380:400–410. www.thelancet.com/journals/lancet/article/PIIS0140-6736(12)60834-4/fulltext.

UN High Commissioner for Human Rights. 2015. "Discrimination and violence against individuals based on their sexual orientation and gender identity." A/HRC/29/23.

United States Agency for International Development. 2014. *LGBT Vision for Action: Promoting and Supporting the Inclusion of Lesbian, Gay, Bisexual, and Transgender Individuals*.

United States Agency for International Development. 2014. *Toolkit for Integrating LGBT Rights Activities into Programming in the E&E Region*, 2014. www.usaid.gov/sites/default/files/documents/1863/LGBT%20Toolkit%20092414.pdf.

World Health Organization. 2013. Executive Board Secretariat. *Improving the health and well-being of lesbian, gay, bisexual and transgender persons*, EB133/6.

30 Striving for reciprocity in electives

Katy Daniels

Introduction

Reciprocity is "the practice of exchanging things with others for mutual benefit, especially privileges granted by one country or organization to another" (Oxford Dictionaries 2016). Although the use of the term "elective" is varied, for our purposes it is defined as part of the curriculum where clinical healthcare students have the flexibility to choose both the study topic and location, which is often in another country.

International electives are a well-established part of curricula at most medical schools in high income countries such as the UK, Australia and Canada (Izadnegahdar *et al.* 2008, Miranda *et al.* 2005, Law *et al.* 2013) and are deemed a desirable component of undergraduate dental education in Europe (Manogue *et al.* 2011). Of the British students undertaking an international medical elective approximately 40 percent of them do so in a developing country (Miranda *et al.* 2005), whereas in Australia this can be as high as 59 percent (Law *et al.* 2013).

With large numbers of students undertaking international clinical electives in under-resourced settings, this potentially exacerbates the lack of resources by consuming staff time (Dowell *et al.* 2014) for tasks such as supervision, translation, and teaching, in addition to tangible (e.g., personal protective equipment, medical supplies) and educational resources (Bozinoff *et al.* 2014). Such electives can also include cultural voyeurism and replicate colonialist practices (Racine and Perron 2012) promoting the "West knows best" attitude, cultural insensitivities, and a power imbalance. Therefore, it is important to explore how striving for reciprocity can minimise these potential negatives and promote benefits for host communities. Key questions include: how reciprocal are current elective practices? What does reciprocity look like and how can it be increased? Who has responsibility for ensuring reciprocity is achieved and how is it measured?

Current clinical elective practices

International electives are included in curricula because of the learning healthcare students gain (Thompson *et al.* 2003, Dowell & Merrylees 2009, Jeffrey *et al.* 2011, Manogue *et al.* 2011 and Racine and Perron 2012), which broadly includes: clinical knowledge and skills, attitudes, personal and professional development, and global perspectives (e.g., cultural differences, healthcare systems, disease patterns). They are also one of the most valued parts of undergraduate medical education, providing significant transformative experiences for many, and reigniting the vocational drive that originally led many to enter the medical profession (Lumb and Murdoch-Eaton 2014) while potentially recruiting trainees to primary care and underserved areas (Thompson *et al.* 2003).

The benefits for students are clearly documented but increasing consideration is now being given to the positive and negative consequences for host communities (Dowell *et al.* 2014, Lumb and Murdoch-Eaton 2014). Host communities in low and middle income countries often experience an imbalance, with burdens potentially outweighing the benefits. There is an awareness of the need for change (Dowell and Merrylees 2009, Racine and Perron 2012) with sending institutions, government reports (Crisp 2007) and importantly, elective host communities in sub-Saharan Africa (Kumwenda *et al.* 2015), South America (O'Donnell *et al.* 2014) and low human development index countries (Bozinoff *et al.* 2014) recognising that reciprocity could be increased in current elective systems.

Addressing this imbalance would increase reciprocity and promote the beneficial learning through electives without creating burdens for host communities.

Characteristics of reciprocity

So, if increasing reciprocity is the aim, what recommendations are there about how to achieve this? Crump, Sugarman and the Working Group on Ethics Guidelines for Global Health Training (WEIGHT) (2010), which notably included individuals from low income countries, and Melby *et al.* (2016) have written guidance regarding ethics and best practices for international electives, while Muir *et al.* (2016) describe a framework for success. Although not exactly the same, it is not surprising that there are significant similarities and overlap.

Two key characteristics of reciprocity are:

1. Cross-cultural effectiveness and cultural humility

Host communities often have very different cultural beliefs and practices, both generally and specifically related to healthcare, while facing a variety of challenges and limitations, all of which students and external parties can be unfamiliar with. An in-depth understanding of these benefits students and host communities as does adopting the attitude that "we all have something to learn and all have something to teach" (Crisp 2010, p.vii). Pre-departure training, which is explored in *Chapter 9*, can address these issues. However, the extent of pre-departure training is varied and sometimes inadequate (Muir *et al.* 2016). Learning about cross-cultural effectiveness and cultural humility largely takes place within the host community and so opportunities to explore these differences during an elective are also crucial. Language barriers, cultural discordance, and unfamiliar clinical environments can decrease a student's independence and standards of ethics and professionalism are relevant irrespective of location (Melby *et al.* 2016), although local culture and beliefs can influence these and students, sending institutions and hosts must appreciate this.

2.   Bi-directional participatory relationships

Sending institutions and host communities need to: discuss expectations, needs, goals, and motivations; identify the benefits and burdens for all stakeholders; establish effective communication and ensure monitoring and evaluation takes place (Crump *et al.* 2010). Strategies are needed to maximise benefits and minimise burdens in a sustainable way, for example:

- Supporting or creating student development opportunities, e.g., promoting equivalent opportunities for local students or identifying and addressing other local student needs that are unable to be met locally.
- Supporting or creating professional development opportunities for host community partners, e.g., provide funding for training, clinical or educational, at an appropriate site or directly sharing the expertise of sending institution staff to address host community identified need(s).
- Formalising exchange partnerships with a regular flow of students and increased duration of placements (Bozinoff *et al.* 2014, Kumwenda *et al.* 2015).
- Offsetting resource consumption (Bozinoff *et al.* 2014, Kumwenda *et al.* 2015).
- Sending institution to support student teaching, supervision, and/or patient care (Kumwenda *et al.* 2015).

Effective leadership will be required which includes positive role modelling, and any partnership will need to be given time to mature (Muir *et al.* 2016).

Without such bi-directional relationship there is a risk of reinforcing the concept that "it is the richer [countries] that have most of the power and who determine the way the world's institutions and relationships work, and the poorer who have to live within a world shaped by others" (Crisp 2010, p.vii).

Having explored these two key characteristics of reciprocity, is anything being done to improve existing practices?

Reciprocity in practice

Having outlined characteristics of reciprocity what might these look like in practice. Unsurprisingly, the outworking of these can look very different so a variety of examples are described below.

Institutional partnerships

Umoren *et al.* (2012) and Muir *et al.* (2016) describe partnerships between institutions in resource rich and resource limited countries. Partnerships grow organically through personal connections of academics or are created for a specific purpose. In North America, an increasing number of partnerships between academic institutions and institutions in low and middle income countries exist (Muir *et al.* 2016). Over 93 percent involve collaborative research and/or educational experiences, such as electives, for North American students. Other forms of health and professional education and health systems development are common. Monroe-Wise *et al.* (2014) and Umoren *et al.* (2014) also describe bilateral exchange opportunities for healthcare staff, largely medical, from low income countries to a high income country.

Alternative types of partnerships also exist. A "responsible elective" programme (Responsible Electives n.d.) was established by the School of Medicine, University of Dundee, Scotland to create a fairer "trade" in electives. Partnerships, with formal agreed memoranda of understanding, exist with two host hospitals in Africa. Instead of creating bilateral exchange opportunities, reciprocity is sought through ongoing relationships, student fund-raising, and limited financial support from the School of Medicine.

A growing number of organisations offer to facilitate the organisation of clinical electives. Many work on a partnership basis and promote benefits to host communities, such as employing local staff and a proportion of fees going to host communities while minimising student burden through pre-departure training and language lessons. Whether or not these reciprocal elements attract students to elective organisations is unknown. They are also commercial organisations, charging for their services, so assessing the extent of reciprocity is challenging. However, the ongoing participation of host communities suggests there is at least some benefit for them. Due to the increasing number of students using such organisations there is potential for meaningful partnerships and trade to exist.

Student–student partnerships

The International Federation of Medical Students Association (2015) has been utilising a network of locally and internationally active students to provide bilateral exchange opportunities through the "SCOPE" programme since 1951. To improve affordability and accessibility, students participating pay costs in their own country for an incoming student. However, even for a bilateral exchange, costs such as exchange fees and international travel make even these programmes unaffordable for the majority of students in low income countries. These partnerships are also more transient than institutional partnerships.

Local students across the world undertake innovative projects that are resulting in change in their own communities and countries (Global Education in Medicine Exchange 2016b). Nawagi, a Ugandan medical student describes asking a local community to share their problems and potential solutions rather than "going and saying this will work and trying to implement it" and discovers that "their suggestions work best in their community, compared to what we would have thought would work" (Global Education in Medicine Exchange 2016c). This highlights how local students recognise they do not have the answers to the problems of other communities in their own country, yet despite this they can help empower local communities to bring about change. With this attitude as a starting point, can incoming elective students partner with and support local innovative projects to promote this type of change? Indeed, encouraging such truly socially accountable activities involving local students who help focus visiting students' activities and learning could be an excellent model of combined, bi-directional learning.

New exchange model

Bilateral exchanges can create opportunities but they are limited in number and organising them on a larger scale is difficult and costly. As such they often remain as a gift from western providers, potentially promote imperialism and concerns exist over encouraging the "brain drain." Recognising this and having an awareness of the lack of international elective opportunities for African medical students resulted in the creation of South–South Medical Eective Exchanges (SSMEEs). This model, inspired from conversations with Dundee Medical School academics and elective host communities in Africa, aims to create international elective opportunities for African medical students in another African country, rather than a high income country. This potentially increases financial sustainability and students should experience healthcare systems similar enough to their own that learning will be transferable to their own context. Interest from African universities was expressed at the Network Conference 2015 in South Africa, and so this model is being piloted with four African universities, one in each of Malawi, Rwanda, South Africa and Uganda, with support from Global Educational Exchange in Medicine and Healthcare Professions (GEMx) (Global Education in Medicine Exchange 2016a). Evaluation data assessing the feasibility and value of this alternative exchange model is not yet available. However, if positive opportunities for individuals, institutions, and organisations are ongoing, this will act to support its continuation.

The challenge of reciprocity

The variety of examples highlights positive features which increase reciprocity; however, challenges also exist.

First, students from the low income countries that host many students from high income countries have limited access to equivalent experiences and consequently miss out on the learning opportunities they provide (Flinkenflögel *et al.* 2015). Many factors may be responsible for this, including: lack of space in curricula, lack of finance, and difficulty obtaining visas. These barriers would need to be addressed if creating direct exchange opportunities.

Many sending institutions do not resource international clinical electives in the same way as other clinical placements so there is rarely any institution providing funding for host communities. Indeed, most international electives are self-funded. If fund-raising is involved, this needs a high level of motivation and engagement which can be difficult to maintain.

While on elective, "culture shock" and stress are experienced by students (Lumb and Murdoch-Eaton 2014) and can create an additional burden for host communities which needs to be addressed. A homestay model provides cultural immersion and social support for students while increasing mutual partnership and moves resources to the local community (Chia *et al.* 2015).

Assessing the true impact of international electives and the extent of reciprocity is challenging, because there is less monitoring, regulation and reporting, compared to other parts of curricula, despite usually being of several weeks' duration (Lumb and Murdoch-Eaton 2014). Even if attempts are made, the perception of the degree of reciprocity can differ. For example, North American institutions described the nature of reciprocity more positively than the low and middle income partner institutions (Muir *et al.* 2016). Challenges such as the lack of bi-directional student exchange and decision making being one-sided and lying with those that provide funding (Muir *et al.* 2016) might be reasons for this difference.

Who is responsible for ensuring reciprocity?

A range of individuals, educational and healthcare institutions and organisations are involved in international electives so where does responsibility lie for ensuring reciprocity?

For long-term partnerships to be successful, all stakeholders must understand a range of associated ethical issues, take into account all perspectives, and implement guidance such as that described by Crump *et al.* (2010) and Melby *et al.* (2016). Through this, long-term reciprocal relationships can be developed and bi-directional learning can take place.

Students are a great resource and source of enthusiasm (Muir *et al.* 2016). Many are proactive in global health and overcoming health inequality issues (Medsin-UK. n.d.). However, they are a transient population and individual electives do not provide the continuity required for the long-term partnerships which host communities seek (Bozinoff *et al.* 2014, Crisp 2007, Kumwenda *et al.* 2015, O'Donnell *et al.* 2014).

Sending institutions are in a position to create these long-term partnerships and have responsibility to facilitate reciprocity. This responsibility is not just because guidance recommends it (Crump *et al.* 2010, Melby *et al.* 2016) and host communities request it (Bozinoff *et al.* 2014, Crisp 2007, Kumwenda *et al.* 2015, O'Donnell *et al.* 2014), but also because they are role models for students. They are in a position to harness and direct student enthusiasm and altruism within an ongoing partnership. Larger collaborative bodies such as the Consortium of Universities for Global Health (2016) and the Working Group on Ethics Guidelines for Global Health Training (2010) also have a role to play in supporting sending institutions and developing guidance.

Evaluating reciprocal arrangements

Evaluation exploring value and impact is an important aspect of any programme and should include all stakeholders (students, sending institutions and host communities). Clearly specified objectives provide a basis for evaluation. In particular, the extent and effectiveness of reciprocity, particularly for host communities in low and middle income countries needs to be evaluated with the value and impact for students widely described already (Dowell and Merrylees 2009, Jeffrey *et al.* 2011, Manogue *et al.* 2011, Racine and Perron 2012).

Meaningful ways of measuring reciprocity need to be found and a variety of factors could be included in an evaluation:

* Net financial transaction per student – this may include impact to the clinical environment and/or wider community;
* Net resources gained, e.g., clinical supplies, equipment, books given;
* Elective related employment, e.g., language, accommodation, meals;
* Host community opinions – clinical staff, administrative staff, patients;
* Numbers of students/trainees being hosted;
* Professional development or training opportunities created for local students/staff;
* Number of direct student exchanges;
* Other means of support, e.g, research collaborations, SSMEEs, local student projects.

Conclusion

Striving for reciprocity in electives is an important issue to be tackled; however, there is not a simple "one size fits all" solution. Instead, each sending institution needs to consider its own elective programmes and explore what steps are appropriate and feasible. This is to ensure that electives are more reciprocal and certainly not a burden to host communities, especially those in low income countries. Involving host communities in this evaluation process and plans for change is likely to be a key to success.

Conflicts of interest

Katy Daniels is the electives lead at the University of Dundee and now runs the responsible elective programme. She is also helping facilitate the setup of the SSMEE pilot and is evaluating it for her medical education masters.

References

Bozinoff, N., Dorman, K.P., Kerr, D., Roebbelen, E., Rogers, E., Hunter, A., O'Shea, T., & Kraeker, C. 2014. "Toward reciprocity: host supervisor perspectives on international medical electives." *Medical Education* 48(4):397–404.

Chia, D., Sadigh, M., Goller, T., Kristiansen, K., Luboga, C., Luboga, S., & Sadigh, M. 2015. "A homestay Model for Global Health and Medical Education in Resource-Limited Settings." *Medical Science Educator* 25(3):317–321.

Consortium of Universities for Global Health. 2016. Retrieved November 25, 2016 from www.cugh.org/.

Crisp, N. 2007. Global Health Partnerships: The UK contribution to health in developing countries.

Crisp, N. 2010. *Turning the world upside down: the search for global health in the 21st century*. CRC Press.

Crump, J.A., Sugarman, J., and the Working Group on Ethics Guidelines for Global Health Training (WEIGHT). 2010. "Ethics and best practice guidelines for training experiences in global health." *The American Journal of Tropical Medicine and Hygiene* 83(6):1178–1182.

Dowell, J., & Merrylees, N. 2009. "Electives: isn't it time for a change?" *Medical Education* 43(2):121–126.

Dowell, J., Blacklock, C., Liao, C., & Merrylees, N. 2014. "Boost or burden? Issues posed by short placements in resource-poor settings." *British Journal of General Practice* 64(623):272–273.

Flinkenflögel, M., Ogunbanjo, G., Cubaka, V.K., & De Maeseneer, J. 2015. "Rwandan family medicine residents expanding their training into South Africa: the use of South-South medical electives in enhancing learning experiences." *BMC Medical Education* 15(1):1.

Global Education in Medicine Exchange. 2016a. Retrieved August 25, 2016 from www.gemxelectives.org/.

Global Education in Medicine Exchange. 2016b. Student projects for Health 2015. Retrieved April 15, 2016 from www.youtube.com/playlist?list=PLn4WjwZY4vPSZ M2GsvmWs7wnmbz4SERXS.

Global Education in Medicine Exchange. 2016c. Student Projects for Health 2015 – Faith Nawagi. Retrieved April 29, 2016 from www.youtube.com/watch?v=uBrdq tmLjcU&list=PLn4WjwZY4vPSZM2GsvmWs7wnmbz4SERXS&index=3.

International Federation of Medical Students Associations. 2015. Retrieved April 1, 2016 from http://ifmsa.org/exchange-the-world/.

Izadnegahdar, R., Correia, S., Ohata, B., Kittler, A., ter Kuile, S., Vaillancourt, S., & Brewer, T.F. 2008. "Global health in Canadian medical education: current practices and opportunities." *Academic Medicine* 83(2):192–198.

Jeffrey, J., Dumont, R.A., Kim, G.Y., & Kuo, T. 2011. "Effects of international health electives on medical student learning and career choice." *Family Medicine* 43(1):21–28.

Kumwenda, B., Dowell, J., Daniels, K., & Merrylees, N. 2015. "Medical electives in sub-Saharan Africa: a host perspective." *Medical Education* 49(6):623–633.

Law, I.R., Worley, P.S., & Langham, F.J. 2013. "International medical electives undertaken by Australian medical students: current trends and future directions." *Medical Journal of Australia* 198(6):324–326.

Lumb, A., & Murdoch-Eaton, D. 2014. "Electives in undergraduate medical education: AMEE Guide No. 88." *Medical Teacher* 36(7):557–572.

Manogue, M., McLoughlin, J., Christersson, C., Delap, E., Lindh, C., Schoonheim-Klein, M., & Plasschaert, A. 2011. "Curriculum structure, content, learning and assessment in European undergraduate dental education – update 2010." *European Journal of Dental Education* 15(3):133–141.

Medsin-UK. (n.d.). Retrieved November 28, 2016 from http://medsin.org/.

Melby, M.K., Loh, L.C., Evert, J., Prater, C., Lin, H., & Khan, O.A. 2016. "Beyond Medical 'Missions' to Impact-Driven Short-Term Experiences in Global Health (STEGHs): Ethical Principles to Optimize Community Benefit and Learner Experience." *Academic Medicine* 91(5):633–638.

Miranda, J.J., Yudkin, J.S., & Willott, C. 2005. "International health electives: four years of experience." *Travel Medicine and Infectious Disease* 3(3):133–141.

Monroe-Wise, A., Kibore, M., Kiarie, J., Nduati, R., Mburu, J., Drake, F., Bremner, W., Holmes, K. & Farquhar, C. 2014. "The Clinical Education Partnership Initiative: An Innovative Approach To Global Health Education." *BMC medical education* 14(1):1.

Muir, J.A., Farley, J., Osterman, A., Hawes, S., Martin, K., Morrison, J.S., & Holmes, K.K. 2016. Global Health Programs and Partnerships: Evidence of Mutual Benefit and Equity. Centre for Strategic and International Studies Global Health Policy Centre and University of Washington. Retrieved August 24, 2016 from: www.csis.org/analysis/global-health-programs-and-partnerships.

O'Donnell, S., Adler, D.H., Inboriboon, P.C., Alvarado, H., Acosta, R., & Godoy-Monzon, D. 2014. "Perspectives of South American physicians hosting foreign rotators in emergency medicine." *International Journal of Emergency Medicine* 7(1):1–7.

Oxford Dictionaries. 2016. Definition of reciprocity in English. Retrieved March 30, 2016 from www.oxforddictionaries.com/definition/english/reciprocity.

Racine, L., & Perron, A. 2012. "Unmasking the predicament of cultural voyeurism: a postcolonial analysis of international nursing placements." *Nursing Inquiry* 19(3):190–201.

Responsible Electives. (n.d.). Retrieved April 1, 2016 from http://blogs.cmdn.dundee.ac.uk/responsible-electives/.

Thompson, M.J., Huntington, M.K., Hunt, D.D., Pinsky, L.E., & Brodie, J.J. 2003. "Educational effects of international health electives on US and Canadian medical students and residents: a literature review." *Academic Medicine* 78(3):342–347.

Umoren, R.A., James, J.E., & Litzelman, D K. 2012. "Evidence of reciprocity in reports on international partnerships." *Education Research International* 2012.

Umoren, R.A., Einterz, R.M., Litzelman, D.K., Pettigrew, R.K., Ayaya, S.O., & Liechty, E.A. 2014. "Fostering reciprocity in global health partnerships through a structured, hands-on experience for visiting postgraduate medical trainees." *Journal of Graduate Medical Education* 6(2):320–325.

Part V
Case studies

31 Making the Links

Helping medical students prepare for global health careers

Ryan Meili

Social accountability of medical schools (*Chapter 17*) refers to the obligation of educational programmes to meet the priority health needs of the communities they serve (World Health Organization 1995). This includes a role in training physicians who will be able to provide care to diverse underserved communities. There has been increased interest in global health teaching, and in particular concentrations in global health among Canadian medical schools (Matthews *et al.* 2015) as a means of offering students the training opportunities to facilitate socially accountable practice.

The Making the Links certificate in global health is a programme that exposes learners to the social determinants of health through classroom teaching and immersive community-service learning. Housed at the College of Medicine in the University of Saskatchewan, the key elements of the programme include exposure to global health experiences in Saskatchewan, Canada and in other countries. Through these experiences, learners develop a greater understanding of global health and gain practical skills for later service as they "make the links" between challenges faced locally and abroad.

In the first years of the programme, Making the Links (MTL) selected four medical students per year to spend 6 weeks in Northern Saskatchewan in the on-reserve community of Buffalo River Dene Nation, also known as Dillon, or in the Métis community of Ile a-la-Crosse. The same students also spent time at the SWITCH student-run clinic in inner-city Saskatoon. They rounded out their MTL experience by spending 6 weeks in Massinga, a small town in Mozambique.

This early version was founded in response to a desire among students and faculty at the College of Medicine to offer a more meaningful global health learning experience. There was growing interest in such experiences, with many students seeking out international electives in low income countries. These were seen to be of varied value for learners and even more questionable value for the host countries. MTL was established with the idea of giving a deeper learning opportunity for student participants and creating continuity of relationships with the communities that welcomed them, allowing for the development of true partnerships and avoiding medical tourism.

The original sites were chosen due to existing community relationships with the College of Medicine. Northern Medical Services (NMS) is a branch of the University of Saskatchewan that provides physician services to the northern regions of the province. NMS doctors located in Ile a-la-Crosse helped make connections with community leaders and identify health-related local projects that students could get involved in. SWITCH, the Student Wellness Initiative Toward Community Health, is a student-run clinic located at the West Side Community Clinic in Saskatoon's core neighbourhoods. Students from nursing, pharmacy, nutrition, medicine, physiotherapy and several other health and non-health-related programmes offer supervised after-hours services to this underserved area of the city. The Mozambique site was selected because of the training for health renewal programme, a train-the-trainers partnership between the Mozambican Ministry of Health and the University of Saskatchewan. This partnership involved community-based participatory action research along with a connection to the local hospital that allowed for clinical rotations. Along with these on-site learning experiences, students participated in seminar discussion on Indigenous and global health and also took training in Portuguese in preparation for their time in Mozambique.

This initial programme proved popular among students and has steadily grown in the number of students it accepts. The early, extracurricular version chose four students per year, that number has now reached 15 students a year out of a class of one hundred. This past year 28 students applied to be part of the programme. With that growth came interest in a more robust academic programme, one that gave students a greater theoretical framework to interpret their experience, and also gave them credit for the significant additional efforts they put in on top of their medical training. In 2011 the University of Saskatchewan established MTL as a certificate in global health, the first of its kind in Canada.

The new certificate model has students completing five for-credit courses. Three of these are practicum classes for the onsite service-learning. The other two are classroom based. In Global Health 1, during their first year of medical school, students learn about specific social determinants of health and their relationship to concepts such as the global burden of disease and international development. There is also a dedicated section for learning about Indigenous health in preparation for time spent in First Nations and Métis communities. During the second year, students take a more practice focused Global Health 2 course, where they work with preceptors to teach their classmates about key communicable and non-communicable diseases relevant to working in global health settings.

Along with the enhanced academic components, Making the Links has also branched out to new sites for students, developing partnerships with Kawacatoose First Nation and the Northern Métis community of Pinehouse in Saskatchewan as well as international sites in Vietnam, Uganda and a second site in Nampula in northern Mozambique. A second student-run clinic,

SEARCH (Student Energy and Action for Regina Community Health), has also been established, offering opportunities for students studying at the College of Medicine campus in Regina.

MTL outlines six learning objectives for students: (1) gain educational experience in multiple contexts; (2) gain exposure to concepts of international, rural and urban health, and community development; (3) experience service-learning; (4) gain language skills and multicultural understanding; (5) improve communication skills; and (6) gain exposure to health systems and health teams.

The way in which these objectives are achieved varies depending on their host communities, and from year to year, as those communities are not static. During the 6 weeks spent in Indigenous communities in Saskatchewan students are involved in a small amount of clinical shadowing (at most one day per week). The rest of the time is spent in health-related community service. These activities include, among many others, planning youth conferences, planting community gardens, hosting local radio programmes, accompanying home care workers, joining in local celebrations and ceremonies and teaching youth about sexual health.

During the urban underserved experience students volunteer for two shifts per month at SWITCH or SEARCH during their first and second year of medical school. They join with students from other health disciplines to provide supervised after-hours care to an underserved inner-city population. Students engage in clinical service appropriate to their level of training and also contribute to health promotion programming, food preparation, child care and volunteer management.

During their international experience, MTL students combine a slightly larger clinical component (approximately 50 percent of their time) with community involvement in health promotion, community-based research, vaccination brigades, and other initiatives led by local healthcare providers and community leaders.

Students are evaluated formally through the coursework and by preceptors during the practicum experiences. They also have opportunities to submit their reflections on their experiences. A 2011 study of these reflections (Meili *et al.* 2011) revealed six theme areas of reflection: (1) the importance of relationships; (2) exposure to the social determinants of health in real life circumstances; (3) the significance of a community development approach for health; (4) the value of interdisciplinary collaboration; (5) the commonalities between international and local communities; and (6) personal learning about their own roles and careers.

The last point is of particular significance, as one of the higher-level objectives for programmes such as MTL is the fostering of a workforce that is prepared to deliver ethical, quality care to underserved communities. Of the 51 students that had completed the programme and gone on to residency as of 2013, 64 percent chose family medicine as their career path. Eighty-one percent of those choosing family medicine matched to rural family medicine programmes. The majority of those that did not choose family medicine chose general specialties (psychiatry, paediatrics, obstetrics and gynaecology).

Of course, seeing students pursue rural family medicine is not the only measure of success for such a programme. Specialists and subspecialists who are able to practice in global health settings and incorporate understandings of the social determinants of health into their practice reflect a valuable outcome as well. However, given the shortfalls in family medicine trainees and rural family practitioners in particular, as well as the unique needs of the Saskatchewan population and Indigenous populations in that province, this result is a hopeful one for the social accountability of the profession.

The same cohort of graduates (2005–13) was surveyed with regard to their current practice location in 2015, and the numbers from residency held true, with 43 percent practising in either a rural or northern setting, and several of those practising in urban settings working directly with inner-city or other underserved populations. Many of the graduates of the programme have also returned as preceptors, accompanying new cohorts of students on international experiences or hosting them in their own practices.

There is likely some selection bias to these high percentages of rural residency and practice, with students more interested in this type of practice more likely to pursue experiences like MTL. However, anecdotal reports, such as this one from one of the earlier participants – "I never thought that I would consider family medicine as a career and I certainly didn't think that I would ever want to do rural family medicine and Northern rural family medicine was completely out of the question. After spending time in a Northern community I can honestly say that rural family medicine in the North is one of my top choices in medicine" – suggest that for some it opens a window into unforeseen possibilities. The more common outcome is likely that students with an interest in this field are exposed to real practice models and lived experiences that make it easier for them to leave the comfort of the urban setting where they trained and strike out to the challenges of global health practice.

Two other questions regarding student impact relate to cost and to academic performance. In terms of cost, given the additional time invested and the travel involved, students could see significant opportunity cost and increased expenses. Not wanting this to be a barrier to participation, the College of Medicine funds the majority of the travel costs and provides a stipend during the Canadian practicum experience. There has also been the question of whether, given the additional class time and independent study, MTL students might find themselves at an academic disadvantage relative to their peers. A study of licensing exam scores compared outcomes from 2007–14 between MTL students and matched cohorts. The MTL students performed significantly better on average, demonstrating that their participation did not disadvantage them, and may even have contributed to better academic outcomes.

Other areas to explore to understand the impact of the programme would be the effect on preceptors and the host communities. Informal discussions with preceptors indicate that they enjoy the experience of working with students and assisting them with gaining practical understanding of global health. In recent years, more of the preceptors are MTL alumni, eager to give back to the programme, maintain connections with the host communities and foster global health leadership among a new generation of colleagues. More formal analysis of the impact of the programme on communities is warranted. However, regular conversations, and the input of community members to the Making the Links advisory board, suggest that the programme is valued. Perhaps the best evidence of this is that the communities continue to support the annual return of students, and local contacts profess that they look forward to meeting and working with each group.

This comprehensive MTL approach to teaching global health has caught the attention of other universities, and similar programmes have begun appearing across the country. Several other Canadian medical schools have sought to establish global health certificates or concentrations in recent years as a means of enhancing the support for students wishing to pursue careers in this field and as part of their social accountability mandate. In order to guide development towards a model of global health education that was ethically and pedagogically sound, global health groups at the Canadian Federation of Medical Students and the Association of Faculties of Medicine of Canada came up with a set of major and minor criteria for such programmes, using the MTL certificate in global health as a model (Matthews *et al.* 2015). The major criteria outlined were: (1) global health course work; (2) local community engagement; (3) student evaluation; (4) a low resource setting elective; and (5) pre-departure training and post-return debriefing. The minor criteria consisted of: (1) global health mentorship; (2) language training; (3) extracurricular global health learning opportunities; and (4) a knowledge translation project. Global health leads at 13 of Canada's 17 medical schools then evaluated these criteria. Agreement was unanimous on the major criteria, with some more divergence of opinion on the minor criteria, including some questioning the necessity of language training in particular.

While there was consensus on the major components of a quality global health concentration, greater variety was to be found in the degree to which each of the major elements were actually present in the various programmes. Hopefully, these criteria, and the discussions that have emerged from them, will serve to advance the efforts of global health leaders at the various faculties, giving them the opportunity to enhance further their global health programming and provide more opportunities for learners.

As the ideas in MTL become more widely understood and integrated into the main curriculum, there is a need for constant innovation in the course content to ensure that the students are truly receiving enhanced learning. MTL also strives continually to offer a better experience for students and their host communities, and to expand the number of positions and types of learning opportunities available for students. 2016 saw an increase from ten to 15 students in the programme. This increase coincides with a new development in the programme, the introduction of an Indigenous health stream. A third of the selected students will identify a focus on Indigenous health as a part of their MTL training. Their classroom work will have a higher emphasis on this topic, and their second year placement will be in an Indigenous community, either within Canada or internationally. The first test of this model begins in summer, 2016, with an experience for students with rural Indigenous communities in Australia. This pilot Indigenous health stream will be evaluated in partnership with Indigenous communities and academics and may lead to the development of an independent certificate in Indigenous health.

The Making the Links certificate in global health has given dozens of medical students an opportunity to build meaningful connections with communities, to gain a deeper understanding of the social determinants of health, and to imagine and pursue careers of meaningful service that meet community needs. By connecting local and international experiences this model brings together the common features of working with communities for health in diverse settings. It is one example of the way in which medical schools can creatively meet their social accountability mandates. Each school must determine their own methods of doing so; develop their own community connections; and support faculty and learners in a way fitting to their circumstance. Making the Links, and the criteria developed from that model, can hopefully serve to inform and inspire new and exciting efforts from schools across Canada and beyond.

References

Matthews DM, Watterson R, Bach P, Halpine M, Kherani I, Meili R. 2015. "Building a framework for Global Health Concentrations – An analysis of Canadian medical schools." *Academic Medicine* 90(4):500–504.

Meili R, Fuller D, Lydiate J. 2011. "Teaching Social Accountability by Making the Links: Qualitative evaluation of student experiences in a service-learning project." *Medical Teacher* 33(8).

World Health Organization. 1995. Reorientation of Medical Education and Medical Practice for Health for All. World Health Assembly Resolution 48.8.

32 Postgraduate medical education in global health

The Yale experience

Tracy L. Rabin

As the demand grows to incorporate global health experiences into clinical training programmes in the Global North, academic institutions that provide these opportunities have become increasingly aware of their responsibility to model ethical and equitable patterns of engagement with partner institutions. This chapter will discuss the philosophical evolution of global health education in the Yale School of Medicine (YSM) Department of Internal Medicine, highlighting the Makerere University–Yale University (MUYU) collaboration as an example of a bilateral medical education capacity building relationship. Specifically, this chapter will detail the development of the collaboration, as well as address concerns related to equity and retention of medical expertise.

From the International Health Programme to the Office of Global Health

The YSM Department of Medicine has been sponsoring ongoing international health elective clinical rotations for residents since 1981, initially under the framework of the International Health Programme (IHP). As described in 1999 by a group that included the founders of the IHP (Gupta *et al.* 1999), this initiative developed in reaction to the desire of Yale medical residents to support a group of Southeast Asian refugees that had been resettled in New Haven, CT. As the authors note:

> [t]he goals of the IHP have been to involve residents in primary care within diverse cultural settings, to encourage cost-consciousness using back-to-basics physical diagnosis without high technologic support, and to engender a sense of social responsibility.

Through this programme, clinical rotations at partner sites in resource limited areas (the International Health Elective; IHE) complemented opportunities for residents to work in a New Haven-based clinic for refugee patients. Although the name includes the word "international," the variety of rotation sites included both international and domestic (Native American reservation and inner-city mobile health van) host partnerships, reflecting the comprehensive IHP goals. The IHP fulfilled the desire of Yale residents for increased opportunities to use their medical training to engage with vulnerable communities in resource limited settings; this desire was held by many, as evidenced by the large percentage who participated in IHE and, in turn, was attractive for residency applicants with similar interests. Additionally, the on-site IHE mentors undertook mini-sabbaticals (funded by Yale) to enhance their skills and, when deemed appropriate, they were awarded adjunct Yale faculty positions.

The IHE rotations ranged in length from 4 to 8 weeks, consisting of a combination of resident elective and vacation time. The rotations were largely clinical, although individual residents were also able to become involved in research (to a limited degree) and educational programming at the host sites. Along the way, both the YSM Department of Medicine and Yale New Haven Hospital (YNHH) have supported the IHE experiences, making an important philosophical statement that residents would continue to receive their salaries and benefits while they are working off-site (a commitment that continues to the present). Additionally, resident airfare and living expenses were offset by funds generated through the Yale International Travelers' and Tropical Medicine Clinic, as well as direct contributions from the Department and YNHH.

In 2001, the IHP successfully obtained grant funding from the charitable arm of Johnson&Johnson to provide both additional financial support for resident IHE rotations, as well as resources for investing in administrative/structural support at international partner institutions. This allowed for a philosophical shift in the degree of engagement between the IHP and partner institutions abroad, ultimately resulting in a focus on a smaller number of global partners with a view towards long-term relationships that are grounded in bilateral capacity building. Thus, the clinical sites available for resident IHE decreased from 18 in the 2006–07 academic year (15 official relationships, and three sites that were independently selected by individual residents), to 12 in the 2007–08 academic year (six official and six independent). By July 2009, residents were no longer able to receive financial support from Yale for rotations at independent sites, and the IHP transitioned under the leadership of Asghar Rastegar to become the Office of Global Health (OGH). A mechanism still exists for residents to obtain approval from the Office of Graduate Medical Education to undertake international clinical rotations at unofficial sites; however, residents need to make the case that there is some specific skill to be developed at that site, or other reason for choosing an alternative site that is critical to their career path, in order to justify engagement with another partner institution. Additionally, there needs to be an appropriate support and supervisory system in place at the unofficial site.

The policy of limiting international clinical rotation sites reflects a specific philosophy of global health engagement: one in which trainees are intentionally steered towards working at sites that have longitudinal relationships with Yale. Through these sites, trainees are exposed to models of international partnership that are developed as bidirectional capacity building relationships, where the initial questions asked (and reassessed periodically thereafter) are, "How does the partner institution benefit from a relationship with Yale?" and "Is the partner satisfied with the degree of benefit provided?" Going back to the original goals of the IHP, the primary intended benefits for residents who participate in international clinical rotations during residency is to broaden their perspectives on clinical care and social responsibility. As the vast majority of these residents will not continue to work abroad in their future careers, this is a critical opportunity to role model equity (and ethical responsibility) in institutional relationships with colleagues in resource limited settings, as detailed elsewhere (Rabin *et al.* 2016).

The transition from IHP to OGH occurred at the time when Michele Barry (who, together with Frank Bia, had founded the IHP) moved from YSM to Stanford University School of Medicine; thus, in recognition of her role in the project, the funding mechanism for clinical rotations abroad evolved to become the Yale/Stanford Johnson&Johnson Global Health Scholars Programme. Importantly, although Johnson&Johnson has continued to fund this programme since 2001, the company has never played a role in selecting the partners, individuals funded, or structure of the programme. OGH submits an annual report to Johnson&Johnson, detailing the number of scholars that have been funded (as well as where they have worked), and providing updates and information about spin-off projects that have developed at each site.

Taking a broader view than the original IHP, the articulated mission of OGH is to confront the disparities in global health through research, education and health services in partnership with institutions serving resource limited communities around the world. This focus on a smaller number of dedicated partnerships has allowed for larger numbers of Yale residents (as well as health professional students and faculty) to become involved with each site, thereby providing a pathway for deeper relationships and the development of collaborative projects with wider impact. The remainder of this chapter will focus on the largest of the six OGH partnerships: the Makerere University–Yale University (MUYU) collaboration, which is a global health medical education capacity building project involving the Makerere University College of Health Sciences (MakCHS) and Mulago National Referral Hospital, in Kampala, Uganda, and YSM in New Haven, CT, USA.

Case study

The idea of MUYU was born in 2002 when former YSM faculty member Majid Sadigh travelled to Kampala to teach about HIV. During that visit, he became acutely aware of the contrast between the numerous high-level clinical and epidemiological research collaborations that had been ongoing through MakCHS, and the resource limited realities of patient care on the wards of Mulago Hospital, the only comprehensive advanced tertiary care facility in the Ugandan public healthcare system. Patient volume at Mulago typically exceeds the 1500-bed capacity; this hospital serves a population of more than 30 million. Mulago Hospital is also the primary clinical training site for the MakCHS undergraduate medical and nursing students, as well as postgraduate medical and surgical specialty trainees.

Drs Sadigh and Rastegar, together with colleagues from MakCHS – notably, Professors Nelson Sewankambo, Harriet Mayanja-Kizza, and Moses Kamya – developed the vision of a mutually beneficial relationship with a focus on improving the quality of patient care on the wards of Mulago Hospital. MUYU was ultimately launched and formalised in 2006 and has evolved into the largest international partnership that is supported by the Yale OGH, with a bidirectional, year-round flow of trainees and faculty. The founding objectives of the MUYU collaboration were as follows:

1. Enhancement of medical education and training for future physicians at Makerere University;
2. Establishment of a comprehensive training site through continued presence, bilateral exchange, and the development of a medical/social studies curriculum for students and residents from developed countries interested in international health;
3. Provision of essential therapeutic modalities at Mulago Hospital, in addition to improving diagnostic capacity, nursing care and patient care through development and strengthening of human resources, leadership and infrastructure; and
4. Development and support of a system of self-deliberation, continuous improvement in the provision of medical training, research and quality healthcare service.

Since its inception, MUYU has evolved to include an organisational structure headed by co-directors (one from MakCHS and one from Yale) and the development of offices to support visiting trainees and faculty at both institutions. These structures are critical to the success of the collaboration, as the robust communication between both partners and degree of support and oversight provided for visiting trainees and faculty at both sites allow for timely and nimble responses in times of crisis (whether an individual issue that is specific to one visitor (e.g., mental or physical health concerns), or something much larger (e.g., university or hospital staff strikes, political strife, or communicable disease outbreaks). Additionally, although MUYU had started as an independent entity, the support of leadership within Uganda has provided stability by enabling MUYU to become incorporated into the MakCHS administrative and financial structure.

Uganda to US exchange

In the first 10 years, MUYU has facilitated the exchange of 17 Ugandan physicians for the purpose of developing their clinical and research expertise in various non-communicable disease subspecialties, cumulatively spending 141 months at YNHH and Yale-affiliated hospitals. The positive impact of this exchange opportunity on the faculty has been described elsewhere (Bodnar *et al.* 2015). Given the strong desire to ensure that faculty are retained within the Ugandan medical system, the selection process has evolved over time such that successful candidates meet the following criteria: (a) are interested in working in a field that is in need of faculty capacity building (as determined by MakCHS leadership); (b) have been employed in that field by either MakCHS or the Ministry of Health for at least 2 years following postgraduate training; and (c) have a desire to contribute to clinical, research, and educational capacity building at MakCHS/Mulago Hospital upon returning to Uganda. Other Ugandans who have come to Yale for skill building through MUYU include one Mulago Hospital nurse (for 3 months of specific training as a diabetes nurse educator) and one MakCHS medical librarian for 3 months.

In addition to the benefits to the Ugandan healthcare system and trainees of exposing faculty and staff to the standards of care and state-of-the-art science that are found in a resource-rich setting, it is also worth noting that the clinical presence of Ugandan faculty who have worked in the Yale system enables visiting US trainees to have frank discussions about systems challenges and comparative standards. Over this same 10-year period of time, 25 MakCHS senior medical students have completed 4-week-long internal medicine rotations at YNHH; these experiences are funded by the Yale School of Medicine in reciprocity for the resources devoted by MakCHS faculty to educating Yale students in Kampala.

US to Uganda exchange: UME to GME to faculty

MUYU facilitates the US to Uganda exchange of health professions trainees for 4–6-week-long clinical rotations (via separate funding mechanisms for YSM medical and physician associate students). Through the Yale/Stanford Johnson&Johnson Global Health Scholars programme, MUYU also facilitates 6-week-long clinical rotations for medical residents (representing internal medicine, emergency medicine, obstetrics/gynaecology, paediatrics, and neurology). These trainees are partnered with Ugandan students and residents for inpatient medical rotations; the goal is that the US trainees are there both to learn from and to teach their colleagues in the course of providing care as a team, but not to be the sole provider of patient care in this foreign system. The US residents are additionally incorporated into ongoing departmental conferences. This exchange contributes to the training of both the Ugandan and US residents, primarily due to the impact of real-time patient care deliberations that encourage critical thinking and the implementation of evidence-based plans.

Trainee research rotations are also an ongoing part of MUYU (primarily involving medical, physician associate, nursing, and public health students); these typically take the form of 8–10-week-long summer research projects that are funded by internal Yale grants. Given that more than half of all Yale medical students will take a tuition-free year off to conduct research in between their third and fourth year (referred to as a fifth year), there are some who also receive fellowship funding to support a one-year project abroad. (Of note, Yale requires all students to complete an MD thesis based on original research, so these projects are typically used to satisfy that requirement.) Additionally, a small proportion of the medical residents have also been involved in research during their clinical rotations; however, this is strongly discouraged unless the resident has previously worked in Uganda or is working closely with local faculty on an ongoing project. With respect to faculty involvement in the collaboration, MUYU facilitates visits from Yale-affiliated faculty that range from 1–2-week-long fact-finding or administrative visits to provide clinical or educational support to a Ugandan faculty member, to longer clinical, educational, and/or research-related visits that last anywhere from 6 weeks to 6 months (which may require external support).

Spin-off initiatives

Over the years, MUYU has given rise to several additional capacity building initiatives that include: the Rainer Arnhold Senior House Officers' Teaching Support (RASHOTS) programme, funded by the US-based Mulago Foundation to support and enhance the education of MakCHS postgraduate internal medicine trainees; the development of the Uganda Initiative for Integrated Management of Non-Communicable Diseases (Schwartz *et al.* 2015), a multisectoral partnership aimed at building Ugandan capacity in the realms of prevention, clinical care, health worker training, and research to enable the provision of effective and integrated management of non-communicable diseases; and medical library support via the ongoing relationship between staff in the Yale School of Medicine Cushing/Whitney Medical Library and the MakCHS Sir Albert Cook Medical Library.

Next steps

The first 10 years of the MUYU collaboration have seen much success with respect to the direct training of Ugandan junior faculty, increased flow of ideas and critical thinking techniques between US and Ugandan postgraduate trainees, and the ultimate impact on Ugandan undergraduate medical trainees and the learning environment at Mulago Hospital. Moving forward, there are two key directions into which MUYU is expanding: (a) development and support of bilateral capacity building relationships outside of internal medicine, beginning with pathology and emergency medicine; and (b) development of a programme to support applied research focused on patient-centred care strategies for patient/community empowerment and the improvement of chronic disease management. By keeping a focus on capacity building within the construct of an equitable relationship, our hope is to continue to grow and evolve the collaboration to meet the changing needs of Mulago Hospital and the Ugandan healthcare system.

Acknowledgements

The author would like to thank the following institutions for providing the support that enables OGH and MUYU to continue this work: Johnson&Johnson, Makerere University College of Health Sciences, the Mulago Foundation, Mulago National Referral Hospital, Yale–Mulago Fellowship Corporation, Yale New Haven Hospital, and the YSM Department of Internal Medicine. Additionally, the author would like to thank the following faculty and administrators in the USA and Uganda, whose contributions and ongoing commitment have played a critical role in making the Yale OGH and MUYU what they are today: Dr Michele Barry, Dr Frank Bia, Mr Michael Bzdak, Mrs Laura Crawford, Mr Mark Gentry, Dr Ralph Horwitz, Dr Robert Kalyesubula, Professor Moses Kamya, Mrs Patricia King, Reverend Professor Sam Luboga, Professor Harriet Mayanja-Kizza, Ms Jamidah Nakato, Ms Susan Nalugo, Dr Kenneth Opio, Dr Asghar Rastegar, Dr Robert Rohrbaugh, Dr Majid Sadigh, Dr Jeremy Schwartz, and Professor Nelson Sewankambo.

References

Bodnar BE, Claassen CW, Solomon J, Mayanja-Kizza H, Rastegar A. 2015. "The effect of a bidirectional exchange on faculty and institutional development in a global health collaboration." *PLoS ONE* 10(3):e0119798.

Gupta AR, Wells CK, Horwitz RI, Bia FJ, Barry M. 1999. "The International Health Program: the fifteen-year experience with Yale University's Internal Medicine Residency Program." *American Journal of Tropical Medicine and Hygiene* 61(6):1019–1023.

Rabin TL, Mayanja-Kizza H, Rastegar A. 2016. "Medical education capacity-building partnerships for health care systems development." *AMA Journal of Ethics* 18:710–717.

Schwartz JI, Dunkle A, Akiteng AR, *et al.* 2015. "Towards reframing health service delivery in Uganda: the Uganda Initiative for Integrated Management of Non-Communicable Diseases." *Global Health Action* 8:26537.

33 By the south, for the south

The Latin American School of Medicine in Cuba

Mena Ramos

In 1999, the Latin American School of Medicine (*Escuela Latinoamericana de Medicina, ELAM*) in Havana, Cuba, was established as an international medical school, recognised by both the World Health Organization (WHO) and the Educational Commission of Foreign Medical Graduates (ECFMG). ELAM's bold mission is to increase the number of healthcare providers in underserved communities globally by targeting and training aspiring students from communities in need whom studies suggest are more likely to remain in practice among the underserved (Walker *et al.* 2010). As of 2015, ELAM graduated 26,842 doctors, the majority of whom come from South and Central America (Gorry 2016).

A year after the school's founding, members of the US Congressional Black Caucus lobbied the Cuban government for medical scholarships, arguing that constituents within their districts were without access to medical care and would benefit from having more doctors, thereby paving the way for scholarship opportunities for US citizens. By 2005, ELAM had graduated its first US student, and by 2015, a total of 113 US students had graduated (Gorry 2016). ELAM's mission addresses the critical shortage of healthcare providers in underserved communities, potentially reversing the global brain drain where doctors trained in the developing world move to practise in high resource settings. Through its mission, recruitment from underserved communities, pedagogy, and context, ELAM provides an alternative model, and in so doing, is uniquely positioned to provide doctors for the underserved by the South and for the South.

A unique study abroad experience

A typical study abroad experience during either medical school or residency in the Global North offers trainees a unique opportunity to catch a glimpse of an alternative healthcare system within a different cultural context as well as exposing students to different types of problems, pathologies and solutions largely defined by the practice setting and resources. Their fundamental limitation is in their length of stay ranging from 2 weeks to 6 months, with the first few weeks spent acclimating to a new setting, developing trusting relationships with local personnel, and by the time students and residents have developed a level of comfort, it is often time to depart. These shorter stay abroad experiences are better framed as introductions and/or contextualised within a well defined time limited project.

In contrast, the ELAM experience is a total of 6 years (7 years for those who require intensive Spanish and pre-medical basic science preparation), which is considerably longer than most study abroad experiences including 2–3 year volunteer placements such as the Peace Corps. Furthermore, unlike study abroad experiences where home institutions have respective satellite offices and/or faculty to support visiting students and volunteers, ELAM is an entirely independent institution run by the Cuban Ministry of Public Health. This is compounded by the limitations in access to information technology beyond medical research as well as limitations on social media and travel restrictions from the United States pose unique challenges for US ELAM students, not just medically but for staying connected with family and friends. Both length of stay as well as total immersion provide ELAM students with unique perspectives as foreigners in a different country, and as foreigners in the unique sociopolitical and economic paradigm that is Cuba. Unlike a short-term "study abroad" experience, where much can be learned but nothing endured, the ELAM experience forces students to embrace the day-to-day challenges of medical school while being immersed in a different cultural context. This type of immersion experience may engender empathy for caring for immigrant populations who face similar challenges like being an outsider, adjusting to a new cultural context, and learning a new language.

While ELAM is a medical school in the Caribbean, it differs from other Caribbean medical schools in several key ways. St George's University School of Medicine in Grenada, the number one international provider of licensed physicians practising in the USA (Young *et al.* 2015), markets itself as a pipeline for doctors into US residencies (Hartocollis 2014). An article from the New York Times entitled "Second Chance Medical School" describes St George's as geared to "catch the overflow of Americans who cannot find a medical school in their home country willing to take them." While a second chance opportunity might not be the case for all students at St George's, the stigma for graduating international medical graduates entering US residency programmes remains.

Institutions such as St George's, Ross University in Dominica, number two on the provider list (Young *et al.* 2015) and American University in Sint Maarten, are for-profit schools, with costs comparable to medical education in the United States. Furthermore, these medical schools aid their students in entering US residencies by paying hospitals to accept their students for clinical clerkships in their third and fourth year of medical school. Due to the sheer diversity of the student body hailing from over 80 countries, ELAM does not directly facilitate clerkship placement to the US. For ELAM grads hailing from the US, the pathway towards residency is largely individually driven and aided by home organisations with a particular interest in increasing providers for underserved communities.

A case can be made that while for-profit Caribbean medical schools are expensive and place considerable financial barriers to education, they also train many doctors who ultimately work in both rural and urban underserved hospitals in the USA through scholarship agreements such as the New York City Health and Hospitals Corporation. ELAM, though, caters specifically to students from underserved communities by providing full scholarships to medical students, the large majority of whom come from and now practise in countries outside of the United States including Central, South America as well as in Africa. The ELAM pipeline was established primarily for the developing world with a Spanish language curriculum and modelled after the Cuban system unlike many schools in the Caribbean, the Philippines, and India who market themselves as schools with a pipeline to the United States.

Addressing barriers

The ELAM model actively addresses the social and economic barriers to medical education in underserved communities in an effort to increase the number of healthcare workers more likely to work and remain in communities of need. This model recognises that education for members of underserved communities not only improves overall economic returns for those communities, but will more likely provide a sustainable, arguably culturally more appropriate, workforce dedicated to addressing the needs of those communities. In a study published in 2010 in the *American Journal of Public Health*, physicians who practised in underserved areas were more likely to report mission-based values such as a sense of responsibility or moral obligation to a particular community or a defined patient population as well as self-identity (including race, language, and personal or family background) as motivators (Walker *et al.* 2010). Furthermore, regardless of race or ethnicity, the majority of physicians who practised in underserved areas reported feeling a unique connection to the particular community in which they practised. Thus, ELAM is uniquely positioned to provide doctors who will continue to practise in underserved communities well beyond graduation.

The student body at ELAM is actively recruited from poor, remote, marginalised and Indigenous populations, reflecting graduates from 84 countries primarily from South and Central America between 2005 and 2015 (ELAM, Department of International Relations 2016). Other countries represented include the United States, and nations from African and Asian countries with bilateral agreements with Cuba. While they do not include costs of transportation to and from countries of origin nor do they cover costs for board certification, full scholarships include tuition, food and lodging. Thus, graduates of ELAM finish medical school with a degree of economic freedom as a result of no or minimal debt compared to the average medical school graduate in the United States and medical school in the Caribbean. As the costs of medical education can result in deterrence from pursuing much needed primary healthcare or working in public sectors that are less well compensated, medical scholarships address these financial barriers to working with the underserved.

The preparation necessary to enter medical school can serve as a significant barrier for most who matriculate through an educational system that either requires funds from an early age to access quality education and to pursue extracurricular activities that make a candidate more competitive for medical school. At ELAM, recruitment from resource limited communities leads to an educationally diverse student body. The educational backgrounds of students at ELAM range from secondary school level to graduates of 4-year universities with or without advanced degrees. To address the educational gap, students are offered a 6–12-month intensive curriculum in basic sciences. For those from non-Spanish-speaking countries, Spanish immersion is also offered as all didactics are in Spanish taught by Cuban professors.

ELAM philosophy and model

Primary care, public health, and the social determinants of health

In addition to recruitment from underserved communities for students with demonstrated commitment to continue serving the underserved, ELAM addresses the critical shortage of healthcare providers for underserved communities through education, training students in an environment that is experientially driven and immersed within local communities, thereby creating a unique connection between learner and local community. Through mission, recruitment, pedagogy and context, the ELAM experience differs from other study abroad experiences and other medical schools in the Global North and the Caribbean.

The philosophy of medical education is exemplified by a curriculum that embodies the strengths of Cuba's healthcare system, combining population health, preventive medicine, and social determinants of health training throughout the 6 years. The 6-year curriculum is divided into 2 years of basic sciences followed by 4 years of clinical rotations including a sixth and final year of internship. These rotations include public health, primary care/community medicine, and a sixth year rotating internship. Students are immersed within a primary care focused model throughout the 6 years, learning physical exam skills and clinical diagnosis in community health clinics to which every community in Cuba is assigned, consisting of a family physician–nurse team that resides in the community (*"El Equipo Basico de Salud"*) charged with providing primary care and chronic disease management. In addition to the family physician and nurse team, a social worker and public health vector control technician complete the basic health team, illustrating the importance of integration through a multisectoral approach.

A robust curriculum on social and economic determinants of health permeates medical student learning through classroom didactics as well as community integration. During this fifth year rotation, students are assigned a local community, usually within walking distance of the teaching hospital in order to conduct a community health diagnosis (*diagnostic de la situación de salud*). This differs from most community health interventions in that they are performed throughout the year on a continuous basis, comprehensive for all households within an assigned community, and structured to identify and address risk factors, both individually and within a household. This system of active case finding and risk stratification allows for comprehensive primary care of a community, centred around a local family medicine clinic. This involves students in door to door household visits, risk stratifying families based on risk factors including economic, social, and environmental risk factors, compiling data for individuals to arrive at a risk assessment known as *dispensarización* for the household, which is then filed at the community health clinic with the family doctor–nurse basic health team. The exercise of active risk assessment and case finding coincides with a larger emphasis on primary care and prevention. Furthermore, ELAM students see their patients within the context of the community, which allows students to gain a better understanding of the social context from where their patients come.

ELAM as an entity of the Ministry of Public Health is also charged with meeting the population health needs of the Cuban community. These lessons are not static; predefined but experiential encounters go beyond the classroom to respond to the current health challenges faced by the community in Havana where the medical school is located, and medical students are integrated into the workings of the larger public healthcare system and play an important role in the workforce needed to respond to epidemics and natural disasters. For example, during epidemics of dengue fever, ELAM students serve as community health workers, going door to door within a community to identify cases of dengue for prompt isolation, testing and treatment. Following the hurricane season, medical students serve as the workforce to go door to door in communities most badly affected by flooding, assessing household access to clean and safe drinking water. In more recent years, the dilemma of Zika virus has been addressed through active case finding and vector control.

The 6-year curriculum allows for more time at the bedside to hone interpersonal skills, interview and physical exam skills, extend public health and family medicine rotations, as well as including mandatory disaster medicine rotations. The Cuban system places strong emphasis on the doctor–patient relationship, the history and physical exam prior to ancillary studies to arrive at a diagnostic impression. This style of medical practice creates a greater consciousness around utilisation of resources, if and when more costly resources are required to establish a diagnosis and/or for treatment ultimately to improve patient care. Third-year medical students spend half of the year learning *Propedeutica Medica*, an introduction to clinical medicine, which is spent almost entirely at the bedside taking detailed histories and performing physical exams. The time spent allows for more extensive bio-psycho-social history taking and interpretation of physical exam findings in order to arrive at a clinical impression prior to any other ancillary studies. Patients often identify students as their treating physicians due to the amount of time spent at the bedside. The time at the bedside with patients allows students to develop the interpersonal skills necessary to build rapport with patients as well as with colleagues and other members of the healthcare team.

Cooperation versus competition

The learning environment at ELAM lends itself to cooperation versus competition as a means of success. As students range from such diverse backgrounds and will ultimately join a health workforce with enormous global need, students do not need to compete with one another for limited spaces in residency or jobs. Furthermore, as ELAM is a relatively young institution founded in 1999 compared to other medical schools with more established reputations, opportunities for residency and views of the quality of ELAM education is largely dependent on the performance of former ELAM graduates.

ELAM classrooms are structured to promote a cooperative and collegial atmosphere for learning. From the first year basic sciences onwards, individual classrooms of 20–30 students are assigned "tutors" among the students in the class who are performing well on written and oral exams. These designated "tutors" are assigned the task of facilitating student learning after hours for peers who encounter more challenges in the subject matter. This team-based approach extends beyond individual classrooms, but also within delegations from respective countries. Graduates from the same country must go through similar challenges of re-integration and board certification that are unique to each country; therefore, they rely heavily on one another for success in practice beyond ELAM.

Challenges

ELAM is not without its challenges. The very diversity of the student body poses a challenge for health educators to support a medical student's transition to residency within their home countries due to the unique requirements for physicians to practise within each respective country. For example, in the USA, medical students are required to pass a series of USMLE exams (Step 1, Step 2 CK and CS) prior to beginning residency. Other countries in Central and South America have their own respective requirements. Due to limited resources, ELAM does not specifically address each and every student's needs for recertification in their own countries, thus leaving the responsibility on individual students themselves. Students have organised into delegations in order to advocate for one another, with resource banks and study groups specifically addressing the hurdles within their own countries to practise upon

graduation from ELAM, once again highlighting the importance of cooperation and partnership to achieve success.

The financial challenges for a resource constrained island country are
real. While Cuba spends 11.1 percent of its gross domestic product (GDP)
on public health expenditure (World Health Organization 2014) it remains
a small island country burdened by a complex history of political isolation
exemplified by the US economic embargo on Cuba that strains an already
struggling economy. This economic strain trickles down to the public health
system where employees of the healthcare system face daily economic challenges for survival and where technological resources for diagnosis are limited. A low infant mortality rate (IMR) and increased life expectancy come at
a cost. While some champions of public health argue that the gains in human
life and quality years gained far outweigh the costs, the issue of compensation remains controversial. What does remain certain is that ELAM graduates training within the economically resource constrained environment of
Cuba lends itself to lessons in resourcefulness, resilience, reliance on history
and physical exam skills, and an eagerness to learn and incorporate the use of
newer technologies best to serve their patients.

Roots in Cuban health and foreign policy

Since the Cuban revolution in 1959, Cuban investment in public health, primary care, and health education have led to staggering improvements in basic
health indicators including life expectancy and IMR. In the 1970s and 1980s,
Cuba strengthened the areas of primary care and prevention, decentralising
basic health services by building polyclinics and factor doctor-and-nurse officers within communities, which provided services ranging from basic health
maintenance screening, management of chronic non communicable disease,
prenatal services, to public health epidemiology and vector control for mos-
quito born illness such as dengue and Zika (Reed, 2008). In 2012, the WHO
reported life expectancy in Cuba to be 79.07 years comparable to 78.74 years
in the United States (World Bank 2015) and the IMR in Cuba is estimated
at 4.76 per 1000 live births in 2013 compared to 5.90 in the United States
(Central Intelligence Agency 2016).

A great deal of Cuba's success is attributed to its capacity to train health
personnel and build a substantial healthcare workforce with 6.7 physicians/
1000 citizens (World Health Organization 2014) compared to 2.5/1000 citizens in the USA (World Health Organization 2013). Furthermore, the commitment to healthcare is evidenced by its public health expenditure, investing
11.1 percent of its GDP compared to 4.7 percent in India (World Bank 2014)
The Cuban health system is unique to its sociopolitical context in that it is a
universal, singular, integrated system that is run by the state. From these perspectives, the Cuban healthcare system serves as one model for a functioning
healthcare system from which lessons can be drawn for both resource limited
and abundant settings.

Cuba's investment in healthcare extends beyond its own national borders. In 1999, an old naval academy was converted into a medical school and ELAM was founded. The founding of ELAM was preceded by decades of Cuban foreign aid delegations, sending doctors to communities in South and Central America devastated by natural disasters such as hurricanes. By training medical students from those respective communities and eliminating the barriers of cost, Cuba created a model for building a sustainable healthcare workforce for the most vulnerable communities globally.

Applications for other medical settings

Now over 10 years since its inception, the ELAM model offers a unique example of medical education strongly rooted in social justice, health equity, cooperation, primary care and community medicine, cultural humility and preferential treatment for the underserved. Central to its success is providing full medical scholarships for students from communities of need expressing the desire to work within those communities upon graduation. This, however, requires the political will to fund medical education and to identify the barriers to quality medical education for vulnerable communities, the willingness to overcome those barriers, and to continue to ensure a pipeline of physicians who are not constrained by mounting financial debts from medical education. Of the US ELAM graduates currently in practice, 90 percent have chosen to pursue primary care specialties including family medicine (61 percent), internal medicine (23 percent), and paediatrics (6 percent) (ELAM, Department of International Relations 2016).

The ELAM student body is a global health community, representing an unprecedented diversity of culture and historical contexts, converging in a medical school environment. Hence the richness of the ELAM experience is drawn not only from its setting within a unique public healthcare system but from the cultural diversity of its student body. The process of adaptation to a new culture and sociopolitical paradigm while living among a global community lays the foundation for lifelong lessons in cultural humility and self-awareness. The balance between balancing one's individual needs versus the collective are challenged daily and reflect but a microcosm of the struggles of more complex healthcare systems with limited resource to address both individual versus collective needs. The ELAM approach strengthens the notion that training in cooperation, humility, and self-reflection are necessary for healthcare workers better to address the complex problems facing global health today and the challenges of sustaining a global health workforce.

References

Central Intelligence Agency. 2016. "Country Comparison: Infant Mortality Rate." The World Factbook. Accessed June 28, 2016. www.cia.gov/library/publications/the-world-factbook/rankorder/2091rank.html.

ELAM, Department of International Relations. 2016. MEDICC Trip, May 2016.

Gorry, Connor. 2016. "Latin American Medical School Class of 2015: Exclusive with Cuban-trained US graduates." *MEDICC Review International Journal of Cuban Health and Medicine* 18(102): January–April.

Hartocollis, Anemona. 2014. "Second Chance Medical School." *New York Times*, July 31, 2014. Accessed June 27, 2016. www.nytimes.com/2014/08/03/education/edlife/second-chance-med-school.html.

Reed, Gail. 2008. "Cuba's Primary Care Revolution: 30 Years On." *Bulletin of the World Health Organization* 86:321–416.

Walker *et al.* 2010. "Recruiting and Retaining Primary Care Physicians in Urban Underserved Communities: The Importance of Having a Mission to Serve." *American Journal of Public Health* 100(11):2168–2175.

World Bank. 2014. "Health expenditure total,% GDP 2014." Accessed June 27, 2016. http://data.worldbank.org/indicator/SH.XPD.TOTL.ZS.

World Bank. 2015. "Life expectancy at birth, total (years)." Accessed June 28, 2016. http://data.worldbank.org/indicator/SP.DYN.LE00.IN.

World Health Organization. 2013. "Physicians density (per 1000 population)." World Health Organization. Accessed May 7, 2017. http://apps.who.int/gho/data/node.main.A1444.

World Health Organization. 2014. "Health expenditure total, % GDP 2014." World Health Organization. Accessed June 27, 2016. http://data.worldbank.org/indicator/SH.XPD.TOTL.ZS.

Young *et al.* 2015. "A Census of Actively Licensed Physicians in the United States, 2014." *Journal of Medical Regulation* 101.

34 Experience of developing a model for responsible electives

The Medicine in Malawi Programme (MIMP)

Jon Dowell and Neil Merrylees

Electives have been a feature of medical education in the UK since the 1970s. Typically they last between 6 and 8 weeks and take place during the final 2 years of a 5–6-year medical course. Approximately 40 percent of British students spend their elective in a developing country (Miranda *et al.* 2005). This means that with around 8000 students a year from the UK participating in medical electives nominally about 500 years of student time annually is spent on elective placement in a resource poor setting from the UK alone. This is by any measure a large commitment in terms of human resources, albeit pre-qualification. In our 2009 paper we explained that neither the potential benefits of this were being capitalised on, nor were real concerns about possible harms being addressed (Dowell and Merrylees 2009).

It was against this background that the Medicine in Malawi Programme (MIMP) was conceived and developed at Dundee Medical School. In this chapter, the programme and its outcomes will be described along with the challenges faced, and lessons learnt. Finally, the legacy will be discussed.

Background

At the time that the MIMP was conceived (around 2005), a number of issues relating to electives were being highlighted.

First, it was clear that they offered valuable educational opportunities; however, it was also clear that there was a number of potential negative aspects. These became apparent when comparing elective outcomes with standard curriculum outcomes and in many ways reflected the value and appeal intrinsic in seeking a highly contrasting clinical and cultural experience. They included culture shock (value of life, disparity of standards), novel levels of clinical opportunity, potential missed learning opportunities, cultural insensitivity (ill prepared), and opportunity cost (absorbing staff time rather than contributing usefully). There was also concern over the personal risks that students were exposed to. In addition, there were other ethical and moral concerns relating to the nature of electives (Miranda and Finer 2005, Radstone 2005). Many of these have been discussed elsewhere in this book and so will not be repeated here.

So although electives appeared a very popular and successful aspect of most western undergraduate courses, the authors suggested at the time that the benefits for students could be substantially increased and negative effects minimised with suitable planning and preparation, ideally assisted by the establishment of long-term partnerships (Dowell and Merrylees 2009).

Key principles

To address these issues, a number of key principles were agreed:

- Partnerships should be at the heart of electives. They should be established between medical schools sending students and those host units where they will be based. These would allow the development of programmes and relationships between faculty and enhance continuity.
- Placements should be longer than typical electives of 6–8 weeks and be based primarily in one clinical area to enhance the potential for student contribution to patient care ideally spaced throughout the year.
- Selection: students should be carefully selected to ensure they "buy in" to the ethos of the programme and have the qualities to allow them to capitalise on what the placement has to offer.
- Preparation before departure should help students maximise the learning opportunities while at the same time protecting their own health and safety and avoiding ethical dilemmas or potentially harming patients.
- Coordination of learning and supervision should be by a senior clinical tutor ideally for both elective and local healthcare students together.
- Practical support for host units should be part of the "package": for instance educational resources or relevant medical equipment provided by project/student fund-raising.
- Reciprocity should allow students in the host country to benefit from elective opportunities.

The MIMP

Based on these principles, the MIMP was established and lasted from 2007 to 2013. It consisted of the following elements.

Partnership

Following initial exploratory visits in January 2006 and August 2007 a memorandum of understanding (MOU) was signed between the College of Medicine (COM) of the University of Malawi based in Blantyre, a central hospital, and Dundee Medical School.

A key determinant was funding. Two grants of £30,000 over 3 years were obtained from NHS Education for Scotland and the Scottish government.

In addition, over the 4 years the student group raised over £13,000. They were involved in identifying areas of need. Examples of items funded were: trolleys for the wards, a projector and a laptop for presentations.

Placements

A programme of placements for senior medical students was established. The normal 6-week elective was extended to 4 months for selected students from Dundee. These rotated throughout the year (apart from exam times) allowing a student presence there for 8 months of the year. The students were based in the medical unit for most of their time.

These placements commenced in July 2008. By the end of the programme in 2013 a total of 34 students had completed extended placements. Each year between seven and nine students took part in groups of three to four.

Selection

Students had to demonstrate suitability through participation in an international health module (or significant previous developing country experience), a sound academic and health record, appropriate understanding of the programme aims, and completion of mandatory preparation. Selection took place approximately 14 months before the placement was due to commence. Students were selected as part of a group and encouraged to work and fundraise together in the year before departure.

Preparation

All students had to attend a number of briefing days before departure. These days covered such topics as culture shock, health and safety and clinical topics.

In addition, they were each required to raise a total of £500 for the hospital. This was kept centrally and the students were encouraged to find out local priorities on how best it should be spent.

Coordination

A local specialist from Malawi who was newly qualified was keen to be involved and visited Dundee to attend a medical education course and meet students.

Practical support/funding

In addition to student exchanges detailed below the opportunity for the development of parallel links with clinical and associated health professionals arose. This involved providing funding for some local training courses for Malawian anaesthetic staff and also visits by two medical physics technicians from Dundee to support maintenance of equipment.

Reciprocity

The College of Medicine was keen for a reciprocal programme through which two of their senior students would spend a 6-week elective in Dundee each year. The exchange programme started in November 2007 and in total 12 COM students undertook an elective in Dundee between 2008 and 2013.

Outcomes of the programme

Evaluations of the electives undertaken by both Dundee students to Malawi and College of Medicine student to Dundee have been carried out.

Dundee student placements

Students' feedback was obtained by face-to-face debriefings with most of the group on return and from their written reports. It was also gathered informally during the attachments by email and phone contact. In addition, both authors made visits and had discussions with local staff.

Findings suggest there have been obvious impacts, largely in terms of clinical examination, practical skills and experience of infectious diseases. However, the experience also seems to have improved confidence, particularly when approaching acutely unwell patients and so have helped the students feel better prepared for the first post qualification year (FY1). They also saw clinical presentations they would never have seen at home and got the opportunity to carry out procedures under appropriate supervision. The latter included lumbar punctures and abdominal and thoracic paracenteses.

The lack of investigations, although frustrating, allowed them to improve their clinical decision-making and they appreciated the greater responsibilities afforded by working in the challenging setting. They also had opportunities to develop their teaching skills to both clinical officers and students. Individually, their experiences afforded them plenty of opportunities to reflect, particularly on contrasting healthcare provision.

Particular problems were highlighted about cost and the provision of support; however, overall the students seem to have enjoyed their experiences, in spite of the challenges faced, and believe the project has been beneficial.

One of the key aims of the programme was to provide opportunities for students to contribute meaningfully to patient care. This worked to some extent. The main mechanism for this seems to have been through attention to detail – for instance following up diligently on laboratory results and making sure they were acted on. Overall the programme proved to be a very powerful experience for some students. No concerning events were reported.

In addition to the clinical work, students were involved in other ways.

Journal club sessions were started and the students had the opportunity to present at these. In addition, they also had the opportunity to develop useful symbiotic relationships with student clinical officers. They could help translate and teach about the local cultural and social context while our students could help them regarding the basic sciences underlying many of the conditions seen and examination techniques.

They carried out a number of small audit projects, which would be of use to the hosting medical department as a whole. These included an audit of HIV drug side effects and a health and safety audit. With groups of students following on from one another, they could follow up on findings and carry out second cycles of audits.

Although based primarily in the medical unit, students also carried out a number of short attachments. These included non-governmental organisations (NGOs) and hospital attachments in other departments for example obstetrics/gynaecoloty, surgery, anaesthesia and paediatrics.

Reciprocal visits by Malawian College of Medicine students

The programme was evaluated by a student doing an intercalated degree and involved interviews with a cross-section of students involved in the programme. Overall the experience was very positive. One concern was that of itself it might encourage students to want to leave the country in the future. However, these concerns did not seem to materialise. One particularly positive aspect was that the both the students and the College of Medicine reported a more patient centred approach by students following the placement, which seemed to extend into their practice after their return.

Challenges

In Dundee

Timetabling for Dundee students was a major issue for Dundee Medical School, due to the extended nature of the elective as it complicated other attachments. One of the main issues for Malawian students visiting Dundee was obtaining the appropriate visas in advance.

In Malawi

These can be grouped into logistical challenges and safety challenges.

a) Logistics

There was a number of local logistical challenges in Malawi to be faced in setting up the programme especially relating to travel and accommodation.

Internet access was a major concern for the students, especially before departure. They were required to complete part of their application for their first post qualification jobs online during a small time window and therefore needed good internet access during this period. In addition, they also needed to submit a number of medical school assignments and carry out some literature searches. In the event, acceptable access was available when required.

Regular power outages had been planned for in advance. However, the location of the accommodation also proved difficult because students could not be accommodated near the hospital and so had to travel. Backpacker accommodation was not really suitable for those who were on longer placements and required to do academic study. For part of the time a house was rented and this proved satisfactory, although costly.

Supervision proved a much greater challenge than had been anticipated. The tutor who had agreed to oversee the students while on placement was seconded away from the hospital at short notice and although replacements were found they did not have the ability to offer the same level of support to the students.

b) Safety issues

Three students suffered exposure to needlestick/splash injuries causing concern. One chose to return to the UK.

Civil disturbances in 2011 resulted in a major disruption to the programme including requiring the movement of two students out of Lilongwe – but to a logistically better rural mission hospital site within Malawi as well as extension of the programme to Zambia to reduce the vulnerability of having a single base. This marked the formal end of the MIMP as such and it evolved into the "Responsible Electives" initiative, which allowed applications from students from other universities.

Lessons learnt

Some of the challenges could not probably have been foreseen. However, overall the programme required a lot of work for a relatively small number of students.

Initially we tried to avoid related overseas staff travel; however, with hindsight this was probably a false economy as potentially some issues might have been resolved with a more frequent presence on the ground.

Legacy

The legacy from the MIMP is somewhat different from what was envisaged when it was established.

Despite the challenges one of the most enduring features has been the partnerships that have been established and the personal contacts made.

The development of a partnership with another centre in Malawi opened the possibility of other activities there. In particular, it has hosted students doing small research projects as part of an intercalated degree in international health. In addition, one of the authors (NM) continues to spend approximately 5 weeks there annually doing some clinical work as well as furthering some academic activities and interests.

In addition, a parallel partnership with another centre in Zambia has evolved based on the same principles facilitating a small but steady "trade" in Responsible Electives student placement from Dundee.

Further work has been done on researching electives. Some of these have been as part of BMSc projects, such as exploring host and student perspectives in depth.

Reciprocity has its challenges and after considering this we are seeking to promote more cost effective regional electives by linking medical schools in South Africa, Malawi, Rwanda and Uganda – to try and maintain the reciprocity aspect in a more sustainable way.

There has been interest nationally in the UK in developing a more coordinated approach to the management of electives. One of the authors (JD) was instrumental in setting up the UK Electives Committee. This is under the auspice of the Medical Schools Council in the UK. It meets regularly and arranges an annual conference presenting work from schools across the UK. In particular, there is an increased focus on elective preparation and sharing best practices. General guidance for the UK is in the process of development.

The MIMP itself ended; however, it has continued in a different and less staff intensive form providing a local "Responsible Electives" initiative which attracts approximately 5 percent of Dundee students each year.

Conclusions

Some 10 years later the picture with electives is much the same but with a number of promising developments across the globe; in particular, improved preparation programmes. Our experience suggests that a lot can be achieved through more considered and long-term partnerships but that these are challenging to maintain and require a consistent "driver" in addition to the goodwill and enthusiasm of staff and students. If such mechanisms can be found or long term support secured then this approach has much to recommend it.

References

Dowell J, and Merrylees N, 2009. "Electives: isn't it time for a change?" *Medical Education* 43:121–126.

Miranda JJ, and Finer S. 2005. "Rethinking your elective." *StudentBMJ* 13:74–75.

Miranda JJ, Yudkin JS, and Willmot C. 2005. "International Health Electives: Four years of experience." *Travel Medicine and Infectious Disease* 3:133–141.

Radstone SJJ. 2005. "Practising on the poor? Healthcare workers' beliefs about the role of medical students during their elective." *Journal of Medical Ethics* 31:109–110.

35 Unite For Sight

Jennifer Staple-Clark

Good intentions are not enough

Despite having good intentions, healthcare participants who do not follow quality global health standards and principles can be wasteful, unethical, and harmful. Worst practices are significant public health concerns which often create new and more substantial barriers to health disparities and perpetuate the cycle of poverty. Short-term missions rarely produce tangible medical benefits in local communities; organisers often fail to research the communities they are entering sufficiently, and without preventive and follow-up care, they cannot provide enduring health improvements. Even the seemingly innocuous distribution of vitamins or over-the-counter pain relievers can lead to overdoses and severe illness. Unintended consequences are especially common when cultural and language barriers exist between visiting healthcare providers and local patients.

A particularly problematic misconception behind some of the worst practices in global health is the idea that providing some care is better than providing none at all. Rachel Bishop and James Litch (Bishop and Litch 2000), co-directors of the Kunde Hospital in Nepal, explain why this philosophy is misguided:

> It is inappropriate arrogance to assume that anything that a Western doctor has to offer his less developed neighbor is progress. These [Western physician] tourists are often working outside their trained specialty or have little concept of how that specialty applies to Nepal. They frequently don't understand local illness presentation, culture, or language. They often offer inappropriate treatment because they think they "must give something." The consultations are often one off, with little possibility for follow up and the local health providers are left to pick up the pieces with no record of the consultation. If an unregistered Nepali doctor on holiday in the United Kingdom offered general medical consultations in a shopping centre there would be a public and professional outcry.
>
> (1017)

Healthcare delivery is complex, and there are numerous barriers that prevent patients from accessing quality care in resource poor settings. The needs of the local community are best known by those who have an understanding of the local situation. Local providers are familiar with the aetiologies and distributions of diseases in their communities. They are also aware of regional aspects of public health such as hospital patterns, who has access to care, and how best to distribute resources. Therefore, programmes are best developed by local medical professionals and social entrepreneurs who understand the barriers to quality care in their communities. Social entrepreneurs are able to develop high-impact social interventions to lift communities out of poverty and, in Unite For Sight's case, to eliminate preventable blindness worldwide. How do we change the landscape in global health to promote entrepreneurship and innovation among local professionals? What resources are needed by those local professionals so that they can best serve the needs of their local communities and populations?

Supporting local innovators

Social entrepreneurship is at the core of Unite For Sight's working philosophy. Social entrepreneurs work to change the landscape in their community or in their field. Perhaps the most coherent and comprehensive definition comes from Roger L. Martin and Sally Osberg (Martin and Osberg 2007) in the Stanford Social Innovation Review, who describe how social entrepreneurs change the landscape in their field. "Imagine that Andrew Carnegie had built only one library rather than conceiving the public library system that today serves untold millions of American citizens. Carnegie's single library would have clearly benefited the community it served. But it was his vision of an entire system of libraries creating a permanent new equilibrium – one ensuring access to information and knowledge for all the nation's citizens – that anchors his reputation as a social entrepreneur."

Unite For Sight supports eye clinics by investing human and financial resources in their social ventures to eliminate patient barriers to eye care. The partner clinics are led by seasoned social entrepreneurs who, like Andrew Carnegie, are working to change the system of eye care delivery for patients living in poverty. The clinics' ophthalmologists organise outreach teams that actively seek out patients who would otherwise not be able to access care. They collaborate with community leaders, governmental bodies, and hospitals to bring high-quality eye care to those living in poverty. This model empowers the local eye clinics to reach high volumes of patients who have significant barriers to care, and the programmes occur on a daily, year-round basis.

Unite For Sight works within the existing infrastructure of local eye clinics to provide quality care by local doctors to patients living in extreme poverty. The programmes empower the local ophthalmologists to develop and lead initiatives that they sustain and direct on a long-term basis. Rather than relying on charitable funding, the partner clinics are economically functional, private businesses that also provide treatment to regular fee-paying customers. A sustainable business model is created with a portion of the revenue generated from their private patients that is used to run outreaches in poor communities, to pay for expenses such as vehicles, supplies for screening patients, fuel for outreach vehicles, and other miscellaneous items.

Unite For Sight has empowered the local clinics to provide eye care for more than 2 million patients living in poverty, including more than 100,000 sight-restoring surgeries through 2016. It is only with Unite for Sight's direct support with human and financial resources that the outreach programmes with phenomenal local doctors were able to employ novel strategies and innovations to reach patients in their villages.

Outreach to provide quality care

Approximately 45 million people in the world are blind, and 87 percent of visually impaired people live in developing countries (World Health Organization 2009). The economic consequences of blindness are staggering, as 90 percent of blind individuals cannot work. Thus, "poverty and blindness are believed to be intimately linked, with poverty predisposing to blindness, and blindness exacerbating poverty by limiting employment opportunities, or by incurring treatment cost" (Kuper *et al.* 2010). As blindness restricts mobility, approximately 75 percent of visually impaired people require assistance, often from family, with everyday tasks. Consequently, blindness affects the community on a practical level, as children cannot attend school when they become caretakers for blind adults. Thus, countless children are denied the opportunity to receive a formal education, and perhaps escape the poverty cycle (Wright *et al.* 2007). Additionally, when a sighted adult becomes the caretaker for a blind individual, he or she must stop working. The long-term economic and educational repercussions are especially felt by community-oriented cultures in the developing world. Unite for Sight Partner DR Seth Wanye, the only ophthalmologist for 2 million people in the Northern Region of Ghana, explains:

> If you have someone who is blind, then someone else will have to forgo his or her activities in order to take care of this person. Oftentimes, you have a child who is supposed to go to school, but he is instead guiding a blind man around the house and directing him wherever he wants to go. This child could have gone to school, studied, and become somebody in the future to help the family.
>
> We often see very young people who are blind, many times younger than the age of 40. They become blind during their productive years; they could have been working and helping to contribute towards building wealth in the country. Instead, the blindness results in a financial loss to the nation because these people are not able to contribute to building the nation.
>
> (Wayne 2010)

With Unite For Sight's support, teams of local ophthalmic nurses and local optometrists from each eye clinic travel daily to remote and impoverished areas up to 7 hours away from the clinic to provide exams, diagnosis, glasses, other treatment and follow-up throughout the year. Patients requiring advanced ophthalmic care or surgery are transported to the local eye clinic for care by the local ophthalmologists.

We focus on local capacity building, and we utilise innovative, evidence-based, and effective healthcare delivery processes. For example, Unite For Sight provides funding to support the salaries of local ophthalmic nurses and local optometrists to be employed by its partner eye clinics in order to provide care each day in the villages, slums, and refugee camps.

Unite For Sight engages local community-based village members as health workers who help the local eye clinics to reach the hardest to reach patients. They identify patients who need to be examined and diagnosed by the visiting local eye doctors each month and accompany the village patients to the eye clinic for their surgery. They also help alleviate fear by educating the patients about surgery and medical care.

Unite For Sight subsidises medically necessary medication (i.e., for infections and other treatable conditions) and eyeglasses and supports the cost for a patient to receive surgical care for patients in villages. The costs include surgical expenses, transportation to and from the eye clinic, overnight lodging near the eye clinic, and postoperative medication expenses. For sight-restoring cataract surgery this cost might be $100.

Visiting volunteers from abroad assist with tasks such as patient intake and visual acuity screening. Through this collaboration with one to two local doctors, the team is able to provide comprehensive care to 100–500 patients each day. While supporting the local doctors in the field, the visiting volunteers learn about barriers to care and realities and complexities of responsible healthcare delivery.

Results

Unite For Sight focuses on outcomes, and not just outputs. We evaluate the number of patients living in poverty who are receiving Unite For Sight-sponsored surgery by the local eye clinics, and we track the number of patients with significantly improved vision after surgery. Unite For Sight requires extensive documentation from each eye clinic partner, including preoperative and postoperative visual acuity data that are analysed to ensure the quality, effectiveness, and social impact of the programmes. We also assess the increase in the cataract surgical rate at each eye clinic, targeted for patients living in poverty.

Unite For Sight has four partners in Ghana, three in India, and one in Honduras, and the programmes are most robust in Ghana. With Unite for Sight's support, four of Ghana's 70 ophthalmologists provide close to 50 percent of all cataract surgeries. For example, prior to Unite For Sight's partnership beginning in 2005, Dr Wanye, mentioned above, lacked operating equipment to provide any cataract surgery and his patients were unable to afford the cost. It is through a decade-long partnership that Dr Wanye and his ophthalmic staff of seven are now able to provide care to more than 65,000 patients annually who live in poverty. In 2011, Ghanaian ophthalmologist Dr Wanye provided 2800 Unite For Sight-supported sight-restoring surgeries for patients living in poverty. In 2012, with Unite For Sight's support, Dr Wanye provided more than 4200 sight-restoring cataract surgeries to patients who were otherwise unable to access or afford care. Similarly, Ghanaian ophthalmologist Dr James Clarke now provides more than 2500 sight-restoring surgeries annually to patients who were otherwise unable to access or afford care.

As an example of the impact of Unite For Sight's programmes, we will share the story of 6-year-old Asana. Born to a family of farmers in northern Ghana, Asana had never known what it meant to see. She suffered from cataracts in both eyes, and her family was not able to access or afford eye care. Since she was unable to see, Asana's sister, Latifa, was unable to go to school so that she could provide full-time care to Asana. For example, Asana needed to be led everywhere by her sighted sister. That all changed when Asana's uncle learned about Ghanaian ophthalmologist Dr Seth Wanye's Friends Eye Clinic outreach programme that is supported by Unite For Sight. With Unite For Sight's support, Friends Eye Clinic was able to provide free sight-restoring surgery to Asana in November 2013. Removing the bandages revealed a new world to Asana, who was seeing for the first time in her life.

International volunteers

Healthcare delivery organisations directly provide care to patients, and there is a variety of examples of leading innovative, outcomes-focused organisations. These organisations typically do not have structured student or volunteer opportunities because they are focused solely on delivering care to their patients. In contrast to the healthcare delivery organisations, there is also a variety of organisations which focus exclusively on student and volunteer educational and learning opportunities. These organisations may partner with local entities to offer educational opportunities, or – in unfortunate instances – implement short-term interventions without regard to the local healthcare providers or local needs. These volunteer-focused organisations are not directly engaged in providing, funding, or advancing the healthcare offered, but instead their goal and mission is to offer visitors opportunities to travel abroad.

In addition to healthcare outcomes, Unite For Sight also focuses on educational outcomes for its visiting participants. Comprehensive training is essential for volunteers. Volunteers who are not both practically and psychologically competent to work abroad can be a burden to a global health organisation and its local partners. On the other hand, well-prepared volunteers can make an immediate, vitally important, high-impact difference. Unite For Sight's research, experience, and evaluation has enabled the organisation to develop its own highly successful pre-service training and orientation process that ensures that volunteers are fully prepared to contribute to the success of the Unite For Sight programmes. Training includes successful online completion of Unite For Sight's global health online course, cultural competency online course, volunteer ethics and professionalism online course, social entrepreneurship overview, community eye health online course, articles about the importance of sustainable development in eye care, effective health education, rumours and word of mouth, overview of spending at the base of the pyramid, and photography and ethics, as well as a TED video about cultural understandings and misperceptions. While assisting and supporting the local ophthalmologists, optometrists, and ophthalmic nurses, Unite For Sight's participants see first hand the global health concepts they studied in their training. Their important skills include acceptance of and respect for different cultures, an aptitude for cross-cultural communication, and a comprehensive understanding of global health. They can synthesise academic knowledge from comparative fields and use an interdisciplinary, culturally appropriate approach when tackling global issues.

Role of trainees

To date, Unite For Sight has directly provided care to more than 2 million patients who were otherwise unable to access or afford care, and developed a model to educate and train current and future leaders in global health while supporting and assisting the local doctors through the provision of human and financial resources. Unite For Sight emphasises the essentials of including eye care in global health priorities, while highlighting the importance of supporting and assisting local professionals in their own social ventures to eliminate disparities in their communities and countries. Unite For Sight trains all of its participants (global impact fellows) in cultural competency, ethics, community eye health, and public health best practices. While assisting the local doctors daily with support tasks such as patient intake, visual acuity testing, and distributing glasses and medication prescribed by the local doctors, the students learn from the doctors about effective strategies to eliminate barriers to care for the hardest to reach patients. Meanwhile, visiting ophthalmologists and optometrists offer ideas exchange and professional development to the local doctors.

Global impact fellows see first hand the global health and human rights concepts that they studied in their pre-departure training. Those interested in global health, for example, learn from the patients and doctors about barriers to care for the hardest to reach patients. They engage with the local doctors to understand sustainable, quality healthcare delivery strategies in resource poor settings. The visiting students interested in non-governmental organisations (NGOs) and sustainability focus their educational opportunities on the realities and complexities of responsible NGO management. They engage with the clinic founders, managers and staff who are dedicated to quality hospital management and sustainability. Students interested in medicine delve the most into the clinical daily work. They are most enthused about testing visual acuity, taking patient histories, dispensing medication and glasses that are prescribed by the local doctors, watching the sight-restoring surgeries performed by the local ophthalmologists, and shadowing and learning from the local doctors.

While each student's interests and goals may vary, all participants are required to explore and contemplate the complexities and realities of global health. What barriers to care affect the patients that they meet, and how are the local doctors modelling best practices to eliminate those barriers? Most critically, Unite For Sight heavily emphasises that healthcare must be delivered by the local healthcare professionals, and the visitor's role is to support and learn from the local experts.

Unite For Sight's thousands of student alumni now range from medical anthropologists and public health professionals with organisations such as Clinton Global Initiative to ophthalmologists and primary care physicians. Our alumni apply to their careers the lessons learned from their immersive community eye health experience. As Abraar Karan – now a medical doctor who had first participated within Unite For Sight as a sophomore in college – explains:

My early experiences with Unite For Sight have shaped the type of care I deliver to patients every day. I think more seriously about the context of their disease within their complex lives, and this allows me to provide more tailored, sensitive care. It is the difference between simply a cured patient and an overall healthier human being. I have since worked in several countries around the world, expanding my understanding of global healthcare systems, but I always remember the lessons I first learned years ago with Unite For Sight.

(Karan 2010)

References

Bishop, Rachel A., and James A. Litch. 2000. "Medical tourism can do harm." *BMJ* 320:1017.

Karan, Abraar. 2010. "Unite For Sight's Alumni Profile Series: Abraar Karan." www.uniteforsight.org/alumni/abraar-karan.

Kuper, Hannah, Sarah Polack, Wanjiku Mathenge, Cristina Eusebio, Zakia Wadud, Mamunur Rashid, and Allen Foster. 2010. "Does Cataract Surgery Alleviate Poverty? Evidence from a Multi-Centre Intervention Study Conducted in Kenya, the Philippines and Bangladesh." *PLoS ONE* 5.

Martin, Roger L., and Sally Osberg. 2007. "Social entrepreneurship: The case for definition." *Stanford Social Innovation Review*, Spring.

Wayne, Seth. 2010. "Module 1: Why Eye Care Is Important." www.uniteforsight.org/community-eye-health-course/module1.

World Health Organization. 2009. "Visual impairment and blindness." Last modified August 2014. www.who.int/mediacentre/factsheets/fs282/en/.

Wright, Heathcote R., Angus Turner, and Hugh R. Taylor. 2007. "Trachoma and poverty: unnecessary blindness further disadvantages the poorest people in the poorest countries." *Clinical and Experimental Optometry* 90:422–428.

36 Foundation for sustainable development

Going beyond do no harm to create mutual benefit

Lisa Kuhn

The Foundation for Sustainable Development (FSD) was founded in 1995 and was recently recognised by the UN when it was granted special consultative status with the Economic and Social Council. It currently partners with more than 250 community organisations in Argentina, Bolivia, India, Kenya, Nicaragua and Uganda working in various sectors ranging from health to agriculture, financial services, income generating activities, and clean energy as appropriate to their communities' needs and priorities.

FSD's mission is to support the achievement of community-driven goals through asset-based community development and international exchange. Because international exchange is a core element of its programming in the community, the achievement of its mission depends in large part on successfully creating the circumstances for public health interns to go beyond "do no harm" to contributing to positive change in the host community.

FSD places students in community organisation settings working broadly on community health issues rather than in clinical settings. For example, an intern placed with a health centre in Nicaragua – a country with one of the highest teen pregnancy rates in the world – might work with local schools to organise peer health educator clubs to address contraception and proper prenatal care. An intern placed with an HIV-AIDS organisation in Uganda might research why fewer men than women consistently take their antiretrovirals.

Each year, FSD hosts 150–200 interns and a similar number of shorter-term volunteers. Approximately 25–30 percent of these work on public health projects. These interns pay a programme fee to FSD to match them with one of FSD's community partners, a host family, and to provide them with training and support in asset-based community development and integration into the work environment of their host community.

FSD's community development model in which the internship is situated incorporates three programmes that support underserved communities in a collaborative and sustainable manner:

- Capacity building: FSD field staff train community partners to create economically, socially, and environmentally sustainable programmes.

- Grantmaking: FSD's grantmaking and giving circles programmes support community-driven projects and capacity building initiatives for its community partners.
- International development training programmes: Provide students and professionals with intensive training in grassroots sustainable development while also providing human resources and technical support to partner organisations.

This combination of complementary and mutually reinforcing programming within the host community provides public health students a rich context in which to learn and work. In each community, FSD partners with organisations addressing public health issues from a variety of angles. These organisations not only host interns but also receive training from FSD on sustainable development approaches and are eligible to receive grants for their projects. FSD's year-round work in the community provides continuity ensuring that one intern's work is built upon by the next.

An example of this integrated, long-term community approach can be found in Kakamega, Kenya. There, FSD not only partners with local hospitals such as Shibwe Sub-District Hospital, but also with 15 community groups and local schools addressing health education, nutrition and income-generating support for HIV-infected persons, food security and environmental health and sanitation. Over the past 10 years, successive interns with Shibwe Hospital have been able to improve patient intake flow, reducing wait times, finish and open a new maternity ward, develop a clean water source, install running water, build a toilet and shower in the maternity ward, train hospital workers to use computers provided by the government, and develop an alert system to trigger a health worker visit when a pregnant woman missed one of her four critical prenatal visits.

FSD's approach also helps interns collaborate across organisations for a more holistic impact on health. For example, an intern with FSD partner ACCES identified that students who were referred from a local school to Shibwe Hospital were not being taken there. FSD's long-term relationship with the hospital facilitated access to the community health extension workers who were able to conduct sensitisation meetings with parents at the school while the intern's project with ACCES focused on setting up a farming club to grow Indigenous vegetables that could be sold by families to pay for the hospital services.

Over its 20-year history working with over 3500 interns and volunteers, FSD has found that it must work extensively with both the students and the community organisations before and during the internship. In particular, FSD places emphasis on the following elements: partnership and relationship management; matching intern interests and strengths with partner needs; managing expectations and building a common understanding of its asset-based community development approach, values around sustainability and internship methodology; providing a framework and tools to interns for listening to the community; and the co-development of a work plan and budget between the intern and host organisation.

Partnership and relationship management

The groundwork for internships through FSD is laid long before an intern applies for the programme. The FSD programme director – a member of the community with expertise in community development as well as international exchange – works with the site team to build and maintain supportive relationships with the community partners throughout the year. The team takes time to get to know a new potential partner to ensure that organisation's operating model and values are compatible with hosting interns and leveraging their efforts for the benefit of the organisation and the community. Once accepted, the FSD team is regularly in touch with the partners to discuss on-going work and priorities in order to identify the needs and opportunities which an intern or volunteer might address. The team monitors the work of any intern on site and visits the partners after the interns leave to review organisation progress and experience.

Matching intern interests and strengths with partner needs

To make a good match, it is important for FSD to understand both the partners' needs, interests and capabilities as well as the students'. FSD asks partners to create and update an organisational profile identifying their priority programming areas and indicating specifically where they see opportunities for interns to add value to their work. Similarly in the application process, students are asked to describe both their experience and their interests as well as to write a short essay about their motivations. All interns are interviewed by the site team to allow them to get a sense of the intern's personality, experience, comfort level, self-sufficiency and support needs. When making a placement, the team considers the organisation's needs and whether the services of an intern would be useful, what projects the intern might work on, the organisation's supervision of and expectations for the intern, the desired outcomes of the completed project, and the capacity of the organisation to provide resources to an intern. Partners receive the CV of the proposed intern and have the opportunity to either accept or reject.

Managing expectations and building a common understanding

FSD has found that it is important to prepare both the host organisations and the students well and to manage expectations on both sides to smooth the way for a successful working relationship. From the beginning during the relationship-building phase, the team talks with each organisation about the FSD programme, challenges and benefits of hosting students, the expectations they have of the students as well as those that the students are likely to have of them.

For all active partners, FSD holds a workshop to prepare them to host the interns. During this workshop, FSD's methodology, programme requirements and timeline are explained. Partners are introduced to the tools that the interns will be using and discuss the appropriate roles for interns and supervisors. Current partners share past experiences hosting interns, and the new partners and supervisors learn from those who have hosted before. The team facilitates a discussion around the expectations, fears, and challenges of hosting an intern. This is especially helpful for new partners so that they think through how they can best organise and prepare to get something positive out of the intern's time with them.

Before departure, students receive their placements and a pre-departure package with information on health, safety, packing, host families, host organisations, and a reading list to help them prepare. Upon arrival, they receive an intensive on-site orientation during which they get a grounding in FSD's asset-based community development approach and the tools and methods they will be using. FSD asks the interns to adopt a role of being more of a facilitator than implementer so as to help communities own the projects for sustainability purposes. To deepen their understanding, students are provided with examples of successful and less successful projects to analyse and may visit successful projects. Giving both students and host organisations the same training helps to create a common language and working approach allowing the students to transition into action more quickly.

Providing a framework and tools to interns for listening to the community

Perhaps one of the most important things that FSD does to set interns up to add value in the community is to equip them with tools that they can use to get to know and listen to the community. All interns receive training on one or more community assessment methodologies such as asset mapping, asset inventory taking, and participatory needs assessments and are expected to spend their first 1–2 weeks in active listening mode. For example, interns with Shibwe Hospital typically spend this time observing hospital operations and interactions with patients and the community as well as interviewing staff and patients. By insisting that all interns engage in a semi-structured assessment of community assets and challenges through observations, field visits and discussions, FSD helps to create space for the community to influence the project. This assessment forms the foundation for work plan development and project design.

Co-development of a work plan and budget between the intern and host organisation

The heart of the FSD internship experience is the co-development of a project between the intern and host organisation. Interns are assigned supervisors at their host organisation who provide mentorship and guidance to their work and integration in the community. The interns' work plans are developed in collaboration with the organisation staff within the organisation's own framework, mission, and philosophy to ensure appropriateness and sustainability. The plans build off what the community is already doing and the skills and experience that the intern brings to the table. Work plans and budgets are developed jointly with the participants, host organisation and the community. The FSD team provides feedback and supervises this process to ensure the incorporation of sustainable development principles. The FSD team also opens spaces for reflection among interns working at different partner organisations where students can discuss their work, their challenges, and their learning.

The challenges and successes of the participants' community projects are always shared and celebrated. At the end of the internship, there is a partner–intern reflection session to review the achievements and the way forward when the interns depart. In this session, the interns officially hand over the community projects to their partner organisations, sharing their challenges as well as their vision for community engagement. This helps ensure partner ownership over the work and increases the likelihood that they will be motivated and equipped to carry it forward.

Positioning and supporting interns to conduct mutually beneficial project-based work requires a bigger investment than shadowing a medical professional, but it provides a rich learning experience for students beginning or contemplating a career in health. It allows interns to observe many social, political, and economic factors that influence health outcomes. They can participate directly in developing strategies to overcome the obstacles and take advantage of opportunities for good health. Moreover, by working on sustainable, community-driven projects, interns have the opportunity to move beyond "do no harm" to contribute to positive gains in health that will live on after they have gone.

Roshan Najafi had the chance to see the long-term impact of her work first hand. Currently a resident in family medicine at the University of Washington, she interned in Kakamega in 2010 while a medical student at the University of Michigan. She writes:

> I had the opportunity to return to Shibwe several years after finishing my internship. It was incredible to witness what had come of our efforts – our collaborations had empowered the community members who had sourced their skills in our hospital initiative to play an active role in developing new initiatives to improve the community as a whole, and the hospital had been able to care for an increased patient load while maintaining quality of care. It was great to reconnect with the community that had left an indelible mark on me.

(Najafi, 2015)

Reference

Najafi, Roshan. 2015. "Voices from the Field: Understanding Our Strengths." April 2015 Bulletin. San Francisco,CA: Foundation for Sustainable Development.

37 CUGH university consortia and the development of educational standards in global health

Anvar Velji, Keith Martin and Thomas Hall

Overview and antecedents

The Global Health Education Consortium (GHEC) was founded as the International Health Education Consortium (IHMEC) in 1991, and "has played a critical role in the evolution of the global health movement. Its accomplishments over 20 years are evident in the growth of interest in the field." (Dr Haile Debas, first Chair CUGH Board) (Velji 2011). The Consortium of Universities for Global Health (CUGH), founded in 2008, merged with GHEC in 2011. The merged organisation adopted a broader mandate and mission to involve all disciplines across many universities to focus on global health education, research, service, advocacy and diplomacy, in an interprofessional manner.

Over the past 25 years, much progress has occurred which includes creating a wide variety of educational products to support global health education: teaching modules, bibliographies, books, developing course curricula for pre-departure and introductory courses, competencies, mentorship programmes and pre-departure courses for global health electives (Velji 2011). CUGH is now participating in close, trans-professional collaborations to further the development of educational tools appropriate for the professional health disciplines and non-health professional schools involved in global health such as law and the environmental and social sciences.

The following section reviews progress made regarding global health education standards for several health professional schools. However, the ultimate contribution by CUGH has been to integrate global health education in an interdisciplinary manner across all schools involved in the field. Furthermore, we make recommendations based on one of the author's (AV) recent experience identifying methods to integrate global health into all medical schools using accreditation standards that require minimum additional curricular hours. The concluding section maps out current and future challenges for CUGH in the rapidly evolving and largely overlapping fields of global health, one health and planetary health.

Global health standards for 21st century global health professionals

To develop educational standards for global health programmes, all professional educators must work together. At CUGH this imperative resulted in developing educational standards for multiple health disciplines while at the same time identifying shared interprofessional competencies.

Developing standards for nursing schools

A list of global health competencies for medical students originally developed by the Association of Faculties of Medicine of Canada and the Global Health Education Consortium was adapted for nurses and translated from English to Spanish and Portuguese (Arthur *et al.* 2011, Wilson *et al.* 2012).

Developing standards for schools of public health

The Association of Schools and Programs for Public Health (ASPPH) recently identified five core competencies: biostatistics, epidemiology, social and behavioural science, health policy and management, and environmental science. In addition, it identified seven interdisciplinary cross-cutting competencies: communication and informatics, diversity and culture, leadership, public health biology, professionalism, programme planning, and systems thinking. All 12 domains are the foundation of graduate public health studies. For global health programmes at schools of public health five additional competencies are required in addition to those of the MPH degree: capacity strengthening, collaborating and partnering, ethical reasoning and professional practice, health equity and social justice, and programme management. As ASPPH states: "They reflect the goal of global health to promote population health, safety, and well-being at local and global levels, as well as eliminate health and social disparities worldwide" (Association of Schools and Programs of Public Health (ASPPH) 2011).

Developing standards for global oral health

The CUGH Interest Group on Global Oral Health has developed competencies in global oral health (Benzian *et al.* 2015). The recent publication of "Competency Matrix for Global Oral Health," lays a critical foundation for the broad discipline of global oral health encompassing professionals in North America and elsewhere (Velji 2015). It is important to note that these competencies were developed to address the interdisciplinary challenges of oral health and share these competencies with other professionals within and beyond the health discipline.

Developing global standards in paediatrics, family medicine and surgery

Many programmes in North America have developed competencies and recommended educational standards in such fields as paediatrics (Howard *et al.* 2011) and family medicine (Redwood-Campbell *et al.* 2011). In contrast, global surgery is an emerging field within general surgery, with primary emphasis on developing academic training and exposure of residents in North America to the massive surgical burden in low to middle income countries. These programmes have their own global health emphasis based on faculty interests, experience, institutional partnerships and resource availability. However, each programme has done so without a broad, unifying set of global health interprofessional competencies (Jogerst *et al.* 2015).

Accreditation standards and integrating global health into medical school curricula: challenges and opportunities

Recent experience at a new medical school in California suggests that the integration of global health into a novel active-learning, system-based and team-driven curriculum, tightly integrated with clinical presentations is a two-step process. First, the identification of cross-cutting competencies related to population health, public health and behavioural health by using the relevant professional accreditation standards required for graduation of both the Liaison Committee on Medical Education (LCME) and the Committee on Accreditation of Medical Education in Canada (CACMAS) (LCME Function and Structure of a Medical School. 2015–16 www.lcme. org). Second, the mapping of these competencies in relation to the principal global health competencies previously identified by a joint US and Canadian committee on global health competencies, convened by GHEC (Arthur *et al.* 2011). Through this approach, the integration of global health in the curriculum is readily accomplished and requires minimal additional teaching time and resources.

Global health electives, field experiences, ethical issues and LCME and CACMAS standards

CUGH is deeply involved in defining the necessary elements of service learning and global health electives. Service learning and global health electives require careful planning, learning outcomes, reflection and assessment. Both these elements require structure and assessment and can be institutionalised as a social accountability mission for the medical school. There was a recent call for the standardisation of short-term experiences in global health, to ensure programme quality by data, ethics that meet both host and sending countries' standards and needs (Melby *et al.* 2015). Several chapters in this volume focus on aspects of standardisation and assessment of this very important part of global health education. CUGH and its partners are deeply committed to developing standards in global health ethics and support the LCME and CACMAS standards.

Interprofessional competencies and LCME standards

The CUGH subcommittee on global health competencies recently identified competencies for preparing global health professionals (Wilson *et al.* 2014, Wilson *et al.* 2015) and interprofessional competencies to prepare 21st century global health professionals (Jogerst *et al.* 2015). A critical part of interprofessional competencies is to develop collaborative skills: "The faculty of a medical school ensure that the core curriculum of the medical education programme prepares medical students to function collaboratively on healthcare teams that include health professionals from other disciplines as they provide coordinated services to patients. These curricular experiences include practitioners and or students from the other health professions" (LCME Element 7.9).

Social accountability of medical schools standard

CACMAS recently proposed social accountability element (1.1.1) (https// www.afmc.ca/pdf/proposedCACMSaccreditationstandards), which will have a significant impact on the mission and function of all medical schools accredited by LCME and CACMAS. The standard will require all medical schools to demonstrate ongoing evidence to show that the schools are socially accountable to the population that they serve. Response to this standard will create great opportunities for medical schools and its global health–public health, social sciences programmes to institutionalise service learning and global health electives. Existing collaborations between institutions in high and low income nations must be re-evaluated to ensure that long-term benefits accrue to the host institution. Students from developed nations benefit from overseas learning experiences but questions exist about the potential benefits to the resource constrained institutions. Collaborations that allow students to acquire learning opportunities in developing country institutions can be a platform for faculty in affluent nations to assist their overseas colleagues to strengthen their training programmes and provide services if desired.

Recommendations for institutionalising global health

We have outlined below ways to identify medical school accreditation standards that can help integrate global health topics into the medical curriculum:

1. Use of the CACMAS and LCME accreditation standards as a framework to map the global health competencies previously identified by GHEC and AFMC.
2. Identify curricular materials and cross-competencies that already exist and are required for graduation in such disciplines as medicine, public health, population health, behavioural health and global health.
3. Specify mode of delivery of the curriculum.
4. Specify modes of formative and summative assessment.

Challenges and successes post-GHEC–CUGH merger: further agenda

Global health education in North America has reached a critical juncture in its evolution over the past two and a half decades. Training in global health has become increasingly important for all undergraduate and graduate healthcare professionals and includes a diverse array of fields including: social justice and accountability, equity, healthcare access, human rights, ethics, cultural competencies, migrant health, and other socioeconomic and behavioural issues. To accelerate progress further in these and other arenas as well as involve a broader collection of inter and trans-university stakeholders the CUGH opened a permanent secretariat in Washington, DC, in 2012. This was deliberately situated close to the centre of political decision-making in the USA and amid a rich array of think tanks, international government organisations, embassies, government departments and funding agencies. Keith Martin, a physician and six-term Canadian member of parliament was chosen to be the founding executive director. The Bill and Melinda Gates Foundation (BMGF) and the Rockefeller Foundation donated seed money to support the beginning of CUGH in 2008. BMGF provided bridge funding in 2012.

Once CUGH opened its doors in Washington, its committees were strengthened to create a mechanism through which members could engage, share information, collaborate and advocate across research, education, advocacy and service. The Education Committee, with the help of supplemental funding, created important products including: a definition of global health competencies; a global health programme advisory service offering mentorship services to academic programmes; curricular and other educational products which are posted on CUGH's website www.CUGH.org; and a trainee advisory committee to help CUGH identify issues important to students and ensure student input into organisational activities. The Enabling Systems Committee focuses on the administration of academic global health programmes and provides high, value-added workshops and webinars. The consortium pursued its own advocacy issues and reached out to university–government relations representatives, non-governmental organisations and other organisations such as the American Cancer Society and Devex to identify other issues. Advocacy efforts included: support for research funding with Research America and the Global Health Council; speeding up the response to the Ebola outbreak; supporting the medical education and nursing education partnership initiatives; advocating for protecting health workers in conflict; addressing the pandemic of fake and substandard drugs in partnership with the American Society of Tropical Medicine and Hygiene; and defending reproductive rights and supporting solutions to reduce gun violence in the USA.

A collaboration with the Pulitzer Center led to communication workshops, an annual global health film festival and a video competition at CUGH's annual conference. Johns Hopkins' Global Health Now and Global Health

Science and Practice provided competitive opportunities for students to be published. An enduring collaboration with the *Lancet Global Health* and the *Annals of Global Health* resulted in these journals publishing the oral and poster abstracts, respectively, from the annual conference. Relationships have deepened with the National Institutes of Health, specifically with the National Cancer Institute, Fogarty Center and the National Heart, Lung and Blood Institute. CUGH has done studies in partnership with the Center for Strategic and International Studies. It also conducted surveys with the Global Health Fellows Programme to identify ways to increase opportunities for minority students and faculty in minority serving institutions.

Looking to the future, global health programmes will continue to blossom as a consequence of the continued interest people have to improve the wellbeing of people and our planet, the recognition that global health diplomacy can address the precursors of human-made and natural threats, and that the skills acquired in this field can be applied to domestic and international challenges. This offers universities many exciting opportunities: building partnerships that focus on creating and retaining training capabilities in low income countries; research in translation and implementation science; building true interdisciplinary training programmes; creating platforms for reverse innovation; improving distance learning; and developing context-relevant curricula. Harnessing the capabilities within universities across research, education, service, advocacy and diplomacy will create new opportunities for institutions and benefits for populations in great need. It will also continue to make a special effort to engage non-medical disciplines to improve the wellbeing of our planet and ourselves.

References

Arthur, M.A., R. Battat, and T.F. Brewer. 2011. "Teaching the basics: core competencies in global health." *Infectious Disease Clinics of North America* 25(2):347–358. doi: 10.1016/j.idc.2011.02.013.

Association of Schools and Programs of Public Health (ASPPH). 2011. Global Health Competency Model – Final Version 1.1 (October 31, 2011). www.aspph.org/educate/models/masters-global-health/accessed 11.07.2016.

Benzian, H., J.S. Greenspan, J. Barrow, J.W. Hutter, P.M. Loomer, N. Stauf, and D.A. Perry. 2015. "A competency matrix for global oral health." *Journal of Dental Education* 79(4):353–361.

Howard, C.R., S.P. Gladding, S. Kiguli, J.S. Andrews, and C.C. John. 2011. "Development of a competency-based curriculum in global child health." *Academic Medicine* 86(4):521–528. doi: 10.1097/ACM.0b013e31820df4c1.

Jogerst, K., B. Callender, V. Adams, J. Evert, E. Fields, T. Hall, J. Olsen, V. Rowthorn, S. Rudy, J. Shen, L. Simon, H. Torres, A. Velji, and L.L. Wilson. 2015. "Identifying interprofessional global health competencies for 21st-century health professionals." *Annals of Global Health* 81(2):239–247. doi: 10.1016/j.aogh.2015.03.006.

Melby, M.K., L.C. Loh, J. Evert, et al. 2015. "Beyond 'Medical Missions' to Impact-Driven Short-Term Experiences in Global Health (STEGHs): Ethical Principles to

Optimize Community Benefit and Learner Experience." *Academic Medicine* Epub ahead of print December 1, 2015.

Redwood-Campbell, L., B. Pakes, K. Rouleau, C.J. MacDonald, N. Arya, E. Purkey, K. Schultz, R. Dhatt, B. Wilson, A. Hadi, and K. Pottie. 2011. "Developing a curriculum framework for global health in family medicine: emerging principles, competencies, and educational approaches." *BMC Medical Education* 11:46. doi: 10.1186/1472-6920-11-46.

Velji, A. 2011. "Global health education consortium: 20 years of leadership in global health and global health education." *Infectious Disease Clinics of North America* 25(2):323–325. doi: 10.1016/j.idc.2011.02.003.

Velji, A. 2015. "Education for global oral health: progress in improving awareness and defining competencies." *Journal of Dental Education* 79(4):351–352.

Wilson, L., B. Callender, T.L. Hall, K. Jogerst, H. Torres, and A. Velji. 2014. "Identifying global health competencies to prepare 21st century global health professionals: report from the global health competency subcommittee of the consortium of universities for global health." *Journal of Law and Medical Ethics* 42 (Suppl 2):26–31 doi: 10.1111/jlme.12184.

Wilson, L., B. Callendar, T. Hall, A. Velji, V. Rowthorn, S. Rudy, K. Jogerst, H. Torres, J. Evert, J. Olsen, J. Adams, J. Shen, E. Fields, and L. Simon. 2015. "Report from the CUGH Global Health Competency Subcommittee." *Annals of Global Health* 81(1):235. doi. org/10.1016/j.aogh.2015.02.1039. Accessed July 7, 2016.

Wilson, L., D.C. Harper, I. Tami-Maury, R. Zarate, S. Salas, J. Farley, N. Warren, I. Mendes, and C. Ventura. 2012. "Global health competencies for nurses in the Americas." *Journal of Professional Nursing* 28(4):213–222. doi: 10.1016/j.profnurs.2011.11.021.

Index

Global North: ethical perspectives 26; global health volunteerism 105–6; health training institutions in 199; and host experiences 165, 169, 176, 177, 178; hubris of 150–1; privilege in 29; *see also* high income countries (HICs); North–South research partnerships
global service learning (GSL) 97
Global South: ethical perspectives 26; and fair trade learning 97; on global health competencies 19–20; global health volunteerism 105, 109; and host experiences 177; volunteerism, global learning 108; *see also* low and middle-income countries (LMICs); North–South research partnerships
globalisation 33, 223
GlobeMed 111, 112
glocal 210
GME *see* graduate medical education (GME)
Goddard, B. 135
graduate medical education (GME): best practices in graduate/postgraduate medical education 42–50; curriculum 44–5; ethical considerations 48; fellowships, global health 45–8; global health pathways 43–4; informal programmes 44; international rotations, ACGME and RRC requirements 44–5; residency training 43–4
Green, T. 109, 168, 170, 174, 176
Guatemala: host organisations 109–10; semistructured interviews with hosts in 168

Hartman, E. 86, 97
Harvey, P. 193
Health Canada 153
Health Education Abroad (HEA) 167
health education, FTL in 99–100
hepatitis 251
herpes infection 251
Herrick, C. 69
HICs *see* high income countries (HICs)
high income countries (HICs) 19, 21; critiques of competency-based education 23–5, 29; global health volunteerism 105; job opportunities (global health), in international settings 205; local clinical personnel dealing with medical electives 166; motivations in global health

training 140; North–South research partnerships 169; student experiences of global health research, ethical challenges 132, 133, 134, 136; *see also* low and middle-income countries (LMICs)
Hippocratic Oath 120
historical and sociocultural dynamics of global health, sustained learning process 112
HIV/AIDs 14, 105, 149, 242, 310; in LGBT population 250, 251, 253
homosexuality 250, 251; *see also* LGBT health
Honduras, STMMs in 194
Hoping to Help (Lasker) 183
host country/community 68, 73, 82, 135, 180; culture and colonial legacies 174–5; dependency 193, 194; discontent, between users of publicly funded healthcare systems 193–4; experiences 165, 165–79, 167, 174, 177; Foundation for Sustainable Development (FSD) 310, 311; gratitude towards STMMs, expressions of 192–3; helping medical students prepare for global health careers 275, 276, 277; host perspectives/non-host goals 170; hubris of Global North 150–1; humility 151; impact of foreigners in a resource constrained environment 170, 174; international volunteer programmes (IVPs) 181–8; IVP participants 184–5; IVP programme providers 185; large multinational NGO sending students to, dealing with 167–8; local clinical personnel dealing with medical electives 165–7; and motivations in global health training 140–2, 144; and participants 184–5; perceptions of international projects and trainees 171–3t; philosophy of life 145–51; power, paternalism or partnership 175–7; and practicums, graduate global health 226, 228, 229; praise for STMMs 192, 193; professional skills adding unique value to host organisations 112; and programme providers 185; and reciprocity, striving for 261–8; seduction of the Other 150–1; sending institution and host community 184; service-learning 95, 97; and

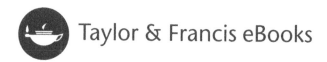 **Taylor & Francis eBooks**

Helping you to choose the right eBooks for your Library

Add Routledge titles to your library's digital collection today. Taylor and Francis ebooks contains over 50,000 titles in the Humanities, Social Sciences, Behavioural Sciences, Built Environment and Law.

Choose from a range of subject packages or create your own!

Benefits for you

» Free MARC records
» COUNTER-compliant usage statistics
» Flexible purchase and pricing options
» All titles DRM-free.

Benefits for your user

» Off-site, anytime access via Athens or referring URL
» Print or copy pages or chapters
» Full content search
» Bookmark, highlight and annotate text
» Access to thousands of pages of quality research at the click of a button.

REQUEST YOUR **FREE** INSTITUTIONAL TRIAL TODAY

Free Trials Available
We offer free trials to qualifying academic, corporate and government customers.

---

eCollections – Choose from over 30 subject eCollections, including:

Archaeology	Language Learning
Architecture	Law
Asian Studies	Literature
Business & Management	Media & Communication
Classical Studies	Middle East Studies
Construction	Music
Creative & Media Arts	Philosophy
Criminology & Criminal Justice	Planning
Economics	Politics
Education	Psychology & Mental Health
Energy	Religion
Engineering	Security
English Language & Linguistics	Social Work
Environment & Sustainability	Sociology
Geography	Sport
Health Studies	Theatre & Performance
History	Tourism, Hospitality & Events

For more information, pricing enquiries or to order a free trial, please contact your local sales team: www.tandfebooks.com/page/sales

 Routledge Taylor & Francis Group | The home of Routledge books

www.tandfebooks.com